A SYLLABUS
for the
SURGEON'S SECRETARY

Jeannette A. Szulec, B.S., RRL

Medical Record Librarian and
Medical Records Consultant
Hospital Administrator

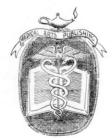

1968

MEDICAL ARTS PUBLISHING COMPANY

P.O. Box 8633 Kensington Station / Detroit, Michigan 48224

Published 1965
Reprinted 1965
Reprinted 1966
Reprinted 1967
Reprinted 1968

This book may be ordered directly from the publisher:

MEDICAL ARTS PUBLISHING COMPANY
P.O. Box 8633—Kensington Station
Detroit, Michigan 48224

Price in U.S.A. $13.18 net prepaid
(12.50 plus .18 postage plus .50 tax)

Price in Canada $14.40 Canadian funds
(Price same as in U.S.A. when paid in U.S.A. funds or
Canadian postal money order)

All non-profit organizations deduct .50 tax

All personal orders must be prepaid

Library of Congress Catalogue Number 65-14908

Printed in the United States of America

Dedicated with love

to the memory of my father

DAMIAN SZULEC

and to my mother

For their loving hearts, their gentle
nobility, and their delicate aesthetic
sensibilities which so enriched my life.

Acknowledgments

An author does not work alone to produce a book of this character and scope. The text develops with the technical assistance and professional guidance of many persons contributing generously of their time and special knowledge. To those persons who have assisted me in making this book possible, I am deeply indebted.

My gratitude is extended to the doctors of St. Joseph Mercy Hospital in Detroit, including Dr. John Lucas, biochemist; Dr. Frank E. Check, Chief of the Department of Obstetrics and Gynecology; Dr. Philip J. Morgan, Chief of the Department of Anesthesia; Dr. Donald R. Simmons, neurologist and neurosurgeon; Dr. J. Anatole Hoski, orthopedic surgeon, Dr. Leo B. Saraf, general surgeon, and Dr. Edward R. Heil, otolaryngologist.

I am further grateful to Dr. Richard E. Straith, Dr. J. Chauncey Hipps and the surgeons of the Straith Memorial Hospital of Plastic and Reconstructive Surgery in Detroit for their kind and generous assistance.

My appreciation is also extended to the many specialty surgeons who contributed descriptions of their operative techniques.

Many persons, known best to me, assisted in the proofreading and arduous secretarial work. My thanks to them are endless.

JEANNETTE A. SZULEC

Preface

Reading maketh a full man; conference, a ready man;
and writing, an exact man.

These words should be dedicated to the secretary whose essential role in business and in the professions is indisputable. In the growing field of medicine she is becoming a particularly important member of the physician's staff and hospital team. As medicine becomes more highly specialized, greater demands are made upon her work. She must be prepared through proper training to meet the challenge of tomorrow as well as that of today.

Fluency with the terminology peculiar to one's professional endeavor is an important element in success. The surgeon's secretary has a responsibility to familiarize herself with the terms describing his highly technical equipment. It is for her and for medical records personnel that this book is intended.

I have long felt the genuine need for a comprehensive reference to assist medical secretaries with technical information not usually found in the medical dictionary. For years they have referred to surgical catalogues for assistance with instrument names. These books are seldom accurate enough for use in a secretary's reference library.

Although A SYLLABUS FOR THE SURGEON'S SECRETARY has been designed primarily as a reference source, the author has used it successfully as a training guide.

It is proposed that the student be assigned sections of this book for study. This should include copying of the operative reports from the book repeatedly until the terminology becomes completely familiar.

Too much emphasis cannot be placed on the importance of having the student see the words spelled correctly. She will learn them by actually typing them. Educators agree that it is far more difficult to change erroneous practices than it is to learn correctly from the outset.

It is further recommended that the student's progress be surveyed through periodic progress tests. Terms and operative reports should be dictated by the teacher from the book. These may be recorded on discs or belts for transcription by the student. If page references are given from the book, the student can check her own work. In so doing, she is actually afforded an additional review. Reports should be dated and saved to compare the progress being made.

Only when a satisfactory degree of proficiency has been achieved should a student be given actual work assignments. She thus learns by POSITIVE TUTELAGE as contrasted with the outmoded method of trial and error.

It is sincerely hoped that medical secretaries, medical record librarians and medical records personnel everywhere will find this a valuable reference which fills a long existing need.

If in some small way this book fulfills the purpose for which it is intended, the many years and countless hours invested in the study and research which have made this work possible will not have been in vain.

JEANNETTE A. SZULEC

Detroit, Michigan
January, 1965

TABLE OF CONTENTS

CHAPTER   **PAGE**

1   The Surgical Secretary   1

2   Punctuation   13

3   Laboratory and X-Ray Examinations   19

4   Pre- and Postoperative Considerations   35
      anesthetics, surgical positions,
      incisions, suture materials,
      suture techniques, bandages and
      dressings

5   Surgical Instruments   47

6   Anatomy of Structure, Circulation and Innervation ..   117

7   General Surgery   149

8   Otolaryngology (E.N.T.)   197

9   Ophthalmology (Eye)   223

10   Neurosurgery   237

11   Gynecology   255

12   Orthopedics   271

13   Plastic Surgery   301

14   Thoracic Surgery   325

15   Urology   333

16   Vascular Surgery   351

17   The Language of Medicine   363

18   A Style Guide   377

GLOSSARY OF OPERATIVE TITLES   381

1 } *The Surgical Secretary*

The surgical secretary is a specialist in the secretarial field and, as such, she is required to be everything that one might expect of an executive secretary and more. In addition to being well versed in the fundamentals of secretarial science, she must have an intelligent concept of her subject matter, whether it be medical terminology in general or, more specifically, the glossology and nomenclature of surgery.

This chapter has been designed to provide a review of the basic considerations in the work of the secretary. It should be of particular value to the student embarking on a medical secretarial career.

Transcription of Dictation

Increasing complexity in the technology of our dictating systems seems to be attended by mounting problems for the secretary. Those of us who have taken dictation directly from the doctor will not argue with the opinion that this is the most satisfactory arrangement. Although shorthand is still used at some facilities, it is fast being replaced by mechanical dictating systems. Without the physician present to whom she might direct her problems with terminology, the secretary must rely on her knowledge of the matter being dictated. It is essential that she be provided with the necessary references to assist her with the more technical phases of her work.

The following books are recommended as basic to the secretary's library.

Webster's Seventh New Collegiate Dictionary.

Medical Dictionary	The large Dorland's or Stedman's are preferred. Taber's Cyclopedic is a good second dictionary.
Anatomy Textbook	Kimber, Gray, Stackpole & Leavell is popular.
PDR (Physician's Desk Reference)	A directory of drugs and biologicals published annually by Medical Economics of Oradell, N.J.

A secretary who is provided with adequate references can be more productive and efficient than the secretary who must seek out the physician for assistance. Each secretary should have her own references, otherwise desk hopping is inevitable.

Regardless of the proficiency of the secretary, problems with recorded dictations will develop due to poor dictating techniques or failure of the equipment.

Partly inaudible dictations should be salvaged to the extent possible and immediately be brought to the attention of the physican concerned. Any portion of the report may assist him in recalling the case, particularly if he is a very busy surgeon.

Blank spaces which represent difficulties encountered in transcribing do not belong in a medical report. When all measures to obtain the information fail, the physician who dictated the report should be contacted for assistance. Physicians seldom insert the required information when a report is furnished to them for signature.

Corrections cannot be detected prior to transcription with some dictating systems. If there are only a few words involved, erasure might be possible. This should be done with an abrasive eraser, lightly. The error may then be covered over with a soft blackboard chalk. Where colored paper is used for the report form, chalk of a similar color may be used. Where a lengthy error is involved, the report should be retyped. If a doctor habitually makes corrections in his dictations, it might be advisable to listen ahead before transcribing his reports.

It is extremely poor secretarial practice to strike out an error or strike over a character without erasing first. Medical records are permanent documents and therefore require the utmost care in preparation. With the patient's authorization, medical reports are furnished to hospitals, physicians, attorneys and various social agencies. They should always be a credit to the facility from which they are issued.

Judging Your Work Volume

A secretary whose test typing speed is 60 words per minute will usually work at the rate of 50 words per minute. To produce one page of single spaced elite type, which consists of an average of 600 words, in addition to a file copy and three additional carbons, she uses her time as follows:

typing time	12 minutes
proofreading	4 minutes
file & 3 carbons	1 minute each

Typing speed is expressed as words per minute. A word is regarded as five strokes. When a secretary types 60 words per minute, she strikes 300 characters and spaces per minute.

A speed of 30 to 60 words per minute is the usual range of commercial touch typists. Fifty to sixty is considered excellent with ranges to 100. Speed specialists type from 140 to 150 words per minute.

When we speak of typing speed in transcription, we are referring to *lines per hour* rather than words per minute. An experienced secretary should be able to transcribe at the rate of 150 to 180 lines per hour.

Setting Up Your Format

Work will flow much more smoothly if your staff will adopt a particular format for their dictations. In order to implement such a system, a note might be placed at important dictating stations including those in the surgical suite.

The information required to completely identify the patient should be itemized to include the patient's name, case number or out-patient status, room number, name of referring physician and attending physician or surgeon.

On operative reports, the surgeon should also include the name of any assistants. The context of the surgical dictation should contain the pre- and post-operative diagnosis, titles of operations performed, anesthetic and position of the patient, findings at surgery and a description of the actual surgical technique. A paragraph containing a complete report of all positive and negative findings dictated before the actual description of the operation will prove most helpful for future reference.

If the secretary is employed in a hospital, forms will be furnished for the various type reports; however, the secretary in the doctor's office may be required to set up her own formats.

A sample operative report is shown in Fig. 1. Such a report form is usually adequate for most operative dictations.

The secretary in the physician's office will usually be asked to send a medical report to the physician by whom the patient was referred. A carbon copy of the report is retained for the office file.

In the hospital, a carbon copy is prepared for the surgeon, referring physician and the assistants and the original report is filed with the patient's hospital record. When house physicians such as internes and residents serve as assistants, carbon copies are placed in their folders. Responsibility for maintaining folders for house staff copies is usually assigned to the medical records office.

The report of surgery is a vital part of the patient's hospital record. It should be dictated within 24 hours after surgery, while the surgeon can still recall the circumstances clearly. Each report must be an individualized account of what was found and what was done. Under no circumstances should a secretary agree to use routine dictations on certain frequently performed cases in lieu of a specifically dictated report. The requirement for an operative report on the patient's chart was designed to protect the interest of the patient. This interest cannot be well served by simply satisfying the chart requirement. This is a point on which there should be no compromise.

ST. JOSEPH MERCY HOSPITAL

DETROIT, MICHIGAN

Operative Report

Date_____

Patient's Name_____ Room _____ Case No. _____

Surgeon _____ CO-SURGEON _____ Assistant(s) _____

Anesthetist _____ Anesthesia _____

PRE-OPERATIVE DIAGNOSIS:

POST-OPERATIVE DIAGNOSIS:

OPERATION (S):

Procedure:

    FINDINGS:

    TECHNIQUE

Figure 1   Operative Report Form

Prescribed Form Used in Business Letters

Attractive and properly spaced letters which conform to prescribed patterns are the responsibility of the secretary. The doctor should be able to dictate a letter fully confident that it will be set up in such a manner as to reflect favorably on his office.

The medical secretary in the doctor's office and the secretary assigned to a particular doctor or group of doctors in the hospital is more likely to do letter writing than is the secretary in the medical steno pool. However, all secretaries should be well trained in the essentials of business letters.

Business letters consist of specific forms and styles of punctuation.

Blocked Form — The date and complimentary closing with writer's identification begin at the center point and appear to the right. The inner address, salutation and each line in the body of the letter are even with the left margin. This style in conjunction with standard punctuation represents the form most often used.

Full Blocked Form — The entire letter with all entries evenly aligned with the left margin is another popular style.

Semi-Blocked Form — Each paragraph of the letter begins with an indentation of five spaces. In all other respects this letter resembles the blocked form.

Indented Form — The date is typed on the right. The inner address is indented in terms of five spaces from the line above, the first line beginning with the left margin. The closing is handled in a similar manner. Each paragraph begins with an indentation of five spaces. This style is seldom used.

Standard punctuation is used most frequently; however, all styles will be defined for those who might have other preferences.

Standard — The only punctuation which appears in the opening and closing of the letter consists of a colon following the salutation and a comma after the complimentary closing. This style is illustrated in Fig. 2 - 4.

Close — Least popular of styles in punctuation, this form requires the use of punctuation after each line in the letter, outside the body of the letter.

Open — No punctuation appears after any portion of the letter outside the body except a period following an abbreviation.

St. Joseph Mercy Hospital

2200 EAST GRAND BOULEVARD

Detroit 11, Michigan

October 22, 1964

Mr. Gerald Towers
Attorney at Law
14 Woodward Avenue
Detroit, Michigan 48226

Dear Mr. Towers:

Pursuant to our telephone conversation of this date, I am
enclosing a release form which your client may sign. This
will serve as my authorization to furnish you with the reports you have requested.

Prepayment of our $ 5.00 service fee is required as a mat-
ter of policy.

Please be assured that your request will receive prompt
attention.

Sincerely yours,

ST. JOSEPH MERCY HOSPITAL

Joan Ferguson
Insurance Office Manager

mm
Enc.

Figure 2   Blocked Form

St. Joseph Mercy Hospital

2200 EAST GRAND BOULEVARD

Detroit 11, Michigan

October 22, 1964

Mr. Gerald Rayburn
Attorney at Law
3605 Woodward Avenue
Detroit, Michigan 48226

Dear Mr. Rayburn:

Pursuant to our telephone conversation of this date, I am
enclosing a release form which your client may sign. This
will serve as my authorization to furnish you with the reports you have requested.

Prepayment of our $5.00 service fee is required as a matter
of policy.

Please be assured that your request will receive our prompt
attention.

Sincerely yours,

Joan Ferguson
Insurance Office Manager

jm
Enc.

Figure 3   Full Blocked Form

St. Joseph Mercy Hospital

2200 EAST GRAND BOULEVARD

Detroit 11, Michigan

October 22, 1964

Mr. Gerald Towers
Attorney at Law
14 Woodward Avenue
Detroit, Michigan 48226

Dear Mr. Towers:

Pursuant to our telephone conversation of this date, I am enclosing a release form which your client, Mr. Roberts, may sign. This will serve as my authority to furnish you with the medical reports you have requested.

Prepayment of our $5.00 service fee is required as a matter of policy.

You may be assured that your request will receive our prompt attention.

Sincerely yours,

Joan Ferguson
CLINIC SUPERVISOR

mm
Enc.

Figure 4   Semiblocked Form

Spacing and Alignment of the Business Letter

Spacing is an important consideration and should be pre-planned to insure an attractive letter.

When we use an 8½ x 11 size letterhead, the body of the letter may be five or six inches wide, the five inch line being preferred for shorter letters with an elite type style. The six inch line is recommended for use with a pica type style.

The elite type style is preferred to pica type for business letters.

ELITE	ELITE
5 inch line	*6 inch line*
Each margin 1¾ inches wide	Each margin 1¼ inches wide
60 spaces per line	70 spaces per line
10 average length words/line	12 average length words/line
Set paper guide at 0	Set paper guide at 0
Set left margin at 20	Set left margin at 15
Set right margin at 80	Set right margin at 85

After the margins have been aligned according to steps enumerated above for a five inch line, the following spacing might be used:

1. Set tabs at 62; to be used for date, complimentary closing, corporation name, name of writer and title.
2. On the 14th line from the top of the paper, at 62 on the scale, begin date.
3. On the fourth line below the date, begin inside address flush with the left margin.
4. On the second line after the inside address, enter the salutation.
5. On the second line after the salutation, begin the body of the letter. In block form, begin at the left margin.
   In semi-block form, begin each paragraph six spaces from the left margin.
   It will be noted that the body of the letter begins on the 24th line from the top edge of the paper.
6. Complimentary close placed on second line after the body of the letter. Align with date by using tab set at 62.
7. Corporation name, if used, is placed on the second line after the close.
8. Name of writer placed on the fourth line after the corporation name.
9. Typist's initials are placed two spaces below, at left margin.
10. Enclosure indication placed immediately below typist's initials.
11. When carbon copies will be sent, place initials cc. two spaces below the typist's and follow with a colon and name of the person who will receive the copy.

A second page is sometimes necessary for a lengthy letter. Each page after the first page of the letter requires a heading which consists of the name of the person to whom the letter is addressed at the left margin, the page number in the center of the line and the date of the letter at the right margin.

The heading is typed six spaces from the top edge of the page and should stand apart from the context of the remaining letter.

All letters should be proofread by the secretary to insure against typographical as well as grammatical errors. A final survey for neatness should also be made. A letter should never be sent out when it contains detectable erasures. Blocked in letters which indicate that the keys need a good cleaning are likewise to be avoided.

Letters convey an impression to their recipients about their senders. Do your letters speak well of you?

Requests for Medical Information

The secretary in the surgeon's office will frequently be requested to obtain medical information regarding patients from other physicians or hospitals. In offices where past medical records are obtained as a matter of policy, a form letter such as that shown in Fig. 5 might be adopted. Form letters are great time savers and their importance should not be overlooked.

Letters requesting medical information must include a provision for the patient's signature. Medical records are regarded as strictly confidential unless the patient signs an authorization form consenting to their release. When the patient is a minor, the parent must sign the release form.

St. Joseph Mercy Hospital

2200 EAST GRAND BOULEVARD

Detroit 11, Michigan

January 24, 1962

PATIENT:
ADDRESS:
BIRTHDATE:

Dear Madame:

Your assistance is requested in furnishing us with the following information regarding the above named patient who is currently under treatment at these facilities.

_____ Medical abstract or photocopy of the medical record particularly _____

_____

_____ Loan of x-ray films

_____ Loan of pathology slides

Your earliest reply in this matter will be appreciated.

Very truly yours,

Jeannette A. Szulec

Jeannette A. Szulec, RRL
MEDICAL RECORD LIBRARIAN

_____

AUTHORIZATION FOR RELEASE OF INFORMATION   (patient to complete)

Permission for release of information from my hospital records in accordance with the above request is hereby granted.

I was treated at the _____ Hospital

in (city and state) _____

on (approximate date) _____ by Doctor _____

SIGNATURE OF PATIENT _____
                              (name under which hospitalized)

Figure 5   Request For Information Form

2 { *Punctuation*

The many rules governing proper punctuation sometimes pose a problem for the secretary. The following guide lists the most frequent circumstances under which punctuation is recommended.

Punctuation Marks   (in common usage)

'	Apostrophe	———	Dash	( )	Parentheses
*	Asterisk	. . . . . .	Ellipsis	.	Period (stop)
[ ]	Brackets	!	Exclamation Point	" "	Quotation Marks
:	Colon	-	Hyphen	;	Semi-colon
,	Comma	?	Interrogation Point	/	Virgule

Apostrophe (')

Contractions

The apostrophe replaces a letter or letters which have been omitted when two words are combined.

EXAMPLE: Don't (do not)
Doesn't (does not)
It's (it is/it has)

*NB: Beware of confusing the contracted *it's* with the possessive pronoun *its*.

EXAMPLE: It's stopped raining.
Its environment was invaded.

Possessive

Singular and plural nouns which *do not* end in an s or z sound take an apostrophe and an s.

EXAMPLE: woman's dress (singular)
women's dresses (plural)

Singular nouns ending in an s or z sound take an apostrophe and an s.

EXAMPLE: boss's   N.Y. Times's editorial
bus's   Burns's poems

---

* NB is used here to mean NOTE WELL (nota bene).

Plural nouns ending in an s or z sound take an apostrophe *without an s.*
    EXAMPLE: Consumers' Digest   The Andrews' home

NB: In plurals where an e follows the s, z or c sound, an apostrophe and an s is used.
    EXAMPLE: mice—mice's

Apostrophe with an s is used after the second possessive *only* when joint ownership is indicated.
    EXAMPLE: John and Joan's bank account

Titles may omit the use of the apostrophe.
    EXAMPLE: St. Marys Hospital

Comma   (,)

The comma is used to prevent misunderstanding by signaling a pause in the sentence. There are many instances in which a comma is recommended as itemized below.

Compound sentences
When two subjects in a compound sentence are different, it is good practice to use a comma to prevent confusion.
    EXAMPLE: I don't recognize anyone, but my mother is expected.

Relative clauses
A clause introduced by WHICH is called a relative clause. When such clauses furnish additional information and can be omitted from the sentence without affecting its meaning, they are called nonrestrictive and require commas around them.
    EXAMPLE: Detroit, which is a large city, faces Windsor, Ontario.

NB: When the words WHO or WHICH are essential parts of the main thought, a comma is not necessary.
    EXAMPLE: The contestant who won the trophy will speak.

Transitional phrases and some conjunctive adverbs such as HOWEVER, THEREFORE, MOREOVER are set off by commas.
    EXAMPLE: The issue, therefore, remains controversial

Statement followed by a question
A comma is always used when a statement is followed by a question in the same sentence.
    EXAMPLE: You weren't guilty, were you?

Numerical Separation
The comma is used between consecutive numbers and identical words.
    EXAMPLE: June 6, 1927
                  That which is, is correct.

Parenthetical Phrases
Interruption of the main thought by phrases such as IN MY OPINION, I THINK, I AM CONFIDENT, are always placed between commas.

EXAMPLE: A larger portion of the funds, in my opinion, should be saved.

Used before OF
A comma is used before OF in phrases indicating residence, position, or title.
EXAMPLE: Dr. Henry Hartwell, of the A.C.S.

Brief questions, maxims or quotations
The comma is used in the following instances:
EXAMPLE: She asked the audience, "What is your pleasure?" "Give us your support," he shouted.

Introduction of an example
Expressions such as THAT IS, i.e., NAMELY, e.g. preceding and introducing an example are placed between commas.
EXAMPLE: The purpose of the operation, namely, to restore function, was achieved.

Specification of place, month, year
EXAMPLE: Dr. Charles Captan opened his office on July 15, 1964, at 31 Willow Blvd., Kalamazoo, Michigan.

Proper names and titles; also titles appearing in succession
EXAMPLE: Dr. Alfred Always, M.D., F.A.C.S.

Quotation marks
Commas appear within quotation marks when used with them.

Colon   (:)

Used after the salutation in a business letter
EXAMPLE: Gentlemen:

Used to introduce a recapitulation of principal points
EXAMPLE: The skeleton might be divided into four gross categories: the bones of the head, the upper extremities, the trunk, and the lower extremities.

Used in expressions of time, numerical formulas, dilutions and bibliographies
EXAMPLE: A dilution of 1:500
At 1:15 P.M.

Semi-Colon   (;)

The semi-colon is a symbol between a period and a comma. It has a number of uses, frequently being used as a strong comma.

Separates clauses of a compound sentence
EXAMPLE: The workers were dissatisfied; their productivity decreased.

Used in the absence of a connective
> EXAMPLE: There must be no compromise; truth will triumph.

Used when a conjunctive adverb serves as the connective
> EXAMPLE: Used before connectives such as THEREFORE, CONSEQUENTLY, HOWEVER, MOREOVER, HENCE, BESIDES, OTHERWISE, IN FACT

Used in lists where a comma would not provide sufficient division

Parentheses and Brackets

In business letters, commas are preferred to parentheses, with dashes being the last choice.

Parentheses are used to inject a thought into a sentence which is not particularly related to the main thought.

Brackets enclose a parenthetical word or expression within the text already in parentheses, or inject a word or phrase as an observation aside from the text.

Quotation Marks   (" ")

Used around all direct quotations
> EXAMPLE: "If my wishes are carried out," said the elderly gentleman, "a shelter will be built for stray animals."

Used around titles of briefer works such as lectures, papers, short plays, paintings, etc.

NB: No quotation marks are necessary when the quoted matter is set in smaller type or is set apart from the remainder of the text with an indentation on either side.

Quotation Marks Used with Other Forms of Punctuation

Commas and periods appear within the quotation marks.

Semi-colons and colons are placed outside the quotation marks.

The interrogation point and exclamation point appear within quotation marks when they are a part of the quotation, otherwise, they appear outside the quotes.

Single Quotation Marks   (' ')

Used for quotations within a quotation
> EXAMPLE: The doctor said: "I heard the patient say, 'The nursing care was excellent'; before he left the hospital."

Brackets ([ ])

Used as parentheses within parentheses.

Exclamation Point (!)

Used to indicate emphatic statements representative of wit, wish, irony, or an otherwise strong feeling.

Interrogation Point (?)

Used after a direct question even when it constitutes a declaration
EXAMPLE: Who will be responsible? today or tomorrow?—with no leadership in the organization.

NB: A request, couched for the sake of courtesy as a question, requires no interrogation point.

Capitals

There are many rules governing the use of capital letters. Some of the more commonly encountered instances are listed here for review purposes. The first letter is capitalized in:

1. Proper nouns and adjectives and their derivatives, in some instances when used in the primary sense.
   EXAMPLE: China   Chino-Russian relations
2. First word of a sentence or an expression used as a sentence.
3. Titles are capitalized when used in conjunction with the name of a specific individual.
4. Holidays and holydays; months of the years; days of the week.
5. Seasons only when they are referred to specifically.
   EXAMPLE: The Spring of 1963
6. Points on the compass when used to refer to specific geographic areas.
   EXAMPLE: The North   The Westerner
   NB: Capitals are not used when points on the compass refer to direction only, such as, *southern* California.
7. Titles and names of specific persons, organizations, agencies, etc.
8. Used in all words appearing in the titles of books, essays, poems, etc., except particles of three letters or less
9. Generic terms when they are a part of a particular geographic name
   EXAMPLE: Detroit River
   NB: The generic term is not capitalized when two or more geographic names precede it.
   EXAMPLE: The St. Clair and Erie lakes

3 { Laboratory and X-Ray Examinations

With advances in our knowledge of physiology and improved technology, laboratory and x-ray examinations have become a valuable diagnostic aid to the physician, helping him to confirm or disprove suspected pathologic conditions. They form an important segment of the diagnostic picture when studied in relation to the clinical findings.

Some of the more commonly used laboratory and x-ray examinations will be discussed in this chapter to provide an understanding for persons engaged in medical secretarial and medical records fields.

Blood

The blood volume of the average person is 5 to 6 quarts (equal to about 5000-6000 ml's or cc.'s). It is broken down and replaced in a healthy individual at a rate of about 50 cc.'s per day. Three types of cells predominate in the composition of the blood; the red corpuscles (RBC's also known as red blood cells or erythrocytes), white corpuscles (also known as WBC's or leukocytes), and platelets. These cells are bathed in a fluid called plasma which serves as a liquid vehicle for their circulation throughout the body.

EXAMINATIONS OF THE BLOOD

Red Blood Count

Normal Values   Male 4,500,000   to 6,000,000 per cu. mm
                        Female 4,300,000   to 5,500,000 per cu. mm

The red blood cells, otherwise known as RBC's or erythrocytes are formed by a cell division in the bone marrow. They are released after approximately seven days into the circulation. The average life of a red blood cell is about 120 days after which it is subjected to a breakdown in the liver and the spleen.

A red pigment known as HEMOGLOBIN is found in the red cells. It possesses the property of carrying oxygen from the lungs to tissues throughout the body.

A lowered red blood count may be seen in the anemias and after a hemorrhage. An increase may result from dehydration or polycythemia.

Hematocrit

Normal values   Male   38–54%
                         Female 36–47%

This is a test on the blood which measures the cells compared to the volume of plasma. It is elevated in polycythemia and dehydration and lowered in the anemias and following hemorrhage. The results are inconclusive after an episode of bleeding or soon after a blood transfusion.

Hemoglobin

Normal Values   Male   14-18 Gm.%
                        Female   12-16 Gm.%
                        Children 12-14 Gm.%

The red cell component of the blood measures about 2000 ml. and consists of about 600 gm. of hemoglobin which can carry 800 ml. of oxygen from the lungs to the tissues of the body.

The hemoglobin is reduced in anemias and hemorrhage and increased in dehydration and polycythemia. It is studied in relation to the red cell count, which does not always vary with the hemoglobin, when the anemias are differentiated.

White Blood Count (WBC)

Normal Value   5,000-10,000

The white blood cells (leukocytes) serve as the body's defense against infection by combating bacterial invaders.

An increase in the white blood cells is seen in infections. It is also seen in some blood disorders and may be very high in the leukemias.

A decreased count may be seen in toxic conditions induced by drugs or chemicals and in blood conditions including the leukopenias.

White Cell Differential

Several types of white blood cells can be differentiated in the white blood count which furnish a valuable index for detecting certain diseases. The differential is usually based on the percentage of particular white cells found in a sample of 100 white blood cells.

Differentiated Cells	per cu. mm.	%	Significance
Band neutrophiles (STABS)	0-500	0-5%	Increased when WBC is elevated as in infections
Basophiles (BASOS)	0-100	0-1%	Increased in certain blood disorders

Eosinophiles .... 50-300 1-3% (EOSINS)		Elevated in parasitic infections
Juvenile neutrophiles ...... 0-100 0-1% (POLYS)		Elevated in very severe infections where WBC is also increased. Also elevated in myelogenous leukemia
Lymphocytes .... 1000-4000 20-40% (LYMPHS) (elevated in children under age 10 yrs.)		Increased in viral infections, measles, pernicious anemia, pertussis, lymphocytic leukemia. Exophthalmic goiter.
Monocytes .... 200-800 4-8% (MONOS)		Increased in SBE (subacute bacterial endocarditis), malaria, typhoid fever, amebic dysentery, trypanosomiasis, Hodgkin's Disease and lipoid storage diseases.
Myelocytes 0 0%		Presence suggests granulocytic leukemia or blood diseases such as pernicious anemia. Metastases to bone in cases of malignancy suggested.
Segmented Neutrophiles 2500-6000 40-60% (SEGS)		Increased in bacterial infections.

Platelets (Thrombocytes)

Normal Value   200,000-500,000

These cells are thought to be important in blood coagulation. An increase is noted in certain of the anemias, polycythemia, injury, emotional stress and thrombocytopenia. Values are decreased in pernicious anemia, acute leukemia, chronic lymphocytic leukemia, aplastic anemia, thrombocytopenic purpura and septicemia.

decrease in platelets

OTHER EXAMINATIONS OF THE BLOOD

The most common examinations performed on the blood have been listed at the beginning of this chapter. Other blood examinations including blood chemistry are listed below in alphabetical order.

EXAMINATION	NORMAL VALUES	SIGNIFICANCE
Albumin	3.5-5.5 Gm./100 cc	Decreased in nephrosis, liver disease, malnutrition.
Amylase	70-200 Somogyi Units	Increased following abdominal surgery, in perforated peptic ulcer, pancreatic diseases, ruptured ectopic pregnancy, mumps, peritonitis and other intra-abdominal conditions.
Ascorbic Acid (Vit. C)	0.4 - 1.0 mg.%	Lowered in Vit. C deficiency manifested clinically by scurvy.

EXAMINATION	*NORMAL VALUES*	*SIGNIFICANCE*
Bilirubin, Immediate (Direct)	0.1 - 0.4 mg.%	Increased in obstructive hepatic disease. It is a measure of the free bilirubin in the blood.
Bilirubin, Total (Indirect) Also: van den Bergh	0.2 - 0.7 mg.%	Increase indicates elevation in destruction of red blood cells.
BSP (Bromsulphalein)	Less than 5% retention	Liver function test.
BUN (Blood Urea Nitrogen)	10 - 20 mg.%	Increased in some of the kidney diseases; preferred to NPN.
Calcium	9 - 11 mg.% 4.5 - 5.5 mEq/l	Decreased in absorptive deficiency conditions of G. I. tract, rickets, Bright's Disease, hypoparathyroidism and kidney diseases. Increase occurs in multiple myeloma, hyperparathyroidism.
Carbon Dioxide (CO_2) combining power	56 - 65 Vol. % 25 - 30 mEq/l	Increased in hypoventilation with alkalosis. Decreased in acidosis.
Cephalin Flocculation	0 - 1+	Test to determine liver function. Used to evaluate patients with cirrhosis of the liver.
Chlorides	350 - 390 mg.% 100 - 110 mEq/l	Decrease seen in Addison's Disease, acidosis, heat prostration. Increase seen in cases of renal malfunction and Cushing's Syndrome.
Cholesterol (total)	110 - 300 mg.%	Increased in liver diseases with hepatic impairment, hypothyroidism. Decreased in anemias, hyperthyroidism.
Cholesterol Esters	75 - 210 mg.%	Decreased in liver damage.
Coagulation Time (clotting time)	6 - 10 min. (Lee & White)	Measurement of ability of blood to clot properly.
Coombs, Direct	negative	Indicates presence of antibody with red blood cells. Used to test newborn blood for erythroblastosis fetalis. Also used in blood cross matching.
Coombs, Indirect	negative	Used to detect possible blood incompatibilities in cross matching. Also used to detect Rh incompatibility in the maternal blood before delivery by demonstrating anti-Rh antibodies.

EXAMINATION	NORMAL VALUES	SIGNIFICANCE
C-Reactive Protein	negative	Shows positive reaction with conditions characterized by inflammation. Seen in the active phase of rheumatic infections, acute myocardial infarction, viral infections, disseminated L.E. and neoplastic diseases.
Creatine (serum)	3 - 7 mg.%	Increases in pregnancy, hyperthyroidism, severe malnutrition.
Creatinine	1 - 2 mg.%	Increased in conditions of impaired kidney function; used as a check on elevated BUN for possible renal factor.
Fibrinogen	150 - 300 mg.%	Helps to localize the defect in clotting deficiencies. It is essential to proper clotting.
Globulin	1.5 - 3.4 Gm/100 cc.	When albumin is lost, compensatory globulin may be formed. Ratio of albumin and globulin (A/G Ratio) decreased in liver impairment, nephrosis, nephritis.
Glucose	80 - 120 mg.%	Test for blood sugar in diabetes, liver disease. Decreased in glycogen storage disease (von Gierke's) , excessive insulin, hypoglycemia.
Glucose Tolerance (Fasting blood Sugar test)	negative	Four blood samples are taken at regulated times to determine how efficiently the body uses glucose. Indication of diabetes where blood sugar does not return to normal in three hours.
Heterophile Antibody	Agglutination in titers up to 1:28	Elevated in infectious mononucleosis and serum sickness.
Icterus Index	3 - 8 Units	Used to discover early jaundice.
Lactic Acid	6 - 20	Increased in diseases where there is a reduced supply of oxygen to the tissues such as congestive heart failure and pneumonia. Metabolic acidosis caused by excesses in the blood.
Latex Slide Agglutination Latex succession Test	1:40 is uppermost serum dilution producing agglutination	Positive in some connective tissue diseases and rheumatoid arthritis.
Lipase	0.2 - 1.5 Units	Increased in pancreatic damage.

EXAMINATION	NORMAL VALUES	SIGNIFICANCE
L.E. Test (Lupus Erythematosus Cell Test)	Absence of L.E. Cell	Used to diagnose disseminated lupus; positive in some cases of rheumatoid arthritis.
Lipids, Total	570 - 820 mg.%	Elevated in uncontrolled diabetes mellitus, ketosis and nephrosis.
Malaria Slide	negative	Used for detection of malarial parasite.
NPN (Non-protein nitrogen)	25 - 40 mg.%	Kidney function test.
Phosphatase, Acid	0 - 1.1 Bodansky U. 0.5 - 3.5 Units (King-Armstrong)	Used to detect metastasizing carcinoma of the prostate.
Phosphatase, Alkaline ★	2 - 4.5 Bodansky U. 4-13 King-Armstrong	Elevated in women in the third trimester of pregnancy and also elevated in children.
Children:	5-14 Bodansky Units 15-20 King-Armstrong	Increased levels seen in bone diseases such as osteomalacia, healing fractures, osteoblastic bone tumors. Hyperparathyroidism. Decreased in malnutrition.
Phosphorus: Adults	3 - 4.5 mg.% (1.8 - 2.3 mEq/1)	Elevated in hypoparathyroidism, uremia, Bright's disease, excessive Vit. D intake.
Children	4 - 6.5 mg.% (2.3 - 3.8 mEq/1)	Lowered in hyperparathyroidism, osteomalacia, rickets.
Potassium (K)	18 - 22 mg.% (3.5 - 5.5 mEq/1)	Elevated levels seen in adrenal cortical deficiency, hypoventilation and shows up on EKG when increased to marked degree. Lowered levels in deficient renal function; hyperactivity of adrenal cortex; marked hyperemesis. (excessive vomiting)
Protein Bound Iodine (PBI)	4.5 - 8 mcg.	Test for thyroid function.
Proteins, Total Total Protein	6.3 - 8.0 Gm./100 cc.	Performed with albumin and globulin. Lowered levels in liver disease, malnutrition, chronic kidney disease.
Prothrombin Time	70 - 110 % of control 12 - 14 seconds with Difco thromboplastin	When anti-coagulant therapy used, prothrombin time kept at from 2 - 2½ times normal.
Red Cell Fragility	96 - 100 % hemolysis with 0.30 % NaCl	Red cells placed in a NaCl (salt) solution and salt in the solution decreased causing water to pass into the blood

EXAMINATION	NORMAL VALUES	SIGNIFICANCE
	0 - 5% hemolysis with 0.50% NaCl	cell which eventually bursts (hemolysis). Cell fragility measured by point at which hemolysis occurs. Increased in aplastic anemia and hemolytic anemias. Decreased in sickle cell anemia, polycythemia vera, iron def. anemia, diseases of the liver, jaundice, and following splenectomy.
Sedimentation Rate	Male 0 - 9 mm/hour Female 0 - 20 mm/hour (Westergren Method)	Increased sed. rate in pregnancy from 12th week to 1 month postpartum. Increased also in Tbc, cancer, rheumatic fever, rheumatoid arthritis and myocardial infarction.
Serology Test for syphilis	Negative	Several tests used such as the Kahn, Kolmer, Wasserman, V.D.R.L. (Venereal Disease Research Lab) Kline, Eagle, Hinton, Mazzini. False positive results sometimes obtained. Positive results may be confirmed with a complement fixation or TPI (Treponema Pallidum Immobilization).

also RPR card test is used.

EXAMINATION	NORMAL VALUES	SIGNIFICANCE
Serum Transaminase (SGOT) or ~~SPGT~~ SGPT	10 - 14 Units	Elevated in liver disease and myocardial infarction.
Sickle Cell Test	sickle-shaped red blood cells *not* seen.	In sickle cell anemia, a red cell is noted which assumes a sickle shape when the oxygen supply is reduced. Sickle cell anemia is found in about 8% of American Negroes. Persons with the sickle cell trait are poor surgical and OB risks.
Sodium (Na)	310 - 340 mg.% 135 - 147 mEq/1.	Decreased in kidney diseases, Addison's Disease and heat prostration.
Takata-Ara Test ?	negative	Liver function test. ?
Thorn Test (eosinophile)	50% drop in eosinophil count 4 hr. after injection of epinephrine or ACTH.	Test for Addison's Disease in which no reduction in eosinophiles occurs.
Thymol Turbidity	0 - 5 Units	Liver function test with increase indicative of liver damage.
Uric Acid	2 - 4 mg.%	Increased in gout, leukemia and toxemia.
Zinc Flocculation (Turbidity)	6 - 12.5 Units	Liver function test.

EXAMINATIONS PERFORMED ON THE URINE

Like the blood, the urine yields valuable information to assist the clinician in further assessing the physiologic status of the patient.

The average sized adult urinary bladder usually can hold about 350 cc. of urine before the urge to urinate becomes manifest. In a 24 hour period an adult may void between ½ and 2 quarts. Throughout the night urine is secreted into the bladder at the rate of about 40 cc. per hour. The intake of fluids throughout the day influences the amount of urine excreted and the frequency of urination. On an average, about a third of the fluid intake is passed within the first hour.

Some of the more common laboratory procedures performed on the urine will be discussed in this chapter in relation to their clinical significance.

EXAMINATION	NORMAL VALUES	SIGNIFICANCE
Acetone	Negative	Used to detect presence of acidosis and possible impending diabetic coma. Acetone may be a normal finding in the urine of children.
Addis Test	Hyaline Casts 0 - 5,000 RBC's 0 - 500,000 WBC's 35,000 - 1,000,000	Comparison of the RBC's, WBC's and hyaline casts helps to differentiate the kidney disease responsible. Casts and RBC's may be greatly increased in nephritis.
Albumin (qualitative)	0 - 15%	Idiopathic albuminuria seen in some persons in the absence of disease. When it is increased it may suggest hypertension, kidney disease or severe heart failure.
Albumin (Quantitative)	Negative	A test to measure the amount of protein being lost in the urine.
Aschheim-Zondek	Negative	Positive in pregnancy and in certain malignant tumors. 98% reliable in detecting pregnancy.
Ascorbic Acid	15 - 20 mg.	Tests Vit. C deficiency in which the amount excreted is below normal.
Bence-Jones Protein	negative	Present in the urine in multiple myeloma and bone neoplasms.
Calcium (Sulkowitch Test)	0.1 - 0.3 gm/24 hr. 9 - 11 mg.% 4.5 - 5.5 mEq./l.	Decreased in hypoparathyroidism.

EXAMINATION	NORMAL VALUES	SIGNIFICANCE
Chlorides	350 - 390 mg.% 100 - 110 mEq./l.	Determines urinary chloride loss.
Creatine	3 - 7 mg.%	Increases in pregnancy, hyperthyroidism and starvation.
Creatinine	1 - 2 mg.%	Elevated in impaired kidney function.
Diacetic Acid (Acetoacetic)	negative	Test for acidosis (ketosis) when present in the urine.
Friedman	negative	Test performed on a female rabbit with urine from a woman suspected of being pregnant. Positive in pregnancy.
Frog Test	negative	Positive in pregnancy and some malignant tumors such as teratomas and chorioepitheliomas as well as in hydatiform mole and chorionic epithelioma where chorionic gonadotrophic hormone is excreted in the urine.
Hippuric Acid (I.V.)	0.7 - 1.0 gm/24 hr.	Liver function test seldom used today. Decreased levels indicate liver disease such as cirrhosis or hepatitis.
17-Ketosteroids Male Female	 8 - 21 mg./24 hr. 4 - 14 mg./24 hr.	Increased levels seen in testicular and adrenal hyperfunction such as Cushing's Disease and adrenogenital syndromes. Very high values suggest carcinoma of adrenal cortex. Decreased levels seen in Addison's Disease, myxedema and pituitary deficiency.
Lead	50 mcg. or less/24 hr.	Used to measure lead content of the urine in suspected lead poisoning.
PSP (Phenolsulfonphthalein)	25% or more/15 min. 40 - 60% / 1 hour 60 - 85% / 2 hours	Elevated in some liver diseases. Reduced in chronic nephritis.
Phenylketonuria (PKU)	negative	Used to detect phenylpyruvic acid in the urine of infants after the 4th week. Performed as a diaper test. Since mental deficiency results from the child's inability to properly metabolize phenylalanine, a diet deficient in this amino acid must be instituted.
Porphyrins	0 - 30 mcg.	Increased in congenital porphyria, pellagra, liver damage and lead poisoning.
Potassium (K)	1.5 - 2.5 gm./24 hr.	Lowered values in Cushing's Disease. Increased in oliguria.

EXAMINATION	NORMAL VALUES	SIGNIFICANCE
Purines	0.05 gm./24 hr.	Increased by ingestion of foods abundant in nucleins such as liver and sweetbreads. Greatest increase occurs in leukemia, destructive liver disease and during absorption of a pneumonic process. Decreased before onset of gout with elevation following onset of an attack.
Sodium	3 - 5 gm./24 hr. 100 mEq./24 hr.	Decreased in Addison's Disease, some kidney diseases, diarrhea and heat prostration.
Urea	25 - 35 gms./24 hr.	Indication of dietary protein intake.
Uric Acid	0.5 - 0.8 gm./24 hr.	Major increase noted in leukemia; also seen in fever, liver damage and during x-ray therapy. It is increased with use of ACTH or 11-oxygenated adrenocortical hormones.
Urobilinogen	0 - 4 mg./24 hr.	Used to differentiate jaundice caused by liver disease where urobilinogen is elevated and obstructive jaundice where no increase occurs. Increased in hemolytic jaundice and some liver diseases.

EXAMINATIONS OF THE CEREBROSPINAL FLUID

In an adult individual, the total cerebrospinal fluid (spinal fluid) amounts to approximately 100-140 cc.'s. It is a clear, colorless fluid which bathes the brain and spinal cord. It is secreted by the choroid plexuses, glandular structures in the lateral ventricles of the brain. The amount secreted in a 24 hour period varies with individuals; however, it is estimated that it may vary from 300 to 1000 cc.'s. The fluid passes through the arachnoidal tissue into the venous circulation.

Samples of cerebrospinal fluid are withdrawn for diagnostic studies by means of a procedure known as a spinal puncture. A long needle is inserted into the vertebral canal through the middle of the space between the third and fourth lumbar vertebrae. Fluid may also be withdrawn by a cisternal puncture by introducing the needle between the first cervical vertebra and the occipital bone.

Pressure readings are usually taken with the patient on his side. In adults such pressure may range from 70-200 mm. of water; in children the range may vary from 50-100 mm. of water and in newborn infants, from 30-80 mm. of water.

EXAMINATION	NORMAL VALUES	SIGNIFICANCE
Sp. Gravity	1.003 - 1.009	
pH	7.35 - 7.40	

Total Cells
  Adults:
  Infants:
	0 - 10 per cu. mm.
	0 - 20 per cu. mm.
		Increased levels seen in encephalitis, neurosyphilis, meningitis.

Chlorides	690 - 750 mg.%	Slightly decreased in purulent bacterial meningitis and even lower in tuberculous meningitis.
Cholesterol	0.05 - 0.20 mg.%	
CO_2 combining power	40 - 60 vol.%	
Colloidal Gold	Negative	When a precipitate of colloidal gold is obtained it may suggest multiple sclerosis, neurosyphilis or other diseases of the CNS. It must be evaluated relative to the entire clinical picture.
Proteins, total Proteins, globulin Proteins, albumin	20 - 45 mg.% 4 - 10 mg.% 16 - 35 mg.%	Increased in hemorrhage. Levels may be elevated as high as 2000 mg.% in meningitis.
Serology	Negative	Positive in neurosyphilis.
Sugar (Glucose)	45 - 75 mg./100 ml.	Absent or low in acute purulent meningitis. Present in ranges from 10 to 20 mg. per 100 ml. in tuberculous meningitis.

OTHER LABORATORY EXAMINATIONS

Basal Metabolic Rate (BMR)	+15 to —15	Elevated in hyperthyroidism and lowered in hypothyroidism. Subject to error.
Protein Bound Iodine	4.5 to 8 mcg.	Lowered values indicate hypothyroidism. Elevated values indicate hyperthyroidism.
Radio-iodine Uptake (I^{131})	15 to 50% uptake	Used as a test for hyperthyroidism.

Triiodothyronine (TBI-Thyrobinding Index)
  Males
  Females
	
	11 to 19%
	11 to 17%
		Levels lowered in hypothyroidism and elevated in hyperthyroidism. Abnormal conditions of the serum proteins may influence results.

X-RAY EXAMINATIONS

The surgeon frequently refers to particular x-ray media and examinations in his dictations and for this reason it will behoove the secretary to become familiar with this information.

X-Ray

Radiologists employ a variety of media which are either injected or taken orally by the patient prior to x-ray examinations. These dyes or contrast media serve to differentiate the organ being examined from the surrounding tissues. Contrast media may be of the radiolucent (permitting some passage of roentgen rays) variety or may be radiopaque (not permitting passage of x-rays) in type. One particular medium may be used for several different exams.

A listing of the more commonly used radiographic contrast media follows:

Baridol	Miokon Sodium
Barium Sulfate	Monophen
Baropaque, A, B or C	Mulsopaque
Barosperse	Neo-Iopax
Basolac	Oragrafin Tablets & Granules
Bismuth Carbonate	Pantopaque
Cholestim	Priodax
Cholografin	Pychokon-R
Conray	Renografin
Diodrast	Rugar
Dionosil	Salpix
Ethiodol	Shadocol
Gastrografin	Sinografin
GBD Tablets	Skiodan
Hippuran	Telepaque
Hypaque Sodium	Teridax
Hytrast	Thixokon
Iodipamide	Thorotrast
Iodochlorol	Umbrathor
Lipiodol	Urokon
Lipomul	Veripaque
Medopaque	Visciodol
Micropaque	X-iodol
Microtrast	

The secretary should be familiar with the specialized procedures performed in the x-ray department and should be acquainted with their significance in the diagnostic work-up.

Aortography

Examination of the aorta and its branches by x-ray during the administration of a radiopaque medium. It is used by the urologist to survey the renal vascular system. This examination is useful in localizing vascular defects and can be used to assess their operability.

Barium Enema

After thorough catharsis, radiopaque media is introduced into the colon by way of an enema. The radiologist observes the filling of the lower G.I. tract under fluoroscopy to detect filling defects. X-ray films are taken following the fluoroscopic examination and the patient is then permitted to expel the barium. When the presence of polyps is suspected, the barium enema is sometimes followed by a double contrast examination consisting of the injection of air into the evacuated colon.

Bronchogram

Fluoroscopic and x-ray examination of the tracheobronchial tree is performed after the injection of a radiopaque medium. This examination is used to detect space occupying lesions as well as foreign bodies, tuberculosis, bronchiectasis and abcesses.

Cardioangiogram

Catheterization of the heart is carried out following which an x-ray medium is injected. X-ray films are made of the heart and large vessels.

Carotid Angiography

X-ray examination of the brain and its circulation is performed in this procedure. Media is injected into the common carotoid artery bilaterally or unilaterally. This technique is used to detect space occupying lesions, displaced vessels, defects and aneurysms of the vessels including thrombi and hematomas.

Cholangiogram

This examination may be carried out preoperatively, during surgery or postoperatively. The operative cholangiogram enables the surgeon to inject media directly into the common duct. This is a particularly useful examination for detecting stones higher in the biliary tree which might have eluded the surgeon during his digital exploration.

The examination may be performed postoperatively by way of a drainage tube left in the wound. X-ray films are made of the dye in the biliary tract.

When the examination is performed preoperatively, the dye is injected intravenously.

Cholecystogram

Following a very light evening meal and catharsis, the patient is given an oral dose of dye in the form of tablets (Priodax). This dye concentrates in the gallbladder which is x-rayed on the following morning. A fatty meal which causes the gallbladder to contract is administered after the first set of films and a film to study gallbladder function is then taken.

Femoral Arteriography

X-ray survey of the femoral artery during injection of radiopaque medium. It affords visualization of the circulation from the inguinal area down the length of the extremity. This examination is employed to discover occlusive phenomena including thrombi, aneurysm, arteriosclerosis, etc.

Hysterosalpingogram

Contrast medium is introduced through the cervical canal into the uterus and fallopian tubes which are then studied by x-ray films. This examination is used to determine the patency of the tubes and uterus.

Myelogram

Air or contrast medium is used in the fluoroscopic and x-ray examination of the spine and subarachnoid space. This study is used to localize and confirm filling defects, herniated nucleus pulposus (ruptured disc), cord tumors, etc.

Pneumoencephalogram

Air is introduced into the subarachnoid space to study the ventricles of the brain.

Pyelogram, I.V.

Dye is injected into the vein and x-ray films taken at spaced intervals to evaluate renal structures and function.

Pyelogram, Retrograde

Dye is introduced by way of ureteral catheters to evaluate renal structure and function. This examination is usually performed with a cystoscopy.

Ventriculogram

Filtered air or oxygen is introduced directly into the lateral ventricles for the study of the brain and ventricles by x-ray. This procedure is preferred over the pneumoencephalogram when there are signs of intracranial pressure.

4 〉 Pre- and Postoperative Considerations

Anesthesia

Modern surgery has developed with an attending surgical specialty, anesthesiology, without which many of the surgical operations performed today would not be possible.

Neither surgery nor anesthesia are the inventions of modern men. Ancient records, predating Christ by thousands of years, describe primitive surgery and attempts to control and alleviate pain.

Anesthesiology, as we know it today, evolved from the discovery of nitrous oxide (laughing gas) in 1772 by an English chemist, Joseph Priestley, who two years later discovered oxygen. Since that time the list of chemicals with anesthesia inducing properties has grown in refinement and variety.

A listing of the more commonly used anesthetics has been prepared here to assist the secretary in her work. Generic names are used as often as trade names in the profession and for this reason this list purports to be only an alphabetical one. Where an anesthetic is variably known by several names, these will be listed in parentheses.

ANESTHETIC AGENTS

Amethocaine (pontocaine, pantocaine tetracaine)
Amytal
Apothesine hydrochloride
Avertin

Benzocaine
Blockain hydrochloride
Brevital
Butadiene

Carbocaine (mepivacaine)
Chloroprocaine (nesacaine)
Cinchocaine (nupercaine, debucaine, percaine)

Cocaine
Cyclaine (hexylcaine)
Cyclohexane (hexamethylene)
Cyclopentane (C_5H_{10})
Cyclopropane (C_3H_6)

Dibucaine (nupercaine, percaine cinchocaine)
Divinyl oxide (vinethene, divinyl ether)
Dyclone

Ethapon (trichloroethanol)
Ether
Ethocaine (procaine, novocain)

ANESTHETIC AGENTS
(continued)

Ethyl chloride
Ethylene
Ethyl ether (ethyl oxide)
Evipan
Fluoromar (trifluoroethyl vinyl ether)
Fluothane (halothane)
Halothane
Hexylcaine (cyclaine)
Lidocaine (xylocaine, lignocaine)
Lignocaine (lidocaine, xylocaine)
Mepivacaine (carbocaine)
Methycaine hydrochloride
 (piperocaine)
Monocaine
Nesacaine (chloroprocaine)
Nitrous oxide (N^2O)
Novocain (procaine, ethocaine)
Nupercaine crystal
Nupercaine hydrochloride (dibucaine
 percaine, cinchocaine)
Orthocaine

Pantocaine (pontocaine, amethocaine,
 tetracaine)
Penthrane
Pentothal (pentothal sodium)
Percaine (nupercaine, dibucaine, cin-
 chocaine)
Piperocaine (metycaine)
Pontocaine hydrochloride (ametho-
 caine, tetracaine, pantocaine)
Procaine hydrochloride (novocain,
 ethocaine)
Surfacaine
Surital sodium
Tetracaine (pontocaine, pantocaine,
 amethocaine)
Trichlorethylene (trilene)
Trifluorethyl vinyl ether (fluoromar)
Vinamar (vinyl ethyl ether)
Vinethene
Vinyl ethyl ether
Xylocaine (lidocaine, lignocaine)

OPHTHALMIC ANESTHETICS
(eye)

Butyn sulfate & Metaphen ophthalmic
 ointment
Metycaine hydrochloride and
 merthiolate

Ophthaine
Ophthetic ophthalmic solution
Tetracaine HCl
Xylocaine hydrochloride 4% solution

PREPARATIONS USED WITH
ANESTHESIA

Anectine .... muscle relaxant
Atropine and
 Scopolamine .... twilight sleep
Carbon Dioxide.. CO_2
Chloral .... hypnotic
Codeine .... analgesic
Curare .... muscle relaxant
Ephedrine .... vasopressor (raises
 blood pressure)
Epinephrine ..... vasopressor and
 cardiac stimulant

Gallamine .... muscle relaxant
Hydralazine ..... anti-hypertensive
 agent
Morphine sulfate. analgesic
Oxygen .... symbol = O
Paraldehyde ..... hypnotic
Syncurine .... muscle relaxant
Tolserol .... muscle relaxant
Tuinal .... hypnotic

MODES OF INDUCTION OF
ANESTHESIA

Basal narcosis

Block

Caudal

Caudal block

Continuous spinal

Endobronchial

Endotracheal

Epidural block (peridural)

Field block

Infiltration (local)

Inhalation

Insufflation

Intercostal block

Intravenous

Local infiltration

Nerve block:
    brachial plexus

    cervical plexus
    lumbar plexus

Open

Open drop ether

Open endotracheal

Paravertebral block

Rectal

Regional spinal

Sacral block

Saddle block

Segmental block

Spinal block (subarachnoid)

Splanchnic block

Sympathetic block

Topical

Transsacral (sacral & caudal)

SURGICAL POSITIONS

Prior to surgery, the chief surgeon on the case decides upon the position in which the patient will be operated. This information is usually included in his surgical report and for this reason the secretary should be familiar with the more commonly used positions.

Arm Extension—Patient flat on his back with the arm extended on an arm board beside him. This position is used for operations on the hand, arm, axilla and breast.

Chest—Patient on his side with his back to the surgeon and his shoulder rotated toward the surgeon to provide access to the chest. This position is used in thoracic surgery and is sometimes called the lateral chest position.

Dorsal (Supine)—Patient placed flat on his back with legs extended before him and arms resting at his sides. This position is used for abdominal surgery.

Dorsal Recumbent—Patient is placed flat on her back with knees drawn up and thighs turned outward. This position is used for examinations of the vagina.

Head Dependent—Patient on his back with a pillow under his neck and the head extended over the end of the table. This position is used for removal of tonsils, operations on the mouth and cleft palate repair.

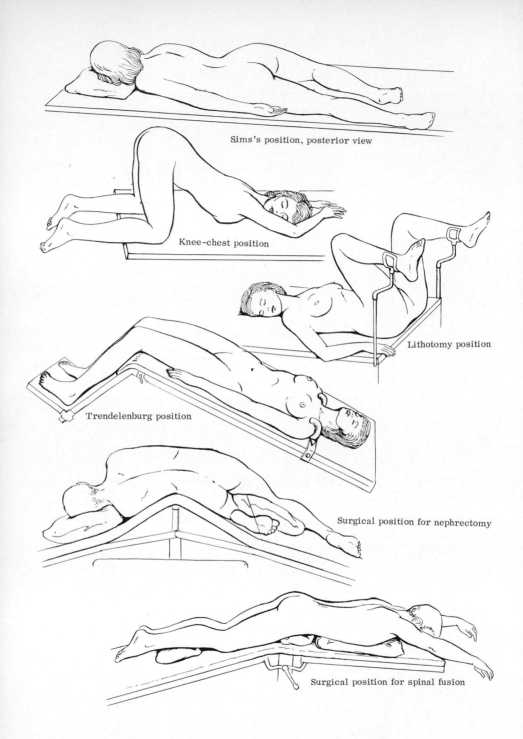

Sims's position, posterior view

Knee-chest position

Lithotomy position

Trendelenburg position

Surgical position for nephrectomy

Surgical position for spinal fusion

POSITIONS

Fowler's—Patient placed flat on his back with foot of the table lowered somewhat and the head raised about 30 degrees.

Jackknife—Patient placed on abdomen with head and foot of table dropped so buttocks are most prominent. This position is used for hemorrhoidectomy.

Kidney—Patient placed on his side, body elevator raised under the patient to hyperextend the side to be operated. Head and foot of table are lowered. This position is used for operations on the kidney and its structures.

Knee-Chest—Patient kneeling on the table, resting on his elbows. This is also called the genucubital position.

Kraske—Same as jackknife.

Lateral Prone—Same as kidney position.

Lithotomy—Patient on back with legs up in stirrups.

Neck Extension—Dorsal position with support under neck. This position is used in removing cervical glands and also for goiter operations.

Prone—Patient positioned flat on abdomen with head turned to one side. Used for operations on the back.

Reverse Trendelenburg—The lower end of the table is dropped to a 45 degree angle. This position is sometimes used in abdominal surgery.

Robson—Patient placed on his back with a sandbag under the hollow of the back.

Rose's—Head lowered for operations on the palate and oropharynx.

Shock—Table inclined with the head lowered.

Sims'—Patient placed on left side with left arm placed in back of the patient causing patient to rest on chest. The right knee is drawn up.

Trendelenburg—Patient placed on her back, table tilted 45 degrees toward the head and broken at the knees. This is a position used in pelvic surgery.

Upright—Patient seated in an operating chair. This position is used for submucous resection and sometimes, for tonsillectomy.

INCISIONS

A properly dictated operative report should contain a reference to the incision. The surgeon may specify the site over which the incision is made. He may indicate whether it is a muscle splitting incision or one carried in the direction of the muscle fibers. He may describe the course of the incision or may specify it by name.

Some of the more commonly referred to incisions are listed here.

Auvray	An incision used in splenectomy.
Banks & Laufman	Transverse popliteal incision of medial aspect of leg.
Bar	An incision used in cesarean sections.
Battle	Same as Battle-Jalaguier-Kammerer incision for abdominal section.
Bergmann	An incision for exposing the kidney.
Bevan	An incision for exposing the gallbladder.
Celiotomy	Incision through the abdominal wall to permit access to the peritoneal cavity.
Circumscribing	Encircling.
Confirmatory	An incision made into an organ for the purpose of confirming a diagnosis.
Crescent	Half-moon shaped.
Crosshatch	An incision consisting of sets of parallel lines crossing parallel lines running crosswise.
Crucial (Cruciate)	Cross shaped incision.
Deaver	An incision for appendicitis through the sheath of the right rectus muscle.
Dührssen	Deep incisions into the cervix uteri to facilitate delivery of an infant.
Endaural	An incision made within the ear.
Exploratory	An incision made for exploratory purposes.
Fergusson	Incision for excision of the upper jaw.
Fowler	Angular incision for anterolateral abdominal section.
Gatellier	Incision over the lateral malleolus of fibula.
Halsted	Inguinal herniorrhaphy incision; also used in radical mastectomy.
Harmon	Incision made on the posterolateral aspect of the leg.
Heerman	Endaural incision.
Hockey-stick	J-shaped incision.
Kehr	Incision used for creating a wide abdominal field.
Kocher	Gallbladder incision.
Kustner	Semilunar abdominal incision.
Langenbeck	Abdominal incision through the linea semilunaris parallel to the fibers of the Rectus abdominis muscle.
Lateral rectus	An abdominal incision.
Lempert	Endaural incision.

Incisions (continued)

Longuet	Incision for transplantation of the testicle.
Mackenrodt	Transverse semilunar abdominal incision.
Mayo-Robson	Right upper quadrant abdominal incision.
McArthur	A vertical upper trans rectus incision with transverse division of the peritoneum and posterior sheath.
McBurney	An abdominal incision used for appendectomy.
Median	A midline incision.
Meyer	Hockey stick incision for entering the lower anterior abdomen.
Ollier	Ankle incision.
Paramedian	An incision just lateral to the midline in the upper abdomen.
Parker	An incision nearly parallel with Poupart's ligament used for appendiceal abscess.
Perthes'	A gallbladder incision.
Pfannenstiel	A curved abdominal incision.
Phemister	An incision along the posterior border of the tibia.
Relief	An incision made to relieve tension in a region.
Saber cut	An inverted U incision.
Semilunar	Half-moon shaped incision.
Visscher	An incision in the lumbo-iliac region.
Wilde	An incision behind the auricle to expose the mastoid region.

SUTURE MATERIALS

Absorbable
Aluminum bronze wire
Ancap silk (braided silk)
Atraumatic

Babcock suture wire
Black silk
Braided
Braided silk
Bronze wire
Bunnell

Cargile membrane
Catgut
Catgut celluloid linen
Champion silk
Chinese twisted silk
Chloramine catgut

Chromic catgut
Circumcision
Cotton
Cuticular
Dacron
Deknatel surgical silk
Dermal

Dermalon monofilament
Dermalon
D & G Kalmerid catgut
Double armed
Double armed retention
Double stop (glass beads & lead shot)

Equisetene silk
Ethicon
Ethicon atroloc

SUTURE MATERIALS (continued)

Ethilon nylon
Ethi-pack steel

Flexon stainless steel

Gastrointestinal surgical gut
Gastrointestinal surgical linen
Gastrointestinal surgical silk
General closure
Gossamer silk
Gut—chromic
Gut—plain

Horsehair

Iodized surgical gut

Kal-dermic
Kangaroo tendon

Linen
Luken's iodized catgut
Mayo iron dyed linen
Medrafil suture wire
Mersilene
Mesh
Monofilament
Multifilament

Non-absorbable
Nylon
Nylon monofilament

OB double armed
Oiled silk
Oyloidin linen
Oyloidin silk

Pagenstecher linen

Pearsall Chinese twisted silk
Plain gut
Pyoktanin catgut

Ramsey County pyoktanin catgut
Retention
Ribbon gut

Silicone treated surgical silk
Silk
Silkworm gut
Silver suture wire
Stainless steel
Steel
Steel mesh
Supramid—Extra (polyfilament synthetic)
Surgaloy mono-strand stainless steel
Surgaloy multi-strand stainless steel
Surgilon (braided nylon)

Tantalum wire—monofilament
Tevdek
Thermo-flex
Twenty day catgut
Twisted cotton
Twisted silk

Unabsorbable

Vascular silk
Vienna wire

White nylon
White twisted silk

Zytor

Suture Techniques

Alternating	Alternating simple interrupted and mattress sutures used to prevent a depressed scar or improper wound contour.
Appolito	A continuous cross stitch.
Argyll-Robertson	Suture for ectropion (turning out of lower eyelid)
Arlt	Suture for entropion (turning of eyelid inward)
Atraumatic	Minimizing traumatic or injurious effects.

Suture Techniques

Back and forth	A continuous suture carried back and forth under the line of incision, thus preventing sutures from lying across the incision line.
Baseball	A continuous suture carried throughout the length of a wound and placed similar to that with which a baseball is stitched.
Bertrandi	A back and forth type continuous suture.
Buried	Sutures placed under the skin and covered over by the skin incision.
Button	Suture placed through buttons situated on either side of the line of incision.
Coaptation	Sutures aligning the wound edges.
Cobbler	Suture with a needle at both ends.
Connell	A suturing technique used on the intestine in anastomosis procedures where a continuous suture is used on one half of the approximation and the other half of the lumen is closed by a suture carried through the entire wall of the intestine.
Continuous	A non-interrupted suture.
Cushing	A continuous suture traversing the line of incision.
Cutaneous	Skin suture.
Czerny	Suturing technique for tenorrhaphy. Intestinal suture carried through mucous membrane layer.
Czerny-Lembert	Intestinal suturing technique.
Emmet	Double Lembert suturing technique used in closure of intestinal wounds.
Figure-of-eight	Suturing technique in which the thread makes a design resembling the number eight.
Gaillard	Suture for entropion of the eyelid.
Gely	A suture technique consisting of cross stitches and made with a suture containing a needle at either end.
Glover	A continuous stitch in which the needle, after each stitch, is passed through the loop of the previous stitch.
Gould	A mattress intestinal suture technique.
Gussenbauer	Closure figure-of-eight stitch used for instrumentation wounds of the intestine.
Halsted	Intestinal closure technique utilizing mattress sutures, interrupted, each one tieing on the opposite side of the incision line from the previous one.
Jobert	Interrupted suturing technique for anastomosis of the intestine.

Suture Techniques

Ledentu	Suturing technique for tenorrhaphy.
LeFort	Suturing technique for tenorrhaphy.
Lembert	Technique for intestinal repair with interrupted sutures taken through the peritoneum and muscular tunic.
Loffler	Intestinal repair technique utilizing wire loops in an interrupted fashion.
Mattress	A stitch carried under the line of incision in the shape of a U and tied to one side of the incisional line where both ends of the stitch can be brought together. These sutures do not cross the line of incision and may be carried as a continuous or interrupted stitch.
Maunsell	Suture used in mesenteric layer following the severing of an intestine.
Palfyn	Suturing technique for intestinal closure with fixation of the sutures to the skin.
Pancoast	A suturing technique utilized in plastic surgery where a groove is cut in one wound edge and a tongue in the opposite edge and the two wound edges sewn together.
Pare	Closure technique using cloth closure strips on either side of the incision which are sewn together to bring the wound together.
Purse-string	A suture carried in a continuous in-and-out manner around a gapping opening in such a manner that when the ends of the suture are drawn taut, the wound closes as would a draw-string bag.
Quilled	An interrupted suture technique in which a double suture is passed deep into the wound with a loop emerging on one side of the incisional line and two thread ends on the opposite side. A soft catheter or bougie is placed under the loops which are then tied over it. The free ends are then tied to each other over a second bougie or quill to relieve tension.
Quilted	Alternating direction, continuous mattress sutures.
Ramdohr	Suturing anastomosis technique of the intestine in which the upper portion of the cut intestine is inverted into the lower part and sutured.
Richter	Closure technique of intestinal wounds utilizing loops of metal which are brought to the surface wound.
Rigal	Harelip suture using rubber bands.
Ritisch	Suturing technique for intestinal repair.
Snellen	Suturing technique for ectropion of the eyelid.

Spiroid	Suturing technique for enterorrhaphy.
Staple	Wound closure technique using metallic U-shaped wires for approximating the wound edges.
Subcuticular	A continuous buried suture taken in the cutis vera on one side of the incisional line and then on the other side and buried from view by the outer skin layer.
Tongue-and-groove	SEE: PANCOAST
Verhoeff	Suture technique for ectropion of the eyelid.
Wolfler	Suturing technique for enterorrhaphy. Suturing technique for tenorrhaphy.
Wysler	Suturing of the peritoneal surfaces of the intestine.

BANDAGES & DRESSING

Ace
Ace Adherent
Ace-Hesive
Ace Longitudinal Strips
Ace Rubber Elastic
Adaptic
Ad-Hese-Away
Aeroplast
Air Pressure
Aureomycin Gauze

Barton
Baynton
Belleview Surgical Wadding
Bias Cut Stockinette
Binocle
Blenderm Surgical Tape
Bolus
Borsch

Castex Rigid
Cilkloid
Cod Liver Oil Soaked Strips
Compression
Contura Medicated
Cotton Balls
Cotton Elastic
Cotton Pledgets
Cotton Wadding
Cottonoid
Crinotene
Cruricast Zinc Oxide Gelatine
Curad Plastic

Demigauntlet

Desault
Elasticfoam Pressure
Elastikon Wristlet
Elastoplast

Fas-Trac Traction Strip
Felt
Figure-Of-Eight
Flex-Aid Knuckle
Flex Foam
Foam Rubber
Foille
Frickes Scrotal
Furacin
Furacin Gauze

Galen
Garrelson
Gauze
Gauztex
Gelfilm
Gelocast
Gibson
Gypsonia Plaster

Hammock
Hueter's Perineal

Ivalon (polyvinyl sponge)

Kerlix
Kling Elastic
Koagamin
Koylon Foam Rubber

Martin's Rubber

46

BANDAGES & DRESSINGS (Continued)

Mechanic's Waste
Merthiolate
Micropore Surgical Tape
Moleskin Traction Hitch

Oiled Silk
Orthoplast
Ostic Plaster
Oxycel

Piedmont All-Cotton Elastic
Plaster
Plaster of Paris
Poly-Flex Traction
Presso-Elastic
Pressoplast Compression
Presso-Superior
Pressure
Priessnitz

Quadro

Red Cross Adhesive
Ribble
Richet
Roller
Rubber

Scan Spray
Scarlet Red Gauze
Scultetus Binder
Sheet Wadding
Sof-Rol Cast Wadding
Spray Band
Steri-Strip Skin Closures
Stockinette

Superflex Elastic
Super-Trac Adhesive Traction
Surgical
Surgicel
Surgipad Combine
Surgitube
Suspensory

T-Bandage
Telfa
Tensoplast Elastic Adhesive
Tensoplast Extension Plaster
Tensor Elastic
Thillaye
Tincture of Benzoin
Tomac Foam Rubber Traction
Tomac Knitted Rubber Elastic
Trac-Grip
Tubegauz

Varick Elastic
Vaseline Gauze
Vaseline Petrolatum Gauze
Velpeau
Velroc Plaster
Ventfoam Traction

Webril

Xeroform

Y-Bandage

Zephyr Rubber Elastic
Zim-Flux
Zimocel
Zoroc Resin Plaster

SLINGS

Acromioclavicular Dislocation
  Harness
Adjustable Strap Arm
Airplane (Aeroplane)

Banjo

Clavicle Strap
Colles
Cradle Arm

Hand Cock-Up

Mason-Allen Universal
Meek Clavicle

Teare Arm

Velpeau

Weil Pelvic

Zimmer Arm
Zimmer Clavicular Cross

5 { *Surgical Instruments and Equipment*

Surgical instruments and equipment listed here have been arranged alphabetically by type and variety. Only such items have been listed which the surgeon is likely to specify in his operative dictation.

ABRADERS

Howard Corneal
Iverson Dermabrader

Lieberman
Montague

ADENOTOMES

Cullom-Mueller
Kelley Direct Vision
LaForce
LaForce-Grieshaber

LaForce-Stevenson
Mueller-LaForce
Myles Guillotine
Shambaugh

AMNIOTOME

Beacham

ANCHORS

Lemoine-Searcy

ANGIOTRIBES

Zweifel

Ferguson

ANOSCOPES

Bodenheimer
Boehm
Brinkerhoff
Buie-Hirschman
Fansler
Goldbacher
Hirschman with obturator
Ives

Muer
Otis
Pratt
Pruitt
Rotating Speculum
Sims
Welch Allyn

APPLICATORS

Allen
Andrew
Brown
Buck
Dean
Ernst Radium
Farrell
Gifford Corneal
Holinger
Ivan Nasopharyngeal
Jackson Laryngeal

Kyle
Lathbury
Ludwig
Playfair Uterine Caustic
Plummer-Vinson Radium (esophageal)
Pynchon
Ralks
Roberts
Sawtell
Strontium-90 Ophthalmic Beta Ray
Uebe

ASPIRATORS

Carmody Electric
Cook County Hospital
Fritz

Stedman Suction Pump
Thorek Gallbladder
Universal

AWLS

Aufranc Trochanteric
Carroll

DePuy
Zuelzer

BANDS

Parham-Martin

BARS

Strut

BASIOTRIBES

Auvard-Zweifel

Tarnier

BOLTS

Barr
Cannulated
DePuy
Fenton
Hexhead

Norman Tibia
Webb
Webb Type Stove
Zimmer

BOUGIES

Bangs
Buerger Dilating
Chevalier Jackson
Dourmashkin Tunneled
Eustachian
Filiform
Fort Urethral
Gabriel Tucker

Guyon Exploratory
Harold Hayes Eustachian
Hurst (mercury filled esophageal)
Jackson Filiform
Jackson Tracheal
LeFort Filiform
Olive Tip
Otis

BOUGIES (Continued)

Phillips Urethral Whip
Ravich
Retrograde
Spiral Tip
Trousseau Esophageal

Tucker Retrograde
Urbantschitsch Eustachian
Wales Rectal
Whalebone Filiform
Whistler

BRACES

Chairback
Forrester Cervical Collar
Hudson
Lyman-Smith Toe Drop
Milwaukee Scoliosis

Murphy
Taylor Spine
Taylor-Knight
Thomas Type Cervical Collar
Von Lackum transection shift jacket

BRONCHOSCOPES

Albert Slotted
Broyles
Bruening
Chevalier Jackson
Davis
Double Channel Irrigating
Emerson
Foregger
Haslinger
Holinger
Holinger-Jackson
Hook-On
Jackson Costophrenic
Jackson Full Lumen
Jackson Standard

Jackson Staple
Jesberg
Kernan-Jackson Coagulating
Michelson Infant
Moersch
Negus
Overholt-Jackson
Pilling
Riecker Respiration
Safar Ventilation
Staple
Tucker
Waterman Folding
Yankauer

BURS

Adson-Rogers Cranial
Allport Eustachian
Bailey Skull
Ballenger-Lillie Mastoid
Burwell Corneal
Cavanaugh-Israel
Cavanaugh Sphenoid
Cushing Cranial
D'Errico
Diamond
Doyen
Ferris-Smith-Halle Sinus

Frey-Freer
Halle Bone
Jordan-Day Fenestration
Kopetzky Sinus
Lempert Fenestration
McKenzie Enlarging
Sachs Skull
Slotting
Somerset
Wachsberger
Wilkerson Choanal
Yazujian Cataract

CALIPERS

Burch Eye
Castroviejo
Green Eye
Jameson

Ladd
Thorpe
Townley Inside-Outside Femur
VM & CO Ruler

CANNULA

Abraham
Adson Brain Exploring
Bellocq
Bishop-Harman Irrigating
Bowers
Bruening
Bucy-Frazier
Carabelli
Casselberry Sphenoid
Castroviejo Cyclodialysis
Coakley Frontal Sinus
Cone-Bucy
Cooper Double Lumen
Day Attic
DeWecker Syringe
Duke
Elsberg Brain Exploring
Ford Hospital Ventricular
Frazier Brain Exploring
Goodfellow Frontal Sinus
Haverfield Brain
Haynes Brain
Hoen Ventricular
Holman-Mathieu
Hudgins
Ingals Antrum
Kanavel Brain Exploring
Killian-Eicken
Killian Antrum
Kos Attic

Krause
Lacrimal
Lillie Attic
Luongo Sphenoid Irrigating
Lukens
Myerson-Moncrieff
Myles Sinus
Neal Fallopian
Paterson Laryngeal
Penn-Neal
Pierce Attic
Pritchard
Pynchon
Randolph Cyclodialysis
Robb Antrum
Rolf-Jackson
Rubin Fallopian Tube
Sachs
Scott Attic
Scott Rubber Ventricular
Sewall Antrum
Skillern Sphenoid
Tenner
Topper
Tracheotomy
Turnbull
Van Alyea Antrum
Von Eicken Antrum
Wolfe Return Flow

CATHETERS

Acmistat
Alcock Return Flow Hemostatic
Bard
Bardex
Bicoude
Blasucci Ureteral

Bozeman
Bozeman-Fritsch
Braasch
Bunts
Campbell
Carlens Bronchospirometric

CATHETERS (Cont.)

Conical Tip
Constantine Flexible Metal
Coude Tip
Councill
Coxeter Prostatic
Cummings Four Wing Malecot
   Retention
Cummings Nephrostomy
Cummings-Pezzer Head
Davol
DeLee Tracheal
de Pezzer
Devonshire
Eustachian
Faucial Eustachian
Filiform
Fogarty Arterial Embolectomy
Foley
Foley-Alcock
Foley Bag, Inflatable
Four-Eye
French
Friend
Friend-Hebert
Furniss Female
Garceau Ureteral
Gouley
Hagner Bag
Hartmann Eustachian
Hatch
Higgins
Indwelling
Itard Eustachian
Jelm Two-Way
Jaeger-Whiteley
Kimball
Lane Rectal
Lloyd Esophagoscopic
LeFort

Lobster Tail
Malecot
McCaskey
McIver Nephrostomy
Mercier
Mushroom
Neal
Nelaton Urethral
Owens
Pezzer
Phillips
Pilcher Bag
Retention
Robinson
Round Tip
Schrotters
Shellac-Covered
Six-Eye
Skene
Solid Tip
Squire
Stitt
Styletted Tracheobronchial
Thompson Bronchial
Tiemann
Tiemann-Coude
Tomac
Touhy
Ureteral
Vertebrated
Walther Female
Whalebone Filiform
Whistle Tip
Winged
Wishard Tip
Wolf Nephrostomy Bag
Woodruff Ureteropyelographic
Yankauer
Zavod Bronchospirometry

CAUTERY

Bovie
Burdick
Downes
Electrocautery

Geiger-Downes
Mueller Currentrol
National
Prince Eye

CAUTERY (Continued)

Wadsworth-Todd Eye
Wappler
Wappler Cold Cautery

Wills Hospital Eye
Ziegler

CHISELS

Adson Laminectomy
Alexander
Andrews
Artmann Disarticulation
Ballenger
Ballenger-Hajek
Bishop
Blair
Bowen Goose Neck
Brown
Bruening
Brunetti
Brunner
Bruns
Burns Guarded
Caltagirone
Cinelli
Cinelli-McIndoe
Clawicz
Cloward
Cloward-Harman
Cloward-Puka
Cloward Spinal Fusion
Converse Nasal
Costotome
Cottle
Councilman
Crane Bone
D'Errico Laminectomy
Eicher Tri-Fin
Faulkner-Browne

Faulkner Trocar
Fomon
Freer
Hajek Septum
Halle
Henderson Bone
Hibbs
Joseph
Katsch
Keyes Splitting
Killian Frontal Sinus
Killian-Reinhard
Kreischer Bone
Lambotte Splitting
Lebsche Sternum
MacAusland
Meyerding
Metzenbaum
Moore Hollow
Murphy
Pick
Rish
Sewall Ethmoidal
Sheehan Nasal
Silver
Stille Pattern Bone
Troutman Mastoid
Virchow
West
Wilmer Wedge
Worth

CLAMPS

Alfred M. Large Vena Cava
Allen Anastomosis
Alyea Vas
A.M. Large Vena Cava
Ann Arbor Double Towel
Ault Intestinal Occlusion
Backhaus Towel

Bainbridge
Beardsley Intestinal
Berens Muscle
Berke Ptosis
Berry Pile
Best Right Angle
Bigelow Calvarium

CLAMPS (Cont.)

Black Meatus
Blalock Stenosis
Blalock-Niedner
Blanchard Pile
Böhler Os Calcis
Boyes Muscle
Bradshaw-O'Neill Aorta
Brock Auricle
Brodny Urethrographic
Buie
Buie-Hirschman Pile
Bulldog
Carmalt
Castroviejo Mosquito Lid
Charnley Bone
Claiborne Lid
Codman Cartilage
Collins
Collins Umbilical
Cottle Columella
Crafoord Coarctation
Crile
Crile Appendix
Crile-Crutchfield
Cruickshank Entropion
Crutchfield
Cunningham Incontinence
Daems Bronchus
Davidson Muscle
Davidson Pulmonary Vessel
Dean MacDonald (W. Dean
   MacDonald) Gastric
DeBakey Bulldog
DeCourcy Goiter
DeMartel-Wolfson Intestinal
Dennis Anastomosis
Derra Anastomosis
Derra Vena Cava
Dieffenbach
Dingman Cartilage
Dixon-Thomas-Smith Intestinal
Doctor Collins Fracture
Donald
Doyen
Earle Pile

Eastman Intestinal
Edebohls Kidney
Erhardt
Falk Vaginal Cuff
Farabeuf-Lambotte Bone Holding
Fehland Right Angle Colon
ferrule (accessory equipment)
Finochietto Artery
Ford
Forrester
Foss Anterior Resection
Frazier-Adson Osteoplastic Flap
Frazier-Sachs
Furniss
Furniss-Clute
Furniss Intestinal Anastomosis
Garland Hysterectomy
Gavin-Miller
Glover Auricular Appendage
Glover Coarctation
Glover Patent Ductus
Gomco Bloodless Circumcision
Goodwin Bone
Gray
Green Lid
Gross Coarctation
Gross Occluding
Gutgeman Auricular Appendage
Guyon-Pean Vessel
Guyon Vessel
Harken Auricle
Harrington-Mixter
Haseltine Umbilical
Haverhill
Hayes Colon
Herbert Adams Coarctation
Herrick Kidney
Hibbs
Hirschman Pile
Hufnagel Valve Holding
Humphries Reserve Curve Aortic
Hunt Colostomy
Hurwitz Intestinal
Hymes Meatus
Jackson Bone Extension

CLAMPS (Continued)

Jacobs
Jahnke-Cook-Seeley
Jarvis Pile
Johns Hopkins Bulldog Occluding
Jones
Joseph Septum
Kane Umbilical
Kanter Circumcision
Kapp-Beck Bronchus
Kapp-Beck Coarctation
Kapp-Beck Colon
Kelsey Pile
Kocher
Ladd Lid
Lahey Thoracic
Lambert-Lowman
Lane Gastroenterostomy
Lem-Blay Circumcision
Lewin Bone
Lilly Rectus Tendon
Linnartz Stomach
Linton Tourniquet
Lockwood
Lowman Bone Holding
Lowman-Hoglund
Martin Cartilage
Mastin Muscle
Mayo
Mayo-Guyon
Mayo-Lovelace Spur Crushing
McCleery-Miller
McDonald
McLean Pile
McNealy-Glassman-Mixter
McQuigg Right Angle
Mikulicz Peritoneal
Mixter Thoracic
Mohr Pinchcock
Moorehead Lid
Moynihan
Muir Rectal Cautery
Myles Hemorrhoidal
Nicola Tendon
Niedner Anastomosis
Nussbaum Intestinal

Ochsner
Ockerblad Kidney
O'Connor Lid
Parham-Martin Bone Holding
Partipilo
Payr Pylorus
Payr Resection
Pean Hysterectomy
Pean Intestinal
Pemberton Sigmoid Anastomosis
Pennington
Phillips Rectal
Poppen-Blalock Carotid Artery
Potts
Potts Coarctation
Potts-Niedner
Potts-Smith Aorta
Price-Thomas Bronchus
Ralks Thoracic
Rankin Anastomosis
Rankin Intestinal
Ranzewski
Reynolds Dissecting
Reynolds Resection
Rhinelander
Richards Bone
Rienhoff Arterial
Rochester Sigmoid
Roeder
Roosevelt Gastroenterostomy
Rubber Shod
Rubin Bronchus
Rubovits
Rumel Myocardial
Rush Bone
Salibi Carotid Artery
Sarnoff Aortic
Sarot Bronchus
Satinsky Vena Cava
Scudder Stomach
Sellors
Selverstone Carotid Artery
Schoemaker Intestinal
Smith Bone
Smith Marginal

CLAMPS (Continued)

Smithwick Anastomosis
Stanton Cautery
Stepita Meatus
Stille Kidney
Stille Vessel
Stockman
Stone-Holcombe
Stone Intestinal
Strauss Meatus
Sztehlo Umbilical
Tatum
Towel
Trendelenburg-Crafoord Coarctation
Vanderbilt, Vessel
Vasconcelos-Barretto
Von Petz (stomach & intestinal)
Walther-Crenshaw Meatus
Walther Kidney Pedicle
Wangensteen Gastric Crushing

Wangensteen Patent Ductus
Warthen Spur Crushing
Watts Locking
Weaver Chalazion
Weck
Wells Pedicle
Wertheim Parametrium
Wertheim Pedicle
Wertheim-Cullen
Wertheim-Reverdin
Wolfson Intestinal
Wolfson Spur Crushing
Young Renal Pedicle
Zachary-Cope-DeMartel
Ziegler-Furniss
Zimmer Cartilage
Zipser Penis
Zutt

CLIPS

Adson Scalp
Autoclips
Children's Hospital Scalp
Duane "U"
Ingraham-Fowler Tantalum
Mayfield
McKenzie Brain
Michel
Olivecrona Silver

Penfield Silver
Pool Pfeiffer Self-Locking
Intracranial Aneurysm
Raney Scalp
Smith Aneurysm
Smithwick Silver
Sugar Aneurysm
Von Petz
Wachtenfeldt

CONTRACTORS

Bailey
Bailey-Gibbon Rib

Effenberger
Graham Rib

COSTOTOME

Tudor-Edwards

Vehmehren

COUNTERBORE

Curry Hip Nail

with Lloyd Adapter

CRANIOCLASTS

Auvard
Braun

Zweifel-DeLee

CRANIOTOMES

Verbrugghen-Souttar

Williams

CURETTE (Curet)

Alvis Foreign Body
Ballenger Ethmoid
Barnhill Adenoid
Billeau Ear
Blake
Bromley Uterine
Bronson-Ray
Brun Ear
Buck Ear
Buck Mastoid
Bumm Uterine
Bush Intervertebral
Carmack Ear
Carroll Hook
Carter
Cloward Cone Ring
Coakley
Cobb
Cone Ring
Converse
DeLee
Dench Uterine
DePuy Bone
Duncan Endometrial
Epstein
Faulkner Ethmoid
Ferguson Bone
Fink
Fox Dermal
Franseen Rectal
Freimuth
Garcia-Rock Endometrial Suction
Gifford Corneal
Goldstein
Green Corneal
Green Uterine

Gross Ear
Gusberg Endocervical
Halle Ethmoid
Hannon Endometrial
Harrison Scarifying
Hayden Tonsil
Heaney Uterine
Heath Chalazion
Hebra Corneal
Hibbs Bone
Holden Uterine
Houtz Endometrial
Lempert
Lounsbury Placenta
Luer Bone
Luongo
Lynch
Mayfield
McCaskey Antrum
Meigs Endometrial
Meyerding Saw Toothed
Meyhoeffer
Middleton Adenoid
Mosher Ethmoid
Myles Antrum
Nolan-Budd Cervical
Novak Uterine Suction
Piffard Dermal with Luer Hub
Pratt Antrum
Randall Endometrial Biopsy
Raney Spinal Fusion
Ray Pituitary
Reiner
Rheinstaedter Uterine
Richards Mastoid
Ridpath Ethmoid

CURETTE (Curet) (Continued)

Rock Endometrial Suction
St. Clair-Thompson Adenoid
Schaeffer Mastoid
Schede
Schroeder Uterine
Scoville
Schwartz Endocervical
Shapleigh Ear
Sheaffer
Simones Spinal
Simpson Antrum
Sims Uterine
Skeele Eye
Skene Uterine Spoon
Skillern Sinus
Spratt Mastoid
Strully Ruptured Disc

Stubbs Adenoid
Thomas Uterine
Thorpe
V.M. & Co. Mastoid
Vogel Adenoid
Volkmann Bone
Voller
Walker Ruptured Disc
Wallich
Walsh Hook Type Dermal
Walton
Weisman Ear
West-Beck Spoon
Whiting Mastoid
Wullstein
Yankauer Salpingeal

CUTTER

Cloward-Dowel

CYSTOSCOPES

Braasch Direct Catheterizing
Brown-Buerger
Butterfield
Kelly
Lowsley-Peterson
McCarthy-Peterson

McCarthy-Campbell Miniature
McCarthy Foroblique Pan Endoscope
McCarthy Miniature
National General Purpose
Nesbit
Ravich Convertible

CYSTOTOMES

Beard
Graefe
Holth
Knapp

Von Graefe
Wheeler
Wilder

DERMABRADERS

Iverson

Sand Paper

DERMATOMES

Bard-Parker
Barker Vacu-Tome
Brown Electro-Dermatome
Manual
Meek-Wall Microdermatome

Padgett
Padgett-Hood
Reese
Stryker
Stryker Rolo-Dermatome

DILATORS

Atlee Uterine
Bakes Common Duct
Bakes-Pearce
Bard Urethral
Beardsley Aortic
Berens Punctum
Black-Wylie
Bowman Lacrimal
Bransford-Lewis Ureteral
Brock Cardiac
Browne-McHardy
Broyles Esophageal
Cardiospasm
Clerf
Crump
Crump-Himmelstein
Delaborde
Derra Cardiac Valve
Dick Cardiac Valve
Einhorn Esophageal
Esophagospasm
Feldbausch
Galezowski Lacrimal
Gohrbrand Cardiac
Goodell Uterine
Guggenheim-Gergoiye
Guyon
Hank Uterine
Hank-Bradley Uterine
Heath Punctum
Hegar Uterine
Hosford
Jackson-Plummer
Jolly Uterine
Kahn Uterine
Kearns Bladder
Kelly's Sphincter
Kollmann
LaBorde Tracheal
Leader-Kollmann

Mantz Rectal
Mixter Common Duct Dilaprobe
Mosher Cardiospasm
Muldoon Lacrimal
Murphy Common Duct
Nettleship-Wilder
Olive Dilator
Ottenheimer Common Duct
Outerbridge Uterine
Palmer Uterine
Patton Esophageal
Plummer Esophageal
Pneumatic
Potts Expansile
Potts-Riker
Pratt Rectal
Pratt Uterine
Ramstedt Pyloric Stenosis
Rapaport
Ritter Meatal
Rolf Punctum
Royal Hospital
Ruedemann Lacrimal
Russell Hydrostatic
Sims Uterine
Sinexon
Sippy Dilating Olives
Starlinger Uterine
Steele Bronchial
Theobold Lacrimal
Trousseau Tracheal
Trousseau-Jackson Esophageal
Turner
Wales Rectal
Walther
Wilder Lacrimal
William Lacrimal
Wylie Uterine
Young Rectal
Ziegler Lacrimal

DIRECTORS

Durnin Angled
Larry Rectal

Pratt

DISSECTORS

Allerdyce
Allis
Aufranc
Brunner Goiter
Butte
Carpenter
Cheyne's Dry
Collin Pleura
Falcao
Hamrick Suction
Harris
Heath Trephine Flap
Herczel
Hurd
Hurd-Wieder
Israel
Judet
Kocher Goiter
Lane
Lewin
Logan

MacAusland
McWhinnie Tonsil
Milligan
Moorehead
Morrison-Hurd
Oldberg
Olivecrona
Penfield
Pierce Submucous
Potts
Rienhoff
Rosen
Sloan Goiter Flap
Smithwick
Stolte Tonsil
Walker Suction
Wangensteen
Watson-Cheyne
Yoshida
Young's

DRAINS

Angle Pezzer
Bardex
Cigarette
Freyer
Hendrickson Suprapubic
Latex
Malecot Four-Wing
Malecot Two-Wing
Marion
Mikulicz
Mosher

Penrose
Pezzer
Ritter Suprapubic Suction
Rubber dam
Soft rubber
Sovally Suprapubic Suction Cup
Stab Wound
T-Tube
Whistle Tip
Wylie

DRILLS

Adson Spiral
Bosworth Crown
Bunnell Hand
Cannulated Cortical Step
Carmody Perforator
Carroll-Bunnell
Cloward Cervical
Collison Body

Collison Cannulated Hand
Collison Tap
Cushing Cranial
DePuy
D'Errico
Dr. Light-Veley Automatic Cranial
Hall Step Down
Harris-Smith Anterior Interbody

DRILLS (continued)

Hudson Cranial
Jacobs Chuck
Jordan-Day
Kirschner Wire
Loth-Kirschner
Lusskin Bone
Magnuson Twist
McKenzie
Modny
Moore Bone
Neill Perforator
Orthopedic Universal
Pease Bone
Ralks Bone
Ralks Fingernail

Raney Cranial
Richter Bone
Sherman-Stille
Smedberg
Stille Pattern Bone
Stille-Sherman
Thornwald Antrum
Twist Drill
Ullrich Drill Guard
Universal Two Speed Hand
Vitallium
Wolferman
Zimalate
Zimmer Kirschner Hand
Zimmer Universal

DRIVERS

Ken
Massie
McNutt

McReynolds
Rush
Zimmer

ELECTRODES

ACMI Retrograde
Arrowsmith
Ballenger Follicle
Bard
Bayonet Tip
Berens Bident
Biopsy Loop
Bugbee
Buie Fulgurating
Collings Fulguration
Conical Tip
Coude
Davis Coagulation
Domed Angle Tip
Flexible Radiothermal
Fulgurating
Galloway
Hamm
Hubbard
Hurd Angular
Hurd Bipolar Diathermy
Hymes-Timberlake
Lane Ureteral Meatotomy

Lynch
McCarthy Coagulation
McCarthy Diathermic Knife
McCarthy Fulguration
McWhinnie
Moersch
Myerson
National Cautery
New's
Platinum Blade Meatotomy
    Fulgurating
Pointed Tip
Retrograde
Riba Electro-Urethrotome
Rychener-Weve
Sluder Cautery
Smith
Timberlake
Turner Cystoscopic Fulgurating
Ureteral Meatotomy
Wappler
Weve

ELECTRODIAPHAKE

LaCarrere

ELECTROTOMES

McCarthy Miniature   Nesbit
McCarthy Punctuate   Stern-McCarthy

ELEVATORS
(also see: Periosteal Elevators)

Abraham   Freer Double
Adson   Freer Septum
Alexander-Farabeuf   Friedrich Rib
Allerdyce   Gillies
Amerson Bone   Graham Scalene
Artmann   Hajek-Ballenger Septum
Ballenger-Hajek   Halle Septum
Ballenger Septum   Hamrick
Bennett   Hatt Golf Stick
Bethune   Hayden Palate
Blair Cleft Palate   Hedblom
Boies Nasal   Henner
Brophy Tooth   Hertzel Raspatory
Brown Bone   Hibbs Costal
Cannon-Rochester Lamina   Hibbs Spinal Fusion Chisel
Carter Submucous   House
Chandler   Howorth
Cobb Spinal   Hurd Septum
Cohen   Joseph-Killian Septum
Converse-MacKenty   Killian Septum
Cooper Spinal Fusion   Kinsella
Cordes-New Laryngeal Punch   Kirmisson
Cottle Septum   Kleesattel
Cottle Skin   Kocher
Crawford Dural   Ladd
Cushing Little Joker   Lane
Cushing Pituitary   Langenbeck
Davidson-Sauerbruch-Doyen   Lee-Cohen Septum
Doyen Rib   Lempert
Dunning   Logan
Farabeuf   Love-Adson
Fay Suction   Luongo Septal
Ferris-Smith'   Matson Rib
File   MacKenty
Fomon Nostril   Moore Bone
Frazier Dura   Moorehead
Frazier Suction   Overholt
Freer   Pennington Septum

ELEVATORS (continued)

Phemister Raspatory
Pierce
Poppen
Rochester
Roger Septum
Rosen
Sauerbruch-Frey Rib
Sayre
Sedillot
Sewall Ethmoidal

Sewall Mucoperiosteal
Shambaugh
Sokolec
Staphylorrhaphy
Sunday
Tarlov Nerve
Tobolsky
Turner Cord
Walker Submucous
Woodson

ENUCLEATOR

Young Prostatic

ERISIPHAKES (also: Erysiphakes)

Bell
Dimitry-Bell
Dimitry-Thomas
Harrington

Kara
Maumenee
Nugent-Green-Dimitry
Viers

ESOPHAGOSCOPES

Ballooning
Boros
Chevalier Jackson
Esophageal Bougies (used with)
Haslinger
Holinger
Jackson Full Lumen
Jesberg

Lell
Mosher
Moure
Roberts Folding
Schindler Optical
Tucker
Yankauer

EVACUATORS

Crigler
Ellik Bladder
Hutch
Kennedy-Cornwell Bladder
McCarthy Bladder

McKenna Tide-Ur-Ator
Snyder Hemovac
Thompson
Timberlake
Toomey Bladder

EXCAVATOR

Lempert

EXPRESSOR

Hess Tonsil

Wilmer-Badgley

EXTRACTORS

Cherry
Cloverleaf Pin
DePuy

Dolan
Eric Lloyd
Jewett Bone

EXTRACTORS (Continued)

McDermott
McNutt
McReynolds
Massie
Moore-Blount
Moore Nail
Murless Head

Rush
Saalfield Comedone
Schamberg Comedone
Smith-Petersen Nail
Unna Comedone
Zimmer

EYE IMPLANTS

Acrylic Ball
Acrylic Conformers
Arruga
Berens Conical
Berens Pyramidal
Berens Sphere
Conventional Shell Type
Corrected Cosmetic Contact Shell
Curl Back Shell
Doherty Sphere
Forty Five Degree Bend Reform
Fox Sphere
Front Build-up
Glass Sphere
Gold Sphere
Guist Sphere
Hemisphere

Hook-Type
Ivalon Sponge
Magnetic
Mules Sphere
Mullers Shield (conformer)
Peanut Eye
Plexiglas
Reverse Shape
Semishell
Shelf Type
Shell
Snellen Conventional Reform
Tantalum Mesh
Vitallium
Wheeler Sphere
Wire Mesh

FACIAL FRACTURE APPLIANCE

Dental Arch Bars
Erich

Joseph Septum Clamp

FASCIA STRIPPER (See: Stripper)

FLANGE

Callahan

Scuderi-Callahan

FORCEPS

A.C.M.I.
Adair-Allis
Adair Uterine
Adson
Alderkreutz
Allen Uterine
Alligator Grasping
Allis
Allis-Adair

Allis-Coakley Tonsil
Allis-Duval
Allis-Ochsner Tissue
Allis-Willauer
Amenabar Capsule
Andrews Tonsil
Arruga Capsule
Arruga-Gill
Arruga-McCool

FORCEPS (continued)

Asch Septum Straightening
Ashby Fluoroscopic Foreign Body
Ayer Chalazion
Babcock
Babcock Intestinal
Babcock Lung Grasping
Baby Lane Bone Holding
Backhaus Towel
Bacon Cranial
Bailey Chalazion
Bailey-Williamson Obstetrical
Bainbridge Thyroid
Baird Chalazion
Ballenger
Ballenger-Forster
Bane
Bane Rongeur
Bardeleben Bone Holding
Barnes-Simpson Obstetrical
Barraquer Cilia
Barrett Placenta
Barrett-Allen Uterine Elevating
Barrett-Murphy
Barrett Uterine Tenaculum
Barton Obstetrical
Bauer Dissecting
Bayonet
Bead
Beaupre Cilia
Beaupre Epilation
Beebe
Beer Cilia
Bennett Epilation
Berens Corneal Transplant
Berens Recession
Bergeron Pillar
Bergh Cilia
Berke Ptosis
Berne Nasal
Berry Uterine Elevating
Billroth Tumor
Bishop-Harman Iris
Blake Ear
Blake Gallstone
Blakesley

Blanchard Hemorrhoid
Bland Cervical Traction
Bland Vulsellum
Blum
Boies
Bolton
Bonaccolto
Bond Placenta
Bonney Tissue
Boston Lying-In Cervical
Botvin Iris
Boys-Allis
Bozeman Uterine Packing
Braasch Bladder Specimen
Bracken Fixation
Bracken Iris
Bradford Thyroid Traction Vulsellum
Braun Uterine Tenaculum
Bridge Deep Surgery
Brigham Brain Tumor
Brown-Adson
Brown Side Grasping
Bruening Septum
Brunner Tissue
Brunschwig Viscera
Buerger-McCarthy Bladder
Buie
Bumpus
Burch Biopsy
Burnham Biopsy
Cairns Hemostatic
Callahan
Cannulated
Carmalt
Carmody Tissue
Carroll-Adson Dura
Castroviejo Transplant Grafting
Cane Bone Holding
Champoniere
Chang Bone Cutting
Cheron Uterine Dressing
Chester
Child
Children's Hospital

FORCEPS (continued)

Cicherelli Rongeur
Citelli
Clark Capsule Fragment
Clark-Guyton
Clark-Verhoeff
Clerf
Cohen Nasal Dressing
Coller
Collins
Collins Mucous
Collins Uterine Elevating
Collins-Duvall
Colver Tonsil
Coppridge Grasping
Corbett Bone Cutting
Cordes-New Laryngeal Punch
Corey Placenta
Corwin Tonsil
Cottle
Cottle-Jansen
Cottle-Kazanjian Nasal
Cottle-Walsham
Cowhorn Tooth Extracting
Crafoord Bronchial & Pulmonary
Craig Septum
Crenshaw Caruncle
Crile Hemostatic
Crossen Puncturing Tenaculum
Cullom Septum
Curtis Tissue
Cushing Brain
Cushing Tissue
Dandy
Dartigues Uterine Elevating
Davidson Pulmonary Vessel
Davis Bayonet
Davis Capsule
D'Errico
Defourmentel Rongeur
DeLee
DeLee-Simpson
Demarest
DeMartel Scalp
Demel Wire Tightening
Dench Ear

Dennis Intestinal
Desjardin Gallstone
Desmarres Chalazion
Devilbiss
Dewees Obstetrical
Dieffenbach
Dieter Malleus
Dingman Bone Holding
Dodrill
Donberg Iris
Dorsey Bayonet
Double Concave Rat Tooth
Douglas Eye
Doyen Uterine Vulsellum
Duplay Uterine Tenaculum
Duval Lung
Duval-Allis
Duval-Crile Lung Grasping
Eastman
Eber
Elliott Obstetrical
Elschnig Fixation
Elschnig-O'Brien Fixation
Elschnig-O'Connor
Elschnig Secondary Membrane
Emmet
Endospeculum
English
Episcleral
Erhardt Eyelid
Erich Biopsy
Essrig Tissue
Ethridge Hysterectomy
Ewald (Hudson)
Ewing
Falcao Fixation
Falk Lion Jaws
Farabeuf Bone Holding
Farabeuf-Lambotte Bone Holding
Farnham Nasal Cutting
Farrington Septum
Fauvel Laryngeal
Feilchenfeld Splinter
Fenestrated Blade
Ferguson Angiotribe

FORCEPS (continued)

Ferguson Bone Holding
Ferguson Tenaculum
Ferris-Smith
Ferris-Smith Fragment
Ferris-Smith-Kerrison Rongeur
Fink Fixation
Fink-Jameson
Finochietto Lobectomy
Fish Grasping
Fisher Advancement
Fisher-Arlt Iris
Fisher Capsule
Fischmann Angiotribe
Fitzwater Peanut Sponge Holding
Fletcher-Van Doren
Foerster Eye
Foley Vas Isolation
Foss Intestinal Clamp
Fraenkel Laryngeal
Francis Chalazion
Freer-Gruenwald
French Pattern
Fry Nasal
Fuchs Iris
Fulpit Tissue
Furniss Polyp
Gabriel Tucker
Garland Hysterectomy
Garrigue Uterine Dressing
Gavin-Miller
Gaylor Biopsy
Geissendorfer
Gellhorn Biopsy Punch
Gelpi Hysterectomy
Gelpi-Lowrie Hysterectomy
Gerald
Gifford Iris
Gilbert
Gill
Gill-Fuchs
Gill-Hess Iris
Gill-Safar
Ginsberg
Glenner Vaginal Hysterectomy
Gold Deep Surgery

Goldman-Kazanjian Nasal
Good Obstetrical
Goodyear-Gruenwald
Gradle Cilia
Graefe Eye
Graefe Fixation
Gray
Gray Cystic Duct
Grayton
Green Fixation
Greenwood
Gross Hyoid Cutting
Grotting
Gruenwald-Bryant
Gruenwald Nasal
Guggenheim Adenoid
Guist Fixation
Gunderson Recession
Gutgemann Auricular Appendage
Gutglass Cervix Hemostatic
Guyton-Noyes
Hajek-Sphenoid Punch
Hajek-Koffler Sphenoid Punch
Halsted Mosquito
Hamilton Deep Surgery
Harman
Harrington Vulsellum
Hartmann Alligator
Hartmann-Citelli Ear Punch
Hartmann-Gruenwald Nasal Cutting
Hartmann Mosquito
Hawks-Dennen
Healy Gastrointestinal
Healy Uterine Biopsy
Heaney-Ballentine
Heaney Hysterectomy
Heaney-Kanter
Heaney-Rezek
Heath Chalazion
Heath Nasal
Hegenbarth
Heise Artery
Heise Vulsellum
Henrotin Uterine Vulsellum
Herman Bone Holding

FORCEPS (continued)

Herzfeld
Hess-Barraquer
Hess Capsule
Hess-Gill Eye
Hess-Horwitz
Hibbs Bone Cutting
Hirschman Hemorrhoidal
Hirst OB
Hirst-Emmet OB
Hoen
Hoffmann Ear Punch
Holmes Fixation
Holth Punch
Horsley Bone Cutting
Hosford-Hicks Transfer
Howard Closing
Howard Tonsil
Hoyt Deep Surgery
Hoytenberger Tissue
Hubbard Corneoscleral
Hudson Cranial
Hufnagel Mitral Valve Holding
Hunt
Hurd Septum Bone Cutting
Hurdner Tissue
Imperatori Laryngeal
Iowa Membrane Puncturing
Jackson Broad Blade Staple
Jackson Cross Action
Jackson Double Concave Rat Tooth
Jackson Double Prong
Jackson Laryngofissure
Jackson's Sister Hook
Jacobs Uterine Vulsellum
Jameson Recession
Jansen Bayonet
Jansen Ear
Jansen-Gruenwald
Jansen-Middleton Septum Cutting
Jansen Nasal Dressing
Jansen-Struycken Septum
Jarcho Uterine Tenaculum
Javerts Polyp
Johns Hopkins Serrefine
Johnson Brain Tumor

Judd-Allis
Judd-DeMartel
Juers Lingual
Jurasz Laryngeal
Kadesky
Kahler Polyp
Kalt Capsule
Kazanjian Nasal Hump Cutting
Kelly Hemostatic
Kelly-Murphy
Kelly Placenta
Kent Deep Surgery
Kern Bone Holding
Kielland Obstetrical
Kielland-Luikart Obstetrical
Killian Septum Compression
King-Prince
Kirby Eye
Kirkpatrick Tonsil
Kittner
Knapp Trachoma
Knight
Knight-Sluder Nasal
Kocher Artery
Koffler Septum
Koffler-Lillie Septum
Kolb Bronchus
Kolodny
Kronfeld Micro Pin
Kuhnt Capsule
Kulvin-Kalt Iris
Lahey
Lahey Goiter
Lahey-Pean
Lahey Thyroid Traction Vulsellum
Lambert Chalazion
Lambotte Bone Holding
Lane Bone Holding
Langenbeck Bone Holding
Larsen Tendon
Laryngeal Sponging
Lauf-Barton OB
Lauf-Piper OB
Laufman
Laval Advancement

FORCEPS (continued)

Lawrence Deep Surgery
Lawton
Lebsche Sternum Punch
Lefferts Bone Cutting
Lempert Rongeur
Leonard Deep Surgery
Lester Fixation
Levenson Tissue
Levora Fixation
Lewin Bone
Lewin Spinal Perforating
Lewis Septum
Lewkowitz Lithotomy
Lillie
Lillie-Killian Septum Bone
Linnartz
Lister Conjunctival
Liston Bone Cutting
Liston-Stille
Litt
Littauer Bone Cutting
Littauer Cilia
Littauer-Liston Bone Cutting
Livingston
Lobenstein-Tarnier
Lockwood
Lockwood-Allis
Lombard-Beyer Rongeur
London Tissue
Long Hysterectomy
Lordan Chalazion
Lore Suction Tube Holding
Lothrop
Love-Gruenwald Alligator
Lovelace Bladder
Lovelace Lung Grasping
Lovelace Thyroid Traction Vulsellum
Lower Gall Duct
Lowis I.V. Disc Rongeur
Luikart Obstetrical
Luikart-McLean
Luikart-Simpson
Lutz Septal Ridge Cutting
MacKenty Tissue
Madden

Maier Uterine Dressing
Mansfield
Marshik Tonsil
Martin Nasopharyngeal Biopsy
Maryan Biopsy Punch
Mathieu Urethral
Matthews
Mayo
Mayo-Blake
Mayo Bone Cutting
Mayo-Harrington
Mayo-Pean
Mayo-Robson
Mayo-Russian
Mayo Tissue
Mayo Ureter Isolation
McCarthy-Alcock Hemostatic
McCarthy-Visual Hemostatic
McCoy Septum Cutting
McCravey
McCullough
McGannon Lens
McGuire Marginal Chalazion
McKay Ear
McKenzie Brain Clip Cutting
McKenzie Grasping
McLean Muscle
McLean Obstetrical
McLean-Luikart
McLean-Tucker-Luikart
McNealy-Glassman-Babcock Viscera
McQuigg
McQuigg-Mixter
Meat
Meeker Deep Surgery
Mendel Ligature
Metzenbaum-Tyding
Michigan Intestinal
Mikulicz Tonsil
Miller Bayonet
Millin Capsule Grasping
Millin Lobe Grasping
Millin T-shaped Angled
Mills Tissue
Mixter

FORCEPS (continued)

Mixter-McQuigg
Moehle Corneal
Moersch Bronchoscopic Specimen
Monod Punch
Montenovesi Cranial Rongeur
Moore
Moritz-Schmidt Laryngeal
Mosher
Mosher Ethmoid Punch
Mosquito Hemostatic
Mount Intervertebral Disc Rongeur
Mouse Tooth
Muck Tonsil
Muldoon Meibomian
Muller-Markham Patent Ductus
Munde Placenta
Murphy Tonsil
Museholdt Nasal Dressing
Museux Uterine Vulsellum
Musial Tissue
Myles
Nelson
Nevins
Newman Uterine Tenaculum
New's Tissue and Biopsy
Niedner Dissecting
Nisbet Eye
Norwood
Noyes Nasal Dressing
Nugent
Nugowski
O'Brien Fixation
Occluding
Ochsner
Ochsner-Dixon
O'Dell Spicule
Ogura
Oldberg
Olivecrona Clip Applying
O'Shaughnessy Artery
Otto Tissue
Overholt
Page Tonsil
Paton Corneal Transplant
Paterson Laryngeal

Payne-Ochsner Artery
Payne-Pean Artery
Payne-Rankin Artery
Pean
Pean G.I.
Peanut Fenestrated
Peapod Intervertebral Disc
Peet
Pelkmann Uterine Dressing
Penfield Suture
Pennington
Percy Intestinal
Perritt
Pfau Polypus
Phaneuf Uterine Artery
Phaneuf Vaginal
Phipps
Pin Bending
Piper Obstetrical
Pischel Micro Pin
Pitha
Pley Capsule
Plondke Uterine Elevating
Poppen
Porter Duodenal
Potter Tonsil
Potts Coarctation
Potts Patent Ductus
Potts-Smith Tissue
Pratt
Pratt T-Shaped
Preston Ligamentum Flavum
Price-Thomas Bronchus
Prince Trachoma
Proctor Phrenectomy
Providence Hospital
Quervain Cranial Rongeur
Quevedo Conjunctival
Raaf-Oldberg Intervertebral Disc
Randall Kidney Stone
Raney
Rankin
Rankin-Crile
Ratliff-Blake Gallstone
Ray Kidney Stone

FORCEPS (continued)

Reese Advancement
Reich-Nechtow Hysterectomy
Reiner-Knight Ethmoid Cutting
Reisinger Lens
Riba-Valeira
Rich
Richard Tonsil Grasping
Richter-Heath
Rienhoff Arterial
Ripstein
Robb Tonsil
Roberts Artery
Roberts Bronchial Biopsy
Robertson Tonsil
Rochester
Rochester-Carmalt
Rochester-Ewald
Rochester-Harrington
Rochester-Ochsner Hemostat
Rochester-Rankin
Rolf
Ronis Cutting
Rowe Bone Drilling
Rowland Double Action Hump
Rugby Deep Surgery
Rugelski Artery
Rumel Lobectomy
Ruskin Bone Cutting
Ruskin-Liston
Ruskin Rongeur
Russell Hysterectomy
Russian
Russian-Pean
Sachs
St. Clair
St. Clair-Thompson
St. Martin Eye
Sam Roberts Bronchial Biopsy
Santy Dissecting
Sarot Pleurectomy
Sauer
Sawtell
Scheinmann laryngeal
Schmidt-Rumpler
Schoenberg Intestinal
Schoenberg Uterine Elevating

Schroeder-Braun Uterine Tenaculum
Schroeder Uterine Tenaculum
Schubert Biopsy Punch
Schwartz
Schweigger Capsule (eye)
Schweizer Uterine
Scobee-Allis
Scudder Intestinal
Scuderi Bi-Polar Coagulating
Searcy Capsule
Segond Tumor
Seletz Foramen Plugging
Semb
Semb-Ghazi Dissecting
Semken
Semmes Dural
Senturia
Shaaf
Shallcross Gallbladder
Shallcross Nasal Packing
Shearer Chicken Bill Rongeur
Sheathed Flexible Gastroscopic
Shuster Tonsil
Simons Stone Removing
Simpson Obstetrical
Simpson-Luikart
Singley Tissue
Skene Uterine Tenaculum
Skillman
Smith-Petersen
Smithwick
Smithwick-Hartmann
Snellen Entropion
Snyder Deep Surgery
Somers Uterine Elevating
Spencer Chalazion
Spero Meibomian
Spicule
Spurling
Stark Vulsellum
Staude-Moore Uterine Tenaculum
Staude Uterine Tenaculum
Stevens Fixation
Stevens Iris
Stille
Stille-Horsley Bone Cutting

FORCEPS (continued)

Stille-Liston Bone Cutting
Stille-Luer Bone Rongeur
Stone Tissue
Storey Hillar Dissecting
Strabismus
Strümpel Ear Punch or Struempel
Struyken Ear
Struyken Turbinate
Suker Iris
Suker Transplant Grafting
Sweet
Szuler
Takahashi Nasal
Takahashi Neuro
Tarnier Obstetrical
Teale Uterine Vulsellum
Terson Capsule
Thoms
Thoms-Allis
Thoms-Gaylor Uterine
Thorpe Corneoscleral
Thumb Forceps
Tischler Cervical Biopsy
Tivnen
Tobold-Fauvel Grasping
Tobold Laryngeal
Tower Muscle
Townley Tissue
Trousseau Dilating
Tucker
Tucker Bead
Tucker McLean
Tucker Reach & Pin
Turell Biopsy
Turnbull Adhesions
Tuttle Obstetrical
Tydings Tonsil
Tydings Lakeside Tonsil
Tuttle Thoracic
Tuttle Tissue
Uterine Vulsellum
Van Buren Sequestrum
Van Doren Uterine Biopsy Punch
Van Struycken

Varco Gallbladder
Vectis (Cesarean Section)
Verbrugghen Bone Holding
Verhoeff
Victor Bonney
Virtus Splinter
Von Graefe
Voris-Oldberg I.V. Disc Rongeur
Waldeau Fixation
Waldron
Walker
Walsham Septum Straightening
Walter (Carmalt) Splinter
Walther Tissue
Wangensteen Tissue
Watson-Williams Nasal
Weil Ear
Weil Ethmoid
Weingartner Ear
Weis Chalazion
Wells
White Tonsil
White-Smith
Wilde Ear
Wilde Ethmoid
Wilde Septum
Wilde-Blakesley
Willauer-Allis
Willett Placenta Previa
Williams Uterine Tenaculum
Wills Hospital
Winter Placenta
Winter-Nassauer Placenta
Wolfe Cataract Delivery
Worth Strabismus
Wound Clip
Wullstein Ear
Wylie Uterine Tenaculum
Yankauer Ethmoid Cutting
Yankauer-Little
Yeomans
Young
Young Uterine Biopsy
Ziegler Cilia

FRAMES (Fracture)

Alexian Brothers Overhead
Balkan
Böhler Reducing
Bradford
Cole Hyperextension
DePuy Rainbow
DePuy Reducing
Doctor Plymale Lift
Foster Turning
Goldthwait

Granberry Hyperextension
Herzmark Hyperextension
Janes
Stryker CircOlectric
Stryker Turning
Thomas
Thomson Hyperextension
Vasocillator
Zimmer

GAGS (See: Mouth Gags)
GASTROSCOPES

ACMI Examining
Benedict Operating
Bernstein Modification
Chevalier Jackson
Eder
Eder-Chamberlin
Eder-Hufford
Eder-Palmer

Ellsner
Herman Taylor
Housset-Debray
Janeway
Kelling
Peroral Chevalier Jackson
Schindler
Wolf-Schindler

GAUZE PACKERS

Allport
Bernay

Kitchen Postpartum
Torpin Automatic Uterine

GONIOMETERS

Conzett
Frykholm

Tomac

GOUGES

Alexander Bone
Andrews Mastoid
Army Pattern Bone
Aufranc Arthroplasty
Ballenger
Bowen
Campbell Arthroplasty
Cave Scaphoid
Cobb
Crane
Dix
Flanagan Spinal Fusion
Freer Nasal
Hibbs Bone
Hoen Lamina
Kuhnt

Lahey Clinic Spinal Fusion
Lillie
Martin Hip
Meyerding
Moore Spinal Fusion
Murphy
Nicola
Putti Arthroplasty
Rowen Spinal Fusion
Smith-Petersen Arthroplasty
Stille Pattern Bone
Trough
Troutman Mastoid
Turner Spinal
Walton Foreign Body
West Bone

GUIDES

Adson-Gigli Saw
Bailey-Gigli Saw
Blair-Gigli Saw
Borchard Bone
Caldwell
Cloward
Cone
Cooper Basal Ganglia
Cottle Cartilage
Cushing-Gigli
Ferciot Wire

Kendrick-Gigli Saw
Modny
Morrissey-Gigli Saw
Mumford-Gigli Saw
Poppen-Gigli Saw
Rand-Wells Pallidothalomectomy
Raney-Gigli Saw
Schlesinger-Gigli Saw
Stille-Gigli Saw
Todt-Heyer Cannula

GUILLOTINES

Lilienthal Rib
Sluder Tonsil

Sluder-Sauer Tonsil
Van Osdel

HALTERS

Cerva Crane
DePuy Head
Diskard Head
Forrester Head

Neck Wrap
Tracto-Halter
Zimfoam Head
Zimmer Head

HEMOSTATS

Boettcher
Broadbill with push fork
Corwin
Crile
Dean

Jackson Tracheal
Mathrop
McWhorter
Sawtell-Davis
Schnidt

HEMOSTATIC BAGS

Aberhart Disposable Urinal
Alcock
Bardex
Brake
Brodny
Coude
Emmet
Foley
Foley-Alcock
Hagner
Hendrickson
Higgins

Nesbit
Owens
Paul Condom
Pearman Transurethral
Pear-shaped Fluted
Pilcher Suprapubic
Severance Transurethral
Short Tip
Soanes
Thackston Retropubic
Two-Way
Wolf

HOOKS

Adson Brain
Adson Knot Tier
Allport
Aufranc
Bane
Barr Crypt
Berens Scleral
Bethune Nerve Hook
Boettcher
Boyes-Goodfellow
Braun Decapitation
Braun Obstetrical
Brown
Carroll Bone
Cloward Dura
Converse
Converse Hinged Skin
Cottle
Cottle-Joseph
Crile Nerve
Culler Rectus Muscle
Cushing Dura
Dailey Fixation
Dandy Nerve
Davis
Day Ear
Dudley Rectal
Dudley Tenaculum
Edwards Rectal
Emmet Uterine Tenaculum
Fink
Frazier Cordotomy
Frazier Dura
Frazier Skin
Freer Skin
Gillies Skin
Goldman Universal Nerve
Graefe Strabismus
Graham Nerve
Gross Ear
Guthrie Skin
Gwathmey
Haven Skin Graft
Henton Tonsil Suture
Hoen Nerve

Iris
Jaeger Strabismus
Jameson Strabismus
Jaw
Johnson
Joseph Tenaculum
Kelly Uterine Tenaculum
Kilner Skin
Kimball Nephrostomy
Kirby Double Fixation
Kirby Intracapsular Lens Expressor
Klemme Dura
Lahey Clinic Dura
Lillie Attic
Lillie Ear
Linton Vein
Lordan Muscle Splitting
Madden Sympathectomy
Martin
Mayo Fibroid
McMahon Nephrostomy
McReynolds Lid Retracting
Muelly
Murphy Ball End
Neivert
Newhart
Nugent Iris
O'Brien Rib
O'Connor
Penn Swivel
Pratt Rectal
Rolf Muscle
Rosser Crypt
Russian Fixation
Sachs Dural
Sadler Bone
Schnitman Skin
Schwartz Expression
Scobee Muscle
Scoville Curved Nerve
Searcy Fixation
Shambaugh Endaural
Sluder Sphenoid
Smellie Obstetrical (& crochet)
Smith Lid Retracting

HOOKS (Continued)

Smithwick
Smithwick Silk Button
Speare Dura
Speer Suture
Steven Traction
Stevens Tenotomy
Stewart Crypt
Strully Dura Twist
Strut Bar

Tauber Ligature
Tyrrell Iris
Tyrrell Skin
Von Graefe Strabismus
Walsh Endaural
Weary
Wiener Corneal
Zoellner

IMPLANT MATERIALS

Also see: Eye Implants & Prostheses

Acrylic
Bone
Cartilage
Celluloid
Ethrone
Homograft
Ivalon (polyvinyl sponge)
Paladon
Paraffin
Plexiglas
Polyether
Polyethylene
Polystan
Polyurethane

Polyvinyl
Shell
Silastic
Silastic Cronin (mammary)
Silastic Medical Adhesive Silicone
Silastic (testicular)
Stainless Steel
Subdermal
Supramid
Tantalum
Tantalum Mesh
Vitallium
Vivosil
Wire Mesh

INVERTERS

Barrett Appendix
Mayo-Boldt

Wangensteen Tissue

KERATOMES

Agnew
Atkinson
Berens
Castroviejo
Czermak
Daily
Grieshaber
Jaeger

Kirby
Lancaster
Landolt
Lichtenberg
McReynolds Pterygium
Rowland
Thomas
Wiener

KNIVES

Abraham
Agnew Canaliculus
Allen-Barkan
Atkin Tonsil
Ayre Cone
Bailey-Glover-O'Neil
  Commissurotomy
Ballenger Mucosa & Cartilage
Ballenger Swivel
Bard-Parker
Barkan Goniotomy
Barker Vacutome Suction
Baron
Barrett Uterine
Beard Lid
Beers Cataract
Berens Sclerotomy
Bistoury
Blair-Brown Skin Graft
Blair Cleft Palate
Bonta Mastectomy
Bosher Commissurotomy
Brock Pulmonary Valve
Brophy Bistoury
Brophy Cleft Palate
Brown Cleft Palate
Buck Ear
Buck Myringotome
Bucy Cordotomy
Caltagirone Skin Graft
Canfield
Carpenter Tonsil
Carter Septum
Castroviejo Ophthalmic
Catling Amputating
Cave Cartilage
Collings
Colver Tonsil
Converse
Cornman Dissecting
Cottle Nasal
Crescent Plaster
Crile Cleft Palate
Crosby
Curdy Sclerotome

Cushing Dura Hook
Davidoff Cordotomy
Daviel Chalazion
Davis F. A.
Dean Tonsil
DeLee Laparotrachelotomy
Dench's Ear
DePalma
Derra Commissurotomy
Derra Guillotine
D'Errico
Desmarres Paracentesis
Deutschman Cataract
Devonshire
Dintenfass Ear
Dintenfass-Chapman
Douglas Tonsil
Downing Cartilage
Dupuytren
Elschnig Cataract
Elschnig Pterygium
Equen-Neuffer Laryngeal
Ferris-Robb Tonsil
Ferris-Smith
Fisher
Fomon
Frazier Cordotomy
Freer-Ingal Submucous
Freer Septum
Freiberg Cartilage
Friesner Ear
Gerzog Ear
Gerzog-Ralks
Gill Corneal
Goldman Guillotine Nerve
Goodyear Tonsil
Graefe Cataract
Graf Cervical Cordotomy
Haab
Harris Tonsil
House
Hufnagel Commissurotomy
Humby
Hymes Scleral
Jackson Tracheal Bistoury

KNIVES (Continued)

Jaeger Keratome
Johnson Evisceration
Joseph Angular
Joseph Bistoury
Joseph Button End
Joseph Cervical
Joseph Double Edge
Joseph Nasal
Joseph-Maltz
Kirby Cataract
Knapp Cataract
Kreissl Meatotomy
Krull Acetabular
Kyle Crypt
Ladd
Lancaster
Lance
Langenbeck Flap
Lanigan Cartilage
Lebsche Sternum
Lee Cartilage
Lee Cohen
Leland Tonsil
Lempert
Liston Amputating
Lothrop Tonsil
Lowe-Breck Cartilage
Lowell Glaucoma
Lundsgaard-Burch
MacCallum P.M.
MacKenty Cleft Palate
Maltz Cartilage
Mandelbaum Ear
Marcks
Mayo
McHugh Flap
McReynolds Pterygium
Mead Lancet
Mercer Cartilage
Metzenbaum Septum
Meyhoeffer
Milette Tonsil
Milette-Tydings
Miltex Ligature
Mitchell Cartilage

Moorehead Ear
Murphy Plaster
Neivert
Newman Uterine
Niedner Commissurotomy
Nunez-Nunez Mitral Stenosis
Pace Hysterectomy
Page Tonsil
Parker Serrated Discission
Paton Corneal
Politzer Angular Ear
Pope Rectal
Potts Expansile
Ralks Reversible
Reese Ptosis
Reiner
Ridlon Plaster
Rish Cartilage
Robb
Robertson Tonsil
Rochester Mitral Stenosis
Rosen Incision (ear)
Royce
Scheie Goniotomy
Schultze Embryotomy
Schwartz Cordotomy
Semilunar Cartilage
Sexton Ear
Shambaugh
Shambaugh-Lempert
Sichel Iris
Sluder
Smillie Cartilage
Smillie Meniscus
Smith Cataract
Smith Cordotomy
Smith-Fisher Cataract
Smith-Green Eye
Somer Tonsil
Speed-Sprague
Stewart Cartilage
Strayer Meniscus
Suker Spatula
Tobold Laryngeal
Tooke

KNIVES (Continued)

Tydings Tonsil
Ulrich Uterine
Vacutome
Vannas Abscess
Vaughan Abscess
Virchow Skin Graft
Von Graefe Cataract
Walb P.M.
Walton Ear

Weber
Weber Canaliculus
Webster Skin Graft
Weiss Pattern
Wheeler Discission
Woodruff Spatula
Wullstein
Ziegler Iris
X-Acto Utility

LARYNGOSCOPES

Adult Reverse Bevel
Albert Andrews Modified Jackson
Anterior Commissure
Atkins-Tucker Shadow-Free
Bizzarri-Giuffrida
Broyles Anterior Commissure
Broyles Optical
Broyles Wasp Waist
Chevalier Jackson
Clerf
Dual Distal Lighted
E.S.I.
Fink
Flagg
Foregger
Guedel
Haslinger
Holinger Anterior Commissure
Holinger Hour Glass Ant.
  Commissure
Holinger Modified Jackson

Holinger Slotted Ant. Commissure
Hook-On Folding
Jackson
Lewy
Lundy
Lynch Suspension
MacIntosh
Miller
Multipurpose
Polio
Roberts Self-Retaining
Rotating
Sam Roberts Self-Retaining
Sanders Intubation
Siker Mirror
Standard
Tucker Anterior Commissure
Welch-Allyn
Wis-Foregger
Wis-Hipple
Yankauer

LENS EXPRESSORS

Arruga
Bagley-Wilmer
Berens
Kirby Intracapsular with curved
  zonal separator
Kirby Intracapsular with cylindrical
  separator

Kirby Intracapsular with double
  ball separator
Kirby Intracapsular with flat
  separator
Rizzuti
Verhoeff
Wilmer-Bagley

LENS LOUPE
Also see: LOOP

Daviel

Levis

LEUKOTOMES

Bailey
Dorsey Transorbital
Freeman Transorbital
Lours

Love
McKenzie
Nosik Transorbital

LID EVERTERS

Berens
Pess
Siniscal-Smith

Vail
Walker

LIGHTS

Co-Axa Lite
Gass Neurosurgical

Goodlite Super Headlight

LITHOTRITES

Alcock
Bigelow
Hendrickson
Keyes

Lowenstein
Ravich
Reliquet

LITHOTRIPTOSCOPE

Ravich with Luer Lock

LOOPS

Amenabar
Arlt Lens
Berens Lens
Billeau Ear

Lewis Lens
McKenzie Leukotomy
Weber-Elschnig
Wilder Lens

MAGNETS

Alnico Magneprobe
Coronet
Equen Stomach
Firlene Eye
Grafco
Holinger Bronchoscopic

Lancaster Eye
Mueller Giant Eye
Ralks
Sweet Eye
Thomas

MALLETS

Bakelite
Boxwood
Carroll Aluminum
Chandler
Crane
Fibre Head
Gerzog

Hajek
Hibbs
Kirk Orthopedic
Lucae
MacAusland Bone
Meyerding
Nylon Head

MALLETS (Continued)

Ralks
Rush
Smith-Petersen

Standard Pattern
White

MASTOID SEARCHER

Allport

MEATOSCOPE

Hubell

MEATOTOMES

Ellik

Riba Electric Ureteral

MECHANICAL FINGER

Quire

MENISCOTOME

Bowen-Grover
Grover

Ruuska

MICROSCOPE, Operating

Shambaugh-Derlacki

Zeiss

MOUTH GAGS

Boettcher-Jennings
Boyle Davis
Brophy
Brown-Fillebrown-Whitehead
Brown-Whitehead
Collis
Danns-Jennings
Davis
Davis-Crowe
Denhardt
Dott with Kilner Modification
Doyen-Jansen
Ferguson-Brophy
Ferguson-Gwathmey
Frohn
Fulton
Green
Green-Sewall
Heister
Hibbs
Jennings Loktite
Jennings-Skillern

Lane
Lewis
Maunder Oral Screw
McIvor
McKesson
Mithoefer-Jansen
Molt
Newkirk
Oral Speculum
Proetz
Proetz-Jansen
Pynchon
Ralks-Davis
Roser
Roser-Koenig
Sluder-Ferguson
Sluder-Jansen
Sydenham
Wesson
Whitehead
Wolf
Wolf Loktite

MUCOTOME

Norelco

NAILS

Augustine Boat Nails
Barr Bolts
Boat Nails
Cannulated
Cloverleaf
Curry Hip
Delitala T-Nails
Diamond
Dooley
Engel-May
Four Flanged
Gissane Spike
Hansen-Street Solid Intramedullary
Hooked Intramedullary
Jewett
Ken
Knowles Pins
Kuntscher Cloverleaf
Kuntscher Intramedullary

Lottes
Lottes Triflange Intramedullary
Massive Sliding
Moore Adjustable
Nylok Self-Locking
Neufeld
Pidcock
Rush
Schneider Intramedullary
Smith-Petersen Cannulated
Temple University
Thatcher
Thornton
Tiemann
V-Medullary
Venable Stuck
Vitallium
Watson Jones
Webb Bolt

NASOPHARYNGOSCOPES

Broyles
Holmes

Meltzer
National

NEEDLES

Abscission
Adson Aneurysm
Adson-Murphy Trocar Point
Agnew Tattooing
Alexander Tonsil
Atraumatic
Barrett Hebosteotomy
Beyer Paracentesis
Blair-Brown
Bowman Iris
Brophy
Brophy-Deschamps'
Brown Staphylorrhaphy
Bunnell
Campbell Ventricular
Carpule

Carroll
Cataract
Charleton Antrum
Cooper Chemopallidectomy
Cournand
Cournand-Grino
Cushing Ventricular
Daily Cataract
Dandy Ventricular
Davis
Dean Iris Knife
Deknatel "K"
Depuy-Weiss Tonsil
Deschamps'
Desmarres Paracentesis
Discission

NEEDLES (Continued)

Dix
Duff Debridement
Durham
Estridge Ventricular
Federspiel
Fein
Fischer Pneumothorax
Fisher Eye
Fish Hook
Floyd Pneumothorax Injection
Flynt Aortogram
Frankfeldt Hemorrhoidal
Frazier Ventricular
Frederick Pneumothorax
French Spring Eye
Gallie Fascia
Gardner
Goldbacher Rectal
Gorsch
Grieshaber 83/4
Hagedorn Suture
Halle Septum
Harken Heart
Hessberg
Hoen Ventricular
Hourin Tonsil
Ingersoll
Jameson Strabismus
Kader Fish Hook
Keith Abdominal
Knapp Iris Knife
Koontz
Kronecker Aneurysm
Lahey
Lane Suture
Lichtwicz Antrum
Linton-Blakemore
List
Loopuyt
Lowsley Ribbon Gut
Luer Lock
Lundy Fascia
Luongo
Maltz

Masson Fascia
Mayo
McCurdy Staphylorrhaphy
Menghini Liver Biopsy
Meyer Cyclodiathermy
Mixter Ventricular Needle
Murphy Intestinal
Nelson
Newman Rectal Injection
Overholt Rib
Pace Ventricular
Parhad-Poppen
Parker Knife
Penfield Biopsy
Poppen Ventricular
Presbyterian Hospital Ventricular
Retter Aneurysm
Reverdin
Rochester-Meeker
Rolf Lance
Ruskin Antrum
Sachs
Sanders-Brown-Shaw Aneurysm
Sheldon-Spatz
Silverman Biopsy
Sluder
Smiley-Williams
Spring Eye
Stocker Cyclodiathermy Puncture
Sturmdorf Cervical
Sturmdorf Pedicle
Swann-Sheldon
Todd Eye Cautery
Trupp Ventricular
Updegraff Staphylorrhaphy
Vim-Silverman
Von Graefe Iris Knife
Walker Tonsil
Ward
Watson-Williams
Wolf Antrum
Yankauer Septum
Ziegler Knife
Zoellner

NEUROTOME

Bradford Enucleation

OPHTHALMODYNAMOMETER

Bailliart   Dial Type

OSTEOCLAST

Phelps-Gocht

OSTEOTOMES

Albee
Alexander Perforating
Army Pattern
Blount Scoliosis
Bowen
Campbell
Carroll
Carroll-Legg
Carroll-Smith-Petersen
Clayton
Cloward Spinal Fusion
Converse
Cottle
Crane
Epstein
Frazier

Hibbs
Hoke
Howorth
Lambotte
Lambotte-Henderson
Legg
Mayfield Bayonet
Meyerding
Miner
Moore
New Lambotte
Rowland
Sheehan
Smith-Petersen
Stille Pattern
U.S. Army Pattern

OTOSCOPES

Bruening Pneumatic
Politzer Air Bag

Siegle Pneumatic

PANENDOSCOPE

McCarthy Foroblique

PELVIMETERS

Breisky
Collyer
DeLee
Hanley-McDermott

Martin
Thoms
Williams

84

PERFORATORS

Bishop Antrum
Cushing Cranial
Joseph Antrum
Lempert

Smellie OB
Wellaminski Antrum
Williams

PERIOSTEAL ELEVATOR (also see: ELEVATOR)

Adson
Allis
Aufranc
Behrend
Bethune
Bowen
Brophy
Cameron
Campbell
Carroll
Cheyne
Cloward
Coryllos
Coryllos-Doyen
Costal
Crego
Cushing-Hopkins
Cushion
Davidson
Davis
D'Errico
Doyen
Federspiel
Fiske
Fomon
Freer
Goodwillie
Harper
Herczel

Hibbs
Hoen
Iowa University
Joseph
Key
Kinsella
Kirmisson
Kocher
Lane
Langenbeck
Love-Adson
Lowis
MacDonald
MacKenty
Massachusetts General Hospital
MGH
Neurological Institute
Overholt
Pace
Raney
Richardson
Rubin-Lewis
Sayre's Double Ended
Scott-MacCracken
Sedillot
Sewall Mucoperiosteal
Spurling
Turner
Urquhart

PERIOSTEOTOMES

Alexander
Alexander-Farabeuf
Ballenger
Brophy
Brown
Ferris-Smith-Lyman
Fomon

Freer
Jansen
Moorehead
Potts
Speer
Vaughan
West-Beck

PESSARIES

Albert Smith
Chambers Intrauterine
Dutch
Findley Folding
Gariel
Gehrung
Gellhorn
Globe Prolapsus
Gold
Gynefold Retrodisplacement
Gynefold Prolapse

Hodge Style
Hollow Lucite
Lever
Menge Stem
Plexiglas Gellhorn
Prochownik
Ring
Safety
Smith Style
Wylie Stem
Zwanck (radium)

PICKS

Burch Ophthalmic
Hoffman Scleral Fixation

House
Wells Scleral Suture

PINS

Beaded Hip
Böhler
Bohlman
Breck
Compere Threaded
Conley
Davis
DePuy
Fahey
Fahey-Compere
Hagie
Hansen-Street
Haynes
Jones
Knowles
Kuntscher
Marble Bone
Modny
Moore Fixation

Oris
Pidcock
Pischel Micro-Pins
Rush
Schneider Self-Broaching
Schweitzer
Shriner
Smith-Petersen Fracture
Steinmann
   calibrated
   with Crowe pilot point
   with pin chuck, ball bearing
   with twist drill points
Strut Type
Turner
Venable-Stuck Fracture
Von Saal Medullary
Zimmer

PLIERS

Fisherman's

Vice-Grip

PLATES

Anchor
Badgley

Blade
Blount

bent blade plate
double angle blade
V-blade plate
Coaptation
DePuy
Eggers
Elliott Femoral Condyle
Finger
Jewett Double Angle Osteotomy
Jewett Slotted
Lundholm
McBride
McLaughlin
Milch Resection
Moe Intertrochanteric
Moore Blade
Neufeld
Newman Toenail
Plain Pattern
Rhinelander

Schweitzer Spring
Serpentine Bone
Sherman
Slotted
Smith-Petersen
SMO
Temple University
Thornton
Townsend-Gilfillan
Trochanteric
Venable Bone
V-Type Intertrochanteric
Vitallium
Wenger Slotted
Wilson Spinal Fusion
Wright Knee Plate
Y-Bone
Zuelzer Hook
Z-Plate

PNEUMOTHORAX APPARATUS

McKesson Pneumothor
R & B Portable

Robinson Artificial
Singer Portable

PROBES

Arbuckle
Anel Lacrimal
Barr Fistula
Bowman Lacrimal
Bresgen Frontal Sinus
Brock
Buck
Buie
Bunnell
Coakley Nasal
Desjardin Gallstone
Earle Rectal
Emmet Uterine
Esmarch Tin Bullet
Fenger Spiral Gallstone
Fish Antrum
Fluhrer Bullet
Fränkel Sinus

French Pattern Lacrimal
Gross
Hotz
Jansen-Newhart
Kistner
Knapp Iris Repositor & Probe
Larry Rectal
Lillie Frontal Sinus
Mayo Common Duct
Mixter Dilaprobe
Myrtle Leaf
Ochsner
Pratt Rectal
Rolf Lacrimal
Rosen Ear
Silver
Sims Uterine
Skillern Sphenoid

PROBES (Continued)

Spencer
Spiesman Fistula
Theobald
Wasko
Welch Allyn

Whale Bone Eustachian
Williams Lacrimal
Yankauer Salpingeal
Ziegler Needle

PROCTOSCOPES

Acmi
Boehm
Fansler
Goldbacher
Hirschman
Hirschman-Martin
Kelly
Lieberman

Montague
National
Newman
Pruitt
Turell
Vernon-David
Welch-Allyn
Yeomans

PROFILOMETER

Cottle

Straith

PROSTHESES

Also see: Implant Material and Eye Implants

Austin-Moore Hip
Bateman Finger Joint
Crimped Dacron
DePalma Hip
DePuy Hip with Scuderi Head
Eicher Hip
House
Judet Type
Lorenzo SMO
Lippman Hip
Matchett and Brown
Minneapolis

Modified Moore Hip
Moore Hip
Neer Shoulder
Sauerbruch
Scuderi
Smith-Petersen Hip Cup
F.R. Thompson Hip
Townley
Two Prong Stem Finger
Ushers Marlex Mesh
Vanghetti
Zimaloy Femoral Head

PUNCHES

Adler Attic Ear
Alexander Antrostomy
Berens Corneoscleral
Beyer Atticus
Brock Infundibular

Brooks
Castroviejo Corneoscleral
Citelli-Meltzer Atticus
Citelli Laminectomy
Cloward-English

88

PUNCHES (Continued)

Cloward-Harper
Cloward Intervertebral
Cone Bone
Cordes-New Laryngeal
Cordes Sphenoid
Corgill Bone
Dorsey Cervical Foramental
Eppendorfer
Faraci
Faraci-Skillern Sphenoid
Gass Cervical
Gellhorn Uterine Biopsy
Goldman Cartilage
Graham-Kerrison
Gruenwald
Gundelach
Gusberg Endocervical Biopsy
Haitz Canaliculus
Hajek Antrum
Hajek-Koffler Sphenoid
Hajek-Skillern Sphenoid
Harper Cervical Laminectomy
Hartmann Nasal
Hartmann Tonsil
Hoffmann Biopsy
Holth Corneoscleral
Ingraham Skull
Jackson
Johnson-Kerrison
Joseph
Kerrison
Keyes Cutaneous
Klause Antrum
Klause-Carmody Antrum
Knighton-Kerrison
Lange Antrum
Lebsche Sternal
Lempert Malleus
Lermoyez Nasal
MacKenty Sphenoid

Meltzer
MGH Glenoid
Mixter Brain Biopsy
Mosher Ethmoid
Mulligan Cervical Biopsy
Noyes Chalazion
Ostrom
Pfau Atticus Sphenoid
Phemister
Raney Laminectomy
Reaves
Ronis Adenoid
Rowe Glenoid
Schlesinger Cervical
Schmeden
Schmithhuisen Ethmoid & Sphenoid
Schnaudigel Sclerotomy
Schubert Biopsy
Seletz Universal Kerrison
Smeden Tonsil
Sokolowski
Spies Ethmoid
Spurling-Kerrison
Stevenson Capsule
Storz Antrum
Takahashi Ethmoid
Thoms-Gaylor Biopsy
Tischer Cervical Biopsy
Turell Angular Rotating
Van Struycken Nasal
Veenema-Gusberg Prostatic
Wagner Antrum
Walton Corneoscleral
Walton-Schubert
Watson-William Ethmoid
Whitcomb-Kerrison Laminectomy
Wittner Cervical Biopsy
Yankauer
Yeomans Biopsy

RASPS

Aufricht
Aufricht-Lipsett
Austin-Moore

Berne Nasal
Brawley Sinus
Brown

RASPS (Continued)

Cohen Sinus
Converse
Cottle
Dean
Eicher
Facet
Fomon
Gallagher Antrum
Gleason
Good Antrum
Israel
Joseph Nasal
Lamont Nasal
Lewis Nasal
Lundsgaard-Burch Corneal

Maliniac Nasal
Maltz
Maltz-Lipsett
Moore
Putti Bone
Ritter
Schantz Sinus
Schmidt
Spratt
Sullivan
F.R. Thompson
Thompson Frontal Sinus
Watson-William Sinus
Wiener Universal Frontal Sinus
Woodward Antrum

RASPATORY

Alexander
Artmann
Babcock
Bacon Periosteal
Ballenger
Bastow's
Berry Rib
Bronchocele Sound
Brunner
Coryllos Rib
Davidson-Mathieu Rib
Davidson-Sauerbruch Rib
Davis
Dolley
Doyen Rib
Farabeuf
Fishtail Spatula (Davis)
Friedrich
Hedbloom Rib
Hein
Herczel Rib
Hoen Periosteal
Hopkins Hospital Periosteal
Jansen Mastoid
Joseph
Kirmisson Periosteal

Kleesattel
Kocher
Kokowicz
Ladd
Lambert-Berry Rib
Lane Periosteal
Langenbeck-O'Brien
Langenbeck Periosteal
Lebsche
Mathieu
Matson
Ollier
Overholt
Phemister
Plenk-Matson
Sauerbruch-Frey
Sayre Periosteal
Scheuerlen
Schneider
Sedillot
Semb
Stillenberg
Trelat
Willauer
Zenker
Zoellner

REAMERS

Aufranc Offset
Cannulated Four Flute
DePuy Cannulated
Gruca Hip
Jergeson
Lorenzo
Lottes
MacAusland
MacAusland Finishing Ball
MacAusland Finishing Cup
Medullary Canal
Moore Bone

Murphy Ball
Norton Adjustable Cup
Norton Ball
Phemister
Rush Awl
Shaft Reamer
Shelf
Smith-Petersen Hip
Sovak
Spiral Trochanteric
Sturmdorf Cervical

RESECTOSCOPES

Bard
Baumrucker
Iglesias
McCarthy Miniature
McCarthy Multiple

Nesbit
Scott Rotating
Stern-McCarthy Electrotome
Thompson Direct Full Vision

RETINOSCOPES

Boilo
Copeland Streak

Welch Allyn Standard
Welch Allyn Streak

RETRACTORS

Adson Cerebellum
Adson Splanchnic
Agricola Lacrimal Sac
Alden
Alexian Hospital Model
Allison Lung
Allport Mastoid
Allport-Gifford
Alm
Alter's Lip
Amenabar
Andrews Tracheal
Ann Arbor Phrenic
Anthony
Apicolysis
Aufranc Femoral Neck (Also: hip; push; psoas)
Aufricht Nasal

Austin
Automatic Skin
Bacon Cranial
Badgley Laminectomy
Balfour
Ballantine Hemilaminectomy
Baron
Barr
Barrett-Adson Cerebellum
Beatty Pillar
Becker
Beckman
Beckman-Adson
Beckman-Weitlaner
Bellfield Wire
Beneventi Self-Retaining
Bennett Tibia
Berens Mastectomy, Skin Flap

RETRACTORS (Continued)

Berens Thyroid
Bergen
Berna Infant Abdominal
Bethune Phrenic
Bicek Vaginal
Blair
Blair-Brown Vacuum
Blakesley Uvula
Bland Perineal
Blount
Boyes Goodfellow Hook
Brantley-Turner
Brawley
Breen
Brewster Phrenic
Brompton Hospital
Brown Uvula
Brunner
Brunschwig Visceral
Buie-Smith Anal
Burford-Finochietto
Burford Rib Retractor
Campbell Lacrimal Sac
Carroll Offset Hand
Carroll Self-Retaining Spring
Carroll-Bennett Finger
Castroviejo
Cave Knee
Chandler Laminectomy
Cloward Self-Retaining
Cloward-Hoen Laminectomy
Colver Tonsil
Cone Scalp
Contour Scalp
Converse Nasal
Cook Rectal
Coryllos
Cottle
Cottle Sharp Prong
Cottle-Neivert
Craig-Sheehan
Crego
Crile
Crotti
Cushing

Cushing Aluminum Cortex
Cushing Vein
Davidson Erector Spinae
Davidson Scapular
Davis Scalp
Deaver
Decker
Delaney Phrenic
DeLee Corner
DeLee Universal
DeLee Vaginal
DeLee Vesical
D'Errico Nerve
D'Errico-Adson
DeMartel Self-Retaining Brain
Desmarres Lid
Downing
Doyen Vaginal
Duryea
Eastman Vaginal
Effenberger
Elschnig Lid
Falk Vaginal
Farabeuf Double Ended
Farr Wire
Federspiel Cheek
Ferguson-Moon
Ferris-Smith Orbital Retractor
Ferris-Smith-Sewall Orbital
Finger Rake
Fink Lacrimal
Finochietto
Finochietto-Geissendorfer Rib
Fisher Lid
Fisher Nugent
Fomon
Foss Gallbladder
Franklin Malleable
Franz Abdominal
Frazier
Frazier Laminectomy
Frazier-Fay
Freer Submucous
Freiberg Hip
Friederich-Ferguson

RETRACTORS (Continued)

Friedman Perineal
Fritsch
Gelpi Perineal
Gelpi Self-Retaining
Ghazi Rib
Gifford Mastoid
Glaser Laminectomy
Glenner
Glenner Vaginal
Goelet Double Ended
Goldstein Lacrimal Sac
Gooch
Goodhill
Goodyear Tonsil
Gosset Abdominal
Gradle Eyelid
Green Thyroid
Groenholm Lid
Gross Patent Ductus
Gross-Pomeranz-Watkins Atrial
Guttmann OB
Guzman-Blanco Epiglottis Forceps
Haight Rib
Hajek
Hamby-Hibbs
Hand
Harken
Harrington Bladder
Harrington-Pemberton
Harrington Splanchnic
Harrison Chalazion
Haslinger Palate
Haslinger Uvula
Haverfield Hemilaminectomy
Hays Hand
Heaney Vaginal
Heaney-Simon
Hedblom
Helfrick Anal
Henner Endaural
Hertzler Baby
Hibbs
Hill-Ferguson Rectal
Hillis Lid
Himmelstein Sternum

Hipps Self-Retaining
Hoen
Holscher Nerve Root
House
Howorth Toothed
Hudson Bone
Hunt Bladder
Hupp Trachea
Iron Interne
Israel
Jackson
Jacobson
Jaeger Lid Plate
Jansen
Jansen Mastoid
Jansen Scalp
Jansen-Gifford
Jansen-Wagner
Johnson Cheek
Johnson Ventriculogram
Judd-Masson
Kalamarides Dural
Kel
Kellig
Kelly-Sims
Kerrison
Killian-King Goiter
Kirkland
Klemme Appendectomy
Klemme Gasserian Ganglion
Knapp
Kocher
Kocher-Crotti Goiter
Kozlinski
Krasky
Kretschmer
Kristeller Vaginal
Kronfeld Eyelid
Lahey
Lange
Langenbeck
Laplace Liver
Latrobe Soft Palate
Leatherman Trochanteric
Legueu Kidney

RETRACTORS (Continued)

Lempert
Lempert-Colver
Levinthal Surgery
Levy Perineal
Lewis
Lilienthal-Sauerbruch
Linton Splanchnic
Little
Lorie Cheek
Lothrop
Love Nasopharyngeal
Love Nerve
Love Uvula
Lowsley
Luer
Lukens
Lukens Epiglottis
Lukens Thymus
Luongo Hand
Luther, Peter
MacAusland Muscle
MacAusland-Kelly
MacKay Contour
Maison
Maliniac Nasal
Maltz
Martin Abdominal
Martin Cheek & Lip
Martin Palate
Masson-Judd
Mathieu
Matson-Mead Apicolysis
Mattison-Upshaw
Mayo-Adams
Mayo-Collins
Mayo-Simpson
McBurney
McCullough Externo-frontal
Meller Lacrimal Sac
Meyerding Finger
Meyerding Laminectomy
Meyerding-Deaver
Middledorpf
Miller
Miller-Senn

Millin-Bacon Bladder
Miltex
Moorehead Cheek
Morrison-Hurd
Mosher Lifesaver
Mott
Mueller Lacrimal Sac
Mueller-Balfour
Muldoon Lid
Munro Self-Retaining
Murphy Rake
Murtagh Self-Retaining Infant Scalp
Myers Knee
Neivert
New York Hospital
O'Brien Phrenic
O'Brien Rib
Ochsner
Oldberg
Ollier
O'Sullivan Self-Retaining Abdominal
O'Sullivan-O'Connor Vaginal
Otto Barkan Bident
Overholt
Parker
Parker-Mott
Paul
Peet Lighted Splanchnic
Pemberton
Percy Amputation
Percy-Wolfson
Phiefer-Young
Pierce Cheek
Piper Lateral Wall
Pryor-Pean Vaginal
Purcell Self-Retaining Abdominal
Quervain-Sauerbruch
Radcliff Perineal
Ragnell
Rake
Rankin
Ribbon
Richardson
Richardson-Eastman
Richter

RETRACTORS (Continued)

Rigby Bi-valve
Rigby Rectal
Rigby Vaginal
Rizzo
Rochester Colonial
Rochester-Ferguson
Rollet Eye
Rose Tracheal
Roux
Rowe Humeral Head
Rowe Scapular Neck Spike
Rudolph Trowel
Ryerson Bone
Sachs
Sachs-Cushing
St. Luke
Sauerbruch
Sauerbruch-Zukschwerdt Rib
Sawyer Rectal
Schwartz Laminectomy
Scoville Nerve Root
Scoville Psoas Muscle
Seletz-Gelpi Self-Retaining
Semb
Senn
Senn-Kanavel
Senturia
Serrefine
Sewall Orbital
Shambaugh Endaural
Shearer Lip
Sheehan
Sheldon Hemilaminectomy
Sherwood
Shriners Hospital
Shriners Interlocking
Shurley Tracheal
Sims Vaginal
Sims-Kelly
Sistrunk Band
Sloan Goiter
Sluder Palate
Smith Anal
Smith-Buie Anal
Smith-Petersen Capsule

Snitman Endaural
Sofield
Splanchnic
Stevenson Lacrimal Sac
Stookey
Strully Nerve Root
Sweet Amputation
Temple-Fay Laminectomy
Theis Vein
Tillary
Tower Interchangeable
Tuffier Rib
Tuffier-Raney
Tyrer Nerve Root
Ullrich Laminectomy
U.S. Army Pattern
Vacher
Vail Lid
Verbrugghen
Volkmann-Rake
Walker Gallbladder
Walker Lid
Walter-Deaver
Webb-Balfour
Weber
Webster Abdominal
Weinberg Vagotomy
Weitlaner
Wesson
Wexler
Wexler-Balfour
White-Proud Uvula
Wieder Pillar
Wieder-Solenberger Pillar
Wilder Scleral Wound
Willauer-Deaver
Wilson Hand
Wolfson Gallbladder
Wort Antrum
Wullstein
Young Bifid
Young Bulb
Young Lateral
Young Prostatic
Zalkind

RIB CONTRACTORS

Adams
Bailey

Bailey-Gibbon
Graham

RIB CUTTERS

See: Rib Shears

RIB SHEARS

Bacon
Bethune
Bethune-Coryllos
Bortone
Brunner
Coryllos-Bethune
Coryllos-Moure
Coryllos-Shoemaker
Doyen
Duval-Coryllos
Eccentric Lock
Giertz-Shoemaker
Gluck
Horgan-Coryllos-Moure
Horgan-Wells
Lebsche Sternum

Moure-Coryllos
Nelson-Bethune
Roberts
Sauerbruch
Sauerbruch-Coryllos
Sauerbruch-Frey
Sauerbruch-Lebsche
Shoemaker
Stille
Stille-Giertz
Stille-Horsley
Thompson
Thomsen Rib
Tudor-Edwards
Walton

RIB SPREADERS

Burford-Finochietto
Finochietto
Gerbode Modified Burford
Haight
Harken
Lefferts
Lilienthal
Lilienthal-Sauerbruch
McGuire
Miltex

Nelson
Overholt
Reinhoff
Reinhoff-Finochietto
Nissen
Sauerbruch-Lilienthal
Sweet
Tuffier
Tudor-Edwards

ROD

Knodt Distraction

RONGEURS

Adson Bone
Andrews-Hartmann
Bacon Bone

Bane
Beyer Bone
Beyer Endaural (Ear)

RONGEURS (Continued)

Blumenthal
Bogle
Bruening-Citelli
Campbell Laminectomy
Cicherelli
Citelli
Cloward Pituitary
Colclough Laminectomy
Converse Nasal
Cranial Bone
Cushing Bone
Dean Bone
Dench
DePuy Pituitary
Devilbiss Cranial
Duckbill
Dufourmental Nasal
Echlin Duckbill
Ferris-Smith Pituitary
Ferris-Smith-Gruenwald
Ferris-Smith-Kerrison
Ferris-Smith-Takahashi
Fulton
Gruenwald Pituitary
Hajek Antrum
Hakansson
Hartmann Bone
Hartmann Ear
Hartmann-Herzfeld Ear
Hein
Henny Laminectomy
Hoen Laminectomy
Hoffman Ear
Horsley Bone
Husks Mastoid
Ivy Mastoid
Jansen
Jansen Bayonet
Jansen-Zaufel
Juers-Lempert Endaural
Kerrison
Kerrison-Costen
Kerrison Mastoid
Lebsche
Leksell

Lempert Bone
Lempert Endaural
Lilly
Littauer
Lombard
Lombard-Beyer
Lombard-Boies Mastoid
Love-Gruenwald Pituitary
Love-Kerrison
Luer
Luer-Hartmann
Meade Bone
Montenovesi Double Action Cranial
Noyes
O'Brien
Oldberg Pituitary
Olivecrona Endaural
Pierce
Poppen Pituitary
Prince
Raney
Reiner
Rowland Nasal
Ruskin Bone
Ruskin Duckbill
Ruskin Mastoid
Ruskin Multiple Action
Sauerbruch
Sauerbruch-Coryllos Rib
Sauerbruch Lebsche
Schlesinger
Schwartz-Kerrison
Selverstone I.V. Disc
Semb
Semb-Sauerbruch
Shearer
Spurling-Kerrison (Colclough)
Spurling Laminectomy
Spurling Pituitary
Spurling-Love-Gruenwald-Cushing
Stille
Stille-Leksell
Stille-Luer
Stookey
Strully-Kerrison

RONGEURS (Continued)

Strümpel or Struempel
Taper Jaw
Tobey Ear
Von Seemen
Voris I.V. Disc
Walton

Watson-Williams I.V. Disc
Weil Pituitary
Weingartner
Whiting Mastoid
Zaufel-Jansen

RULERS

Berndt Hip
Chernow Notched
Joseph Measuring
Metal

Millimeter
Pischel Scleral
Walker Scleral

SAWS

Bailey Gigli
Becker-Joseph
Bishop Oscillatory Electric Bone
Bosworth
Brown
Charriere Aseptic Metacarpal
Clerf Laryngeal
Converse
Crego-Gigli
Electric Laryngofissure
Engel Plaster
Gigli
Gigli Wire
Hetherington Circular
Hey Skull
Joseph Bayonet
Joseph-Maltz Angular
Joseph Nasal
Lamont Nasal

Langenbeck Metacarpal
Lell Laryngofissure
Luck Bone
Magnuson Circular Twin
Magnuson Double Counter-rotating
Magnuson Single Circular
Maltz Bayonet
Mueller
Satterlee Amputating
Satterlee Aseptic
Seltzer
Silver
Slaughter Nasal
Stille-Gigli Wire Saw
Stryker
Tyler Spiral Gigli
V.M. & Co. Amputating
Wigmore Plaster
Woakes Nasal

SCISSORS

Ada
Adson
Aebli
Alligator
Atkinson-Walker
Baltimore Nasal
Bantham Wire Cutting
Barraquer-DeWecker

Baruch Circumcision
Beaded Tip
Becker Septum
Berens Iridocapsulotomy
Blum Arterial
Boettcher Tonsil
Bowman Strabismus
Boyd Dissecting

SCISSORS (Continued)

Braun Episiotomy
Brooks Gallbladder
Brophy
Brown
Buerger-McCarthy
Buie Rectal
Bull Dog
Burnham
Busch Umbilical
Castroviejo
Caylor
Chevalier Jackson
Church
Church Pediatric
Classon Pediatric
Converse
Cottle Bull Dog
Cottle Dorsal
Cottle Nasal
Crafoord Lung
Craig
Crown & Collar
Dandy Trigeminus
Dean Tonsil
Deaver
DeBakey Stitch
Dewecker Iris
Doyen Abdominal
Dubois Decapitation
Duffield
Dumont Thoracic
Emmet Uterine
Enucleation
Essrig Dissecting
Federspiel
Ferguson Abdominal
Finochietto
Fomon Saber Back
Frazier Dura
Fulton Pediatric
Gauze
Gillies Suture
Good Tonsil
Graham Pediatric
Guggenheim

Guist Enucleation
Guyton
Haimovici Arteriotomy
Harrington
Heath Suture and Wire Cutting
Heyman Nasal
Hoen Laminectomy
Hooper Pediatrics
Iris
Irvine
Jackson Turbinate
Jorgenson
Joseph-Maltz
Kahn
Katzeff Cartilage
Katzin Corneal
Kelly
Knapp Iris
Knight Nasal
Knowles
Kreuscher
LaGrange
Lahey
Lakeside
Lawton Corneal
Lexer Dissecting
Lillie Tonsil
Lincoln Pediatric
Lister
Littauer
MacKenty
Maclay Tonsil
Malis Neurological
Martin Ballpoint
Martin Cartilage
Martin Throat
Mattis
Maunoir
Mayo Dissecting
Mayo-Harrington
Mayo-New
Mayo-Noble
Mayo-Potts Dissecting
Mayo-Stille
McAllister

SCISSORS (Continued)

McClure Iris
McGuire Corneal
McLean Capsulotomy
McReynolds
Metzenbaum
Miller Rectal
Mixter Operating
Morse Backward Cutting Aortic
Munro Brain
Nelson Lobectomy
Noble
Northbent Suture
Noyes Iris
Nugent-Gradle
Ochsner Ball Tipped
Ochsner Diamond Edge
Olivecrona Angular
Olivecrona Guillotine
Panzer Gallbladder
Potts
Potts-Smith
Pratt Rectal
Prince-Potts
Prince Tonsil
Quimby Gum
Reinhoff Thoracic
Resano
Reynolds Dissecting
Rochester-Ferguson
Sadler Cartilage
Satinsky Vena Cava
Schmeden

Schroeder Operating
Seiler Turbinate
Serratex
Sims Uterine
Sistrunk Dissecting
Spencer Stitch
Stevens Tenotomy
Strabismus
Strully Hook
Sweet Esophageal
Taylor Dural
Tenotomy
Thorek
Toennis
Vannas Capsulotomy
Verhoeff Dissecting
Vezien Abdominal
Walker-Apple
Walker-Atkinson
Walker Corneal
Walton
Weber Tissue
Westcott Tenotomy
Westcott-Schele
White
Willauer
Wilmer Iris
Wincor Enucleation
Wullstein
Wutzler
Yankauer
Zoellner

SCLEROTOMES

Alvis-Lancaster
Curdy
Lancaster

Lundsgaard-Burch
Walker-Lee

SCOOPS

Arlt Fenestrated Lens
Beck Abdominal
Berens Lens
Daviel Lens
Desjardin Gall Duct

Elschnig Lens
Ferguson Gallstone
Green Lens
Hess Lens
Knapp Lens

SCOOPS (Continued)

Lewis Lens
Luer Fenestrated Lens
Luer-Korte Gallstone
Mayo Common Duct
Mayo-Robson Gallstone

Moore Gallstone
Moynihan Gallstone
Pagenstecher Lens
Wells Enucleation
Wilder Lens

SCREWS

Basile Hip
Bosworth Coracoclavicular
Carpal Scaphoid
Carrell-Girard
Collison
Coracoclavicular
Cruciform Head Bone
Cubbins
Demuth Hip
Doyen Tumor
Eggers
Jewett Pick-up
Johannsen Lag
Lag
Leinbach Olecranon
Lorenzo

Lundholm
Marion
Morris Bi-phase
Phillips Recessed Head
Sherman Bone
Sherman Molybdenum
Stryker
Thatcher
Townley Bone Graft
Townsend-Gilfillan
Virgin Hip
Vitallium
Wood
Woodruff
Zimmer

SCREW DRIVERS

Automatic
Becker
Collison
Cubbins Bone
DePuy
Lane
Lever Type
Lok-It
Massie
Master

Plain
Richter Bone
Sherman
Sherman-Pierce
Stryker
Trinkle
V.M. & Co.
White
Zimmer

SEPARATORS

Benson Pylorus
Davis Nerve
Dorsey
Frazier Dura
Grant
Hoen Dura

Horsley Dura
Hunter
Rosen Bayonet (Ear)
Sachs Dura
Sachs Nerve

SHEARS
Also See: Rib Shears

Clayton Laminectomy
Esmarch Plaster
Diertz
Gluck
Lebsche Sternum
Liston

Sauerbruch-Frey
Seutin Plaster
Semb
Stille Plaster
Weck

SIGMOIDOSCOPES

Boehm
Buie
Frankfeldt
Kelly
Lieberman with Swinging Window
Montague

Solow
Turell
Tuttle
Vernon David
Welch Allyn

SKIDS

Davis
Meyerding
Murphy Bone

Murphy-Lane
Ryerson Bone
Scudder

SNARES

Alfred
Banner Enucleation
Beck-Shenk Tonsil
Boettcher-Farlow
Bosworth Nasal
Brown Tonsil
Bruening Ear
Buerger
Crapeau Nasal
Douglas Nasal
Douglas Tonsil
Eves Tonsil
Farlow Tonsil
Farlow-Boettcher
Foerster Enucleation
Frankfeldt Rectal
Krause Ear
Krause Nasal
Laryngeal
Lewis Tonsil

Martin
Myles Tonsillectome
Neivert-Eves
Nesbit Tonsil
Newhart-Casselberry
Norwood
Pynchon Ear
Quires Mechanical Finger
Reiner-Beck Tonsil
Robert Nasal
Sage Tonsil (automatic ratchet)
Stutsman Nasal
Storz-Beck Tonsil
Tydings Tonsil
Weston Rectal
Wilde-Bruening Ear
Wilde-Bruening Nasal
Wright Nasal
Wright Tonsil

102

SOUNDS

Campbell Miniature
Davis Interlocking
Dittel Urethral
Fowler Urethral
Gouley Tunneled Urethral
Guyon Urethral
Guyon-Benique Urethral Sound
Hunt Metal
Jewett Urethral
Kocher Bronchocele

LeFort Urethral
McCrea Infant
Otis
Pratt Urethral
Schroeder Interlocking
Simpson Uterine
Sims Uterine
Von Buren Urethral
Walther Urethral
Woodward

SPATULAS

Castroviejo Cyclodialysis
Cave Scaphoid
Children's Hospital Brain
Culler
Cushing Brain
Davis
D'Errico Brain
Elschnig Cyclodialysis
Freer
Garron
Green
Gross
Kirby Iris
Knapp Iris
Laird
Lindner Cyclodialysis
Meller Cyclodialysis
O'Brien
Olivecrona Brain

Paton
Peyton Brain
Raaf Flexible Lighted
Sachs
Scoville Brain
Segond Vaginal
Smith-Fisher Cataract
Smith-Fisher Iris
Smith-Green Double End
Smith-Petersen
Suker Cyclodialysis
Tauber Vaginal
Thomas
Weary Brain
Wecker Iris
Wheeler Cyclodialysis
Wullstein Transplant
Wurmuth

SPECULA (Speculum)

Adson
Allen-Heffernan Nasal
Allingham Rectal
Arruga Eye
Aufricht Septum
Auvard Weighted Vaginal
Barr Anal
Barr Rectal
Barr-Shuford
Beard Eye
Beckman

Beckman-Colver Nasal
Berens Eye
Berlind-Auvard
Bodenheimer
Bosworth Nasal
Boucheron Ear
Brewer Vaginal
Brinkerhoff Rectal
Bruner Vaginal
Buie-Smith Rectal
Carter Septum

SPECULA (Speculum)

Castroviejo Eye
Chelsea Eaton Anal
Chevalier Jackson Laryngeal
Coakley Nasal
Coldlite
Coldlite-Graves Vaginal
Collins Vaginal
Converse Nasal
Cook Eye
Cook Rectal
Cottle Septum
Cusco Vaginal
David Rectal
DeLee
De Roaldes
Devilbiss Vaginal
Devilbiss-Stacey
Douglas Mucosa
Doyen Vaginal
Dudley-Smith Rectal
Duplay Nasal
Duplay-Lynch Nasal
Eaton Nasal
Erhardt Ear
Fansler Rectal
Farkas Urethral
Fergusson Tubular Vaginal
Flannery Ear
Flint Glass
Foster-Ballenger
Fox Eye
Garrigue Vaginal
Gerzog Nasal
Gilbert-Graves
Gleason
Goldbacher Anoscope
Goldstein Septum
Graefe Eye
Graves Vaginal
Gruber Ear
Guild-Pratt Rectal
Guist Eye
Guist-Black Eye
Guttmann Vaginal
Guyton-Park Eye

Halle Nasal
Halle-Tieck Nasal
Hartmann Nasal
Heffernan Nasal
Henrotin Vaginal
Higbee Vaginal
Hinckle-James Rectal
Hood-Graves Vaginal
Ingals Nasal
Ives Rectal
Jackson Vaginal
Jonas-Graves Vaginal
Kahn-Graves Vaginal
Killian Septum
Klaff Septum
Knapp Eye
Kogan Endospeculum
Kramer Ear
Kristeller Vaginal
Kyle Nasal
Lancaster Eye
Lancaster-O'Connor
Lang Eye
Lillie Nasal
Lister-Burch Eye
Luer Eye
Macon Hospital
Mason-Auvard Weighted Vaginal
Mahoney Intranasal Antrum
McKinney
McLaughlin
Mellinger Eye
Metcher Eye
Miller Vaginal
Montgomery Vaginal
Montgomery-Bernstine
Mosher Nasal
Mosher Urethral
Mueller
Murdock Eye
Murdock-Wiener Eye
Myles Nasal
Myles-Ray
National Ear
Nott Vaginal

SPECULA (Speculum)

Nott-Guttmann Vaginal
Noyes
O'Sullivan-O'Connor Vaginal
Park Eye
Park-Guyton Eye
Patton Septum
Pederson Vaginal
Pennington Rectal
Picot
Pilling-Hartmann
Plain Wire
Pratt Bi-Valve
Pratt Rectal
Preefer Eye
Pynchon Nasal
Ray Nasal
Richard Gruber
Roberts Esophageal
Rosenthal Urethral
Sauer Eye
Senturia Pharyngeal
Shoe Horn
Simrock
Sims' Rectal
Sims' Vaginal
Sluder Sphenoidal
Smith Anal

Smith Eye
SMR
Sonnenschein
Stearns
Storz Septum
Steiner-Auvard
Tauber
Taylor Vaginal
Tieck
Tieck-Halle
Toynbee Ear
Trelat
Troeltsch Ear
Vernon-David Rectal
Vienna Nasal
Voltolini
Von Graefe
Watson
Weeks Eye
Weisman-Graves Vaginal
Welch Allyn
Wiener Eye
Williams Eye
Worchester City Hospital Vaginal
Yankauer
Ziegler Eye
Zower

SPHINCTEROTOME

Doubilet

SPLINTS

Abduction Finger
Abduction Thumb
Adam & Eve Rib Belt
Airfoam
Airplane (Aeroplane)
Aluminum Fence
Aluminum Finger Cot
Anterior Acute Flexion Elbow
Ball-peen
Banjo
Basswood
Baylor Adjustable Cross

Böhler Wire
Böhler-Braun (King's Traction)
Brant Aluminum
Bunnell Knuckle Bender
Bunnell Outrigger
Cabot Leg
Calibrated Clubfoot
Campbell Airplane
Campbell Traction Humerus
Carl P. Jones Traction
Coaptation
Cock-Up Hand

SPLINTS (Continued)

Colles
Cramer Wire
Culley Ulna
Curry Walking
Davis Metacarpal
Denis Browne Clubfoot
Denis Browne Hip
DePuy
DePuy Aeroplane
DePuy Any Angle
DePuy Coaptation
DePuy Open Thimble
DePuy-Pott's
DePuy Rocking Leg
DePuy Rolled Colles
Easton Cock-Up
Eggers Contact
Erich Nasal
Ferciot Tip Toe
Fillauer Night
Forrester Head
Frejka
Fruehevald
Funsten Supination
Granberry's
Gunning (Jaw)
Hart Extension Finger
Haynes-Griffin Mandible
Hinged Thomas
Hirschtick Utility Shoulder
Hodgen Hip
Hodgen Leg
Jelenko
Jonell Countertraction Finger
Jonell Thumb
Jones Arm
Jones Forearm & Metacarpal
Joseph Septum
Keller-Blake Half Ring Leg
Kerr Abduction

Keystone
Lambrinudi
Lewin Baseball Finger
Lewin Finger
Lewin-Stern Thumb & Finger
Love Nasal
Lytle Metacarpal
Magnuson Abduction Humerus
Mason-Allen Universal Hand
Mayer Nasal
Mohr Finger
Murray-Jones Arm
Murray-Thomas Arm
Neubeiser Adjustable Forearm
O'Donaghue Knee
O'Donaghue Stirrup
Opponens
Orthopedic Strap Clavicle
Ponseti
Pott's
Putti
Roger Anderson Well Leg
Safety Pin
Scott Humerus
Simpson Sugar Tong
Speed Hand
Spigelman Baseball Finger
Strampelli Eye
Teare Arm
Thomas Full Ring
Thomas Hinged
Thomas Leg
Thompson Modification of
    Denis Browne
T-Finger
Yucca Wood
Zimmer
Zimmer Clavicular Cross
Zim-Zip Rib Belt
Zucker

SPOONS

Bunge Exenteration
Coyne
Culler Lens

Cushing Pituitary
Daviel Lens
Elschnig Lens

SPOONS (Continued)

Falk Appendectomy
Fisher
Gross Ear
Hess Lens
Hoke-Roberts
Kalt Eye
Kirby Lens

Knapp Lens
Kocher Brain
Moore Gallbladder
Ray Brain
Royal
Skene Uterine
Wells Enucleation

SPREADERS

Also see: RIB SPREADERS
Gross Ductus
Inge Lamina
Kimpton Vein

Lemmon Sternal
Millin-Bacon Bladder Neck
Tudor-Edwards
Ventura

SPUDS

Alvis
Bennett Foreign Body
Corbett Foreign Body
Davis Foreign Body
Dix Foreign Body
Ellis Foreign Body
Fisher
Francis Knife

Gross Ear
Hosford Foreign Body
LaForce Knife
Levine Foreign Body
Nicati Foreign Body
O'Brien Foreign Body
Walter Corneal
Whittle

SPUR CRUSHERS

Baby
Berger
DeWitt-Stetten Colostomy
Garlock
Gross
Mayo-Lovelace
Mikulicz

Ochsner-DeBakey
Pemberton
Stetten
Warthen
Wolfson's
Wurth

STAPLES

Zimaloy Epiphyseal

STONE DISLODGERS

Councill
Creevy Calyx
Davis Modification of Councill
Dormia
Howard Spiral
Howard-Flaherty Spiral
Johnson Stone

Johnson Ureteral Basket
Levant
Morton
Ortved
Robinson
Woven Loop
Wullen

STRIPPERS

Babcock Jointed Vein
Bartlett Fascia
Bunnell Tendon
Cannon Type
Carroll Forearm Tendon
Clark Vein
Cole Polyethylene Vein
Crile Vagotomy
Doyle Vein
Dunlop
Emerson Vein
Friedman Vein
Joplin Tendon
Kurten Vein
Lempka Vein
Linton Vein
Masson Fascia
Matson Rib

Matson-Alexander Rib
Matson-Mead Periosteum
Mayo Vein
Mayo-Myers
Myers Spiral Vein
Nabatoff Vein
Nelson Rib
Nelson-Roberts
Phelan Vein
Price-Thomas Rib
Rib Edge
Roberts-Nelson Rib
Shaw Carotid Artery Clot
Smith Posterior Cartilage
Trace Hydraulic Vein
Webb Vein
Wurth Vein

SUCTION TUBES

Andrews Pynchon
Anthony
Buie
Fitzpatrick
Gwathmey
Humphrey Coronary Sinus Sucker
Lore
Mosher Life Saving

O'Hanlon-Poole
Poole Abdominal
Poole Pediatric
Pynchon
Weck
Yankauer
Yeder

TAMP

Kiene Bone

TELESCOPES

Best Direct Forward Vision
Foroblique
Kramer Direct Vision
McCarthy Foroblique Operating

McCarthy Miniature
Retrospective
Transilluminating
Walden

TENACULUMS

Adair
Barrett Uterine
Braun Uterine

Brophy
Corey
Cottle

TENACULUMS (Continued)

Duplay Uterine
Emmet
Jacobs Uterine
Jarcho
Kahn Traction
Lahey Goiter
Potts
Revots Vulsellum

Ritchie Cleft Palate
Schroeder
Skene Uterine
Staude-Moore
Thoms
Watts
Weisman

TENOTOME

Ryerson

TENDON PASSERS

Carroll
Joplin

Ober
Withers

TENDON STRIPPER

See: STRIPPER

TENDON TUCKER

See: TUCKER

THERMOPORE

Shahan

THORACOTOME

Bettman-Forvash

THORACOSCOPES

Coryllos
Cutler Forceps
Jacobaeus

Jacobaeus-Unverricht
Moore
Sarot

TONG, Traction

Böhler
Crutchfield Skull

Raney-Crutchfield Skull

TONGUE DEPRESSORS

Andrews
Andrews-Pynchon
Balmer
Beatty
Blakesley
Boebinger
Bosworth
Chamberlain
Colver-Dawson
Dorsey
Farlow
Granberry

Hamilton
Israel
Jobson-Pynchon
Kellogg
Layman
Lewis
Mullins
Pirquet
Proetz
Pynchon
Titus
Weder

TONOMETERS

Bailliart
McLean
Mueller Electronic

Schiotz
Sklar

TONSILLECTOMES

Ballenger-Sluder
Beck-Mueller
Beck-Schenck
Brown
Daniels
Hemostatic
LaForce
Meding Tonsil Enucleator
Moltz-Storz
Myles

Sauer
Sauer-Sluder
Searcy
Sluder
Sluder-Ballenger
Sluder-Demarest
Sluder-Sauer
Tydings
Van Osdel Tonsil Enucleator
Whiting

TOURNIQUETS

Adams Modification of Bethune
Bethune Lung
Campbell-Boyd
Carr Lobectomy
Conn Pneumatic
Esmarch
Linton

Pneumatic
Robbins Automatic
Roberts-Nelson Lobectomy
Rumel Cardiovascular
Rumel-Belmont
Weiner

TRACTION BOWS

Bendixen-Kirschner
Boehler
Crego-McCarroll
Granberry Finger
Keys-Kirschner

Logan
Pease-Thomson
Beaded Wires
Petersen Skeletal

TRACTORS

Blackburn Skull Traction
Bucks Extension
Freiberg Traction
Gerster Traction Bar
Handy-Bucks Extension
Hoke-Martin
Kestler Ambulatory Head
Kirschner Wire
Lowsley Prostatic
Moleskin Traction

Nauth Os Calcis Apparatus
Orr-Bucks Extension
Rankin Prostatic
Rocking Chair Truck
Russell Traction
Russell-Bucks Extension
Steinmann Traction
Vinke Skull
Young Prostatic
Wells Tractor

TRANSILLUMINATORS

All Purpose
Briggs
Finnoff
Hooded
National All-Metal

National Opal Glass
Rotating
Speculum Illuminator
Tatum Ureteral
Widner

TREPHINES

Arruga Eye
Barraquer Corneal
Blakesley Lacrimal
Boiler Septum
Brown-Pusey Corneal
Castroviejo Corneal
Cross Scleral
Damshek Sternal
D'Errico
Devilbiss Skull
Dimitry Chalazion
Dimitry Dacryocystorhinostomy
Elliot Eye
Galt
Gradle Corneal
Green Automatic Corneal
Grieshaber Corneal

Jentzer
Lichtenberg Corneal
Lorie Antrum
Michele
Mueller Electric Corneal
Paton Corneal
Paufique Corneal
Polley-Bickel
Searcy Chalazion
Sidney Stephenson Corneal
Stille
Thornwald Antrum
Turkel
Walker
Wilder
Wilkins

TROCARS

Allen Cecostomy
Arbuckle-Shea
Babcock Empyema
Barnes Internal Decompression
Beardsley Cecostomy

Birch
Boettcher Antrum
Charlton Antrum
Coakley Antrum
Davidson

TROCARS (Continued)

Dean Antrum
Denker
Diederich Empyema
Douglas Antrum
Duke
Durham Tracheotomy
Emmet Ovarian
Faulkner
Fein Antrum
Frazier Brain Exploring
Gallagher
Hargin Antrum
Hunt
Hurwitz
Intercostal
Judd
Kreutzmann
Lichtwicz Antrum
Lillie Antrum
Livermore
Myerson Antrum
Neal Catheter Trocar

Nelson
Nested
Ochsner Gallbladder
Patterson
Pierce Antrum
Pierce-Kyle
Plain Vesical
Potain Aspirating
Poole
Ruskin
Sewall Antrum
Singleton's Empyema
Southey Anasarca
Southey-Leech
Sweet Antrum
Van Alyea
Walther Aspirating Bladder
Wangensteen Internal Decompression
Wiener-Pierce Antrum
Wilson Amniotic
Wright-Harloe Empyema
Yankauer Antrum

TUBES
Also see: SUCTION TUBES

Abbott
Abbott-Rawson
Adson Brain Suction
Alesen
Bardic
Beardsley Empyema
Bellocq
Bettman Empyema
Blakemore
Bouchut
Buyes Air-Vent Suction
Cantor
Cattell Forked Type T-Tube
Cattell T-Tube
Chaussier
Colton Empyema
Coupland Suction
Davol
Deaver T-Tube
Debove

Denker
DePaul
Dr. Twiss Duodenal
Greiling Gastroduodenal
Duke
Durham
Einhorn
Frazier Brain Suction
Honor-Smathers Double Lumen
Humphreys Coronary Sinus Sucker
Johnson Intestinal
Jutte
Kaslow
Killian
Kozlowski
Lahey Y-Tube
Levin Duodenal
Linton
Lyon
Mackler Intraluminal

TUBES (Continued)

McGowan-Keeley
Miller-Abbott Double Lumen
  Intestinal
Mixter
Morch Type Swivel Tracheostomy
Mosher
Nachlas Gastrointestinal
Neuber Bone
O'Beirne Sphincter
Ochsner Gallbladder
O'Dwyer
Polyvinyl
Polyethylene
Poole Abdominal Suction

Puestow-Olander G.I.
Rehfuss Duodenal
Ryle Duodenal
Sachs
Sengstaken Nasogastric
Souttar
T-Tube
Toynbee Diagnostic
Turkel
Valentine Irrigation
Voltolini
Wangensteen
Yankauer
Zyler

TUCKERS

Also see: TENDON TUCKERS
Bishop
Bishop-Black
Bishop-DeWitt
Bishop Peter
Burch-Greenwood

Fink
Green Strabismus
Harrison
Smuckler
Wayne

TURNBUCKLE

Giannestras

VALVULOTOMES

Brock
Derra
Dogliotti
Gohrbrand
Harken
Himmelstein Pulmonary
Longmire

Longmire-Muller Curved
Malm-Himmelstein Pulmonary
Niedner
Potts Expansile
Potts-Riker
Sellor
Universal Malleable

VULSELLUM

See: FORCEPS

WHISTLES

Barany Noise Apparatus

Galton Ear

WRENCHES

Hexagonal
Kurlander Orthopedic
Petersen Fracture

Thomas
Waldon

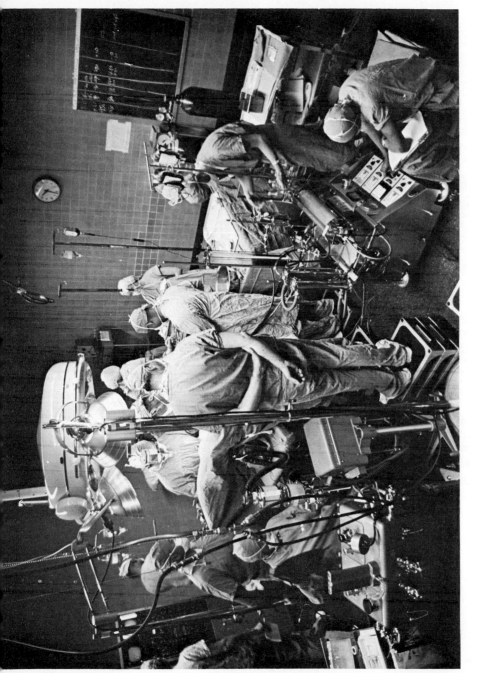

Operating room scene during open heart surgery at the Montefiore Hospital and Medical Center, New York City. Note modern heart and lung machine in right foreground.

Section II-Anatomy

6 { *The Anatomy of Structure, Circulation and Innervation*

Regional anatomy is alphabetically listed under the specialty sections in this book to assist the secretary with transcription of anatomic terms. The anatomy of the musculoskeletal system, circulatory system and peripheral nervous system cannot be limited to any one specialty exclusively. In order to obviate duplication, alphabetically arranged tables of ARTERIES, VEINS, BONES, JOINTS, LIGAMENTS, MUSCLES AND NERVES are listed in this chapter. These tables are designed to provide a ready reference for transcription purposes.

NB: Although the tables listing anatomic structures in the following pages show the first letter of each item capitalized, in context the English version of anatomic terms is used with the lower-case. Structures named after individuals in these tables are used with the upper-case as are the proper (B.N.A.) names of muscles.

CIRCULATION

A survey of the circulatory system in the body provides an appreciation of the role of the arteries and veins in this circuit. Venous blood enters the right atrium (auricle) of the heart, passes to the right ventricle, is pumped to the lungs by way of the pulmonary artery and into the pulmonary capillaries. In the capillaries of the lung, carbon dioxide is given off and oxygen is absorbed. The oxygenated blood is returned to the left atrium of the heart by the pulmonary veins. The blood then passes into the left ventricle from which it is pumped out into the aorta, arteries and capillaries. In the arterial capillaries, oxygen is given up to the tissues and carbon dioxide is absorbed. The blood then passes into the venous system and with its collection of carbon dioxide and metabolic wastes, is returned by the veins to the venae cavae. It is then carried back into the heart through the right atrium.

Blood Circuit:

right atrium — right ventricle — pulmonary artery — pulmonary capillaries — pulmonary veins — left atrium — left ventricle — aorta — arteries — capillaries throughout the body and into the venous system — venae cavae — right atrium of heart.

The circuit from the heart, through the lungs and back to the heart is called the pulmonary (lesser) circulation. The course of the blood from the left ventricle out into the tissues and back to the right atrium of the heart is termed the systemic (greater) circulation. The systemic circulation time in an adult is about 23 seconds.

The volume of blood in the body is related to body weight. The blood volume, in pints, may be approximated by dividing the body weight in pounds by 14.

Blood pressure is a measure of the pressure of the blood on the walls of the arteries and is expressed as the systolic (maximum) pressure over the diastolic (minimum) pressure. The systolic arterial blood pressure rises during excitement or activity and falls during sleep. In a normal relaxed adult it is between 110 and 145 mm. of mercury.

ARTERIES

Acetabular
Acromial
Acromiothoracic
Alar (nose)
Alveolar
Angular
Anterior, superior, dental
Aorta, arch
Aorta, ascending
Aorta, thoracic
Appendicular
Arciform
Arcuate, of foot
Arcuate, of kidney
Auditory
Auricular, anterior
Auricular, posterior
Axillary
Azygos, of vagina
Basilar
Brachial
Bronchial
Buccal
Buccinator

Calcaneal
Calcarine
Caroticotympanic
Carotid, common
Carotid external
Carotid, internal
Carpal
Cavernous
Cecal
Celiac
Central, of retina
Cerebellar, inferior, anterior
Cerebellar, superior
Cerebral, anterior
Cerebral, middle
Cerebral, posterior
Cervical, ascending
Cervical, deep
Cervical, transverse
Charcot's
Choroid
Ciliary
Circumflex, of fibula
Circumflex, of humerus

ARTERIES (Continued)

Circumflex, iliac
Circumflex, lateral of thigh
Circumflex, medial of thigh
Circumflex, of scapula
Clitoral
Colic
Collateral
Common carotid
Communicating
Conjunctival
Coronary
Cortical
Costocervical
Cricothyroid
Crural
Cystic
Deferential
Dental
Digital, of fingers
Digital, of toes
Diploic
Dorsal, of clitoris
Dorsal, of feet
Dorsal, of nose
Dorsal, of penis
Epigastric
Episcleral
Esophageal
Ethmoidal
External carotid
Femoral
Frontal
Gastric
Gastroduodenal
Gastroepiploic
Genicular
Glaserian
Gluteal
Hemorrhoidal
Hepatic
Hepatic, proper
Humeral
Hypophyseal
Ileal
Ileocolic
Iliac, common

Iliac, external
Iliac, internal
Iliolumbar
Inferior dental
Inferior hemorrhoidal
Inferior mesenteric
Inferior pancreatic
Infraorbital
Infrascapular
Innominate
Intercostal
Interlobar, of kidney
Interlobular, of kidney
Internal carotid
Interosseous, common
Interosseous, dorsal
Interosseous, recurrent
Interosseous, volar
Interventricular
Intestinal
Jejunal
Labial
Lacrimal
Laryngeal
Lateral nasal
Lateral striate
Lenticular
Lenticulostriate
Lienal
Lingual
Lumbar
Macular
Malleolar
Mammary, internal
Mandibular
Marginal
Masseteric
Mastoid
Maxillary
Medial striate
Median
Mediastinal
Medullary
Meningeal
Mental
Mesenteric

ARTERIES (Continued)

Metacarpal, dorsal
Metacarpal, volar
Metatarsal, dorsal
Metatarsal, plantar
Musculophrenic
Neubauer's
Nutrient, of femur
Nutrient, of fibula
Nutrient, of humerus
Nutrient, of tibia
Obturator
Occipital
Omphalomesenteric
Ophthalmic
Ovarian
Palatine, ascending
Palatine, descending
Palmar
Palpebral, lateral
Palpebral, medial
Pancreatic
Pancreaticoduodenal
Perforating, of thigh
Pericardiacophrenic
Perineal
Peroneal, of tibia
Pharyngeal
Phrenic, inferior
Phrenic, superior
Plantar
Pontine
Popliteal
Posterior dental
Posterior pancreaticoduodenal
Principal, of thumb
Principal, of pterygoid canal
Pubic
Pudendal
Pulmonary
Pyloric
Quadriceps
Radial
Radicular
Ranine
Recurrent, radial
Recurrent, tibial

Recurrent, ulnar
Renal
Sacral
Scapular
Scrotal
Septal, of nose
Sigmoid
Somatic
Spermatic
Sphenopalatine
Spinal
Spiral
Splanchnic
Splenic
Stapedial
Sternal
Sternocleidomastoid
Sternomastoid
Striate
Stylomastoid
Subclavian
Subcostal
Sublingual
Submental
Subscapular
Sulcal
Supraorbital
Suprarenal
Sural
Tarsal
Temporal
Terminal
Testicular
Thoracic, long
Thoracoacromial
Thoracodorsal
Thymic
Thyrocervical
Thyroid
Tibial
Tonsillar
Transverse, scapular
Transverse, of face
Transverse, of neck
Tympanic
Ulnar

ARTERIES (Continued)

Umbilical
Urethral
Uterine
Vaginal
Vertebral
Vesical
Volar, digital, common

Volar, digital, proper
Volar, radial, index finger
Wilkie's
Willis
Zinn's
Zygomatico-orbital

VEINS

Accessory, cephalic
Accessory, hemiazygos
Accessory, saphenous
Angular
Anterior auricular
Anterior bronchiole
Anterior coronary
Anterior facial
Anterior jugular
Anterior mediastinal
Anterior parotid
Anterior tibial
Anterior vertebral
Articular, of knee
Articular, of mandible
Ascending lumbar
Axillary
Azygos
Basilic
Basivertebral
Brachial
Bronchial
Cephalic
Cerebellar
Cerebral
Choroid
Colic
Comitans lateralis
Comitans medialis
Common digital
Common facial
Common iliac
Coronary
Coronary, of the stomach
Costoaxillary
Cystic
Deep

Deep cervical
Deep circumflex iliac
Deep femoral
Deep iliac circumflex
Deferentiales
Dental
Digital
Diploic
Dorsal digital of hand
Dorsal digital of foot
Dorsal metacarpal
Dorsal metatarsal
Dorsal, of penis
Ductus venosus
Duodenal
Emissary
Esophageal
External iliac
External jugular
External nasal
External pudic
Femoral
Femoropopliteal
Frontal
Galen
Gastroepiploic
Gluteal
Great cardiac
Great saphenous
Hemiazygos
Hepatic
Hypogastric
Ileocolic
Iliolumbar
Inferior epigastric
Inferior gluteal
Inferior mesenteric

VEINS (Continued)

Inferior ophthalmic
Inferior palpebral
Inferior petrosal sinus
Inferior phrenic
Inferior thyroid
Inferior vena cava
Innominate
Intercapitular
Intercostal
Internal auditory
Internal circumflex
Internal iliac
Internal jugular
Internal mammary
Internal maxillary
Internal pudendal
Internal pudic
Internal vertebral
Intervertebral
Jugular, external
Labial
Lateral circumflex femoral
Lateral plantar
Lateral sacral
Left coronary
Lienal (splenic)
Lingual
Long thoracic
Lumbar
Marginal, right
Medial plantar
Median
Median antebrachial
Median temporal
Mediana cubiti
Meningeal
Metacarpal
Middle cardiac
Middle colic
Middle hemorrhoidal
Middle sacral
Musculophrenic
Nasofrontal
Obturator
Occipital
Ophthalmic, inferior

Ophthalmic, superior
Orbital
Ovarian
Palatine
Palmar digital
Palmar metacarpal
Pancreatic
Pancreaticoduodenal
Paraumbilical
Pericardial
Peroneal
Pharyngeal
Plantar digital
Plantar metatarsal
Popliteal
Portal
Posterior auricular
Posterior bronchiole
Posterior external jugular
Posterior facial
Posterior mediastinal
Posterior parotid
Posterior scrotal
Posterior tibial
Prostatic
Pubic
Pudendal
Pyloric
Radial
Renal
Short gastric
Short saphenous
Sigmoid
Small cardiac
Small saphenous
Spermatic
Sphenopalatine
Sphenoparietal
Splenic
Stylomastoid
Subclavian
Subcutaneous abdominal
Subcutaneous thoracic
Superficial circumflex iliac
Superficial epigastric
Superficial, of penis

VEINS (Continued)

Superficial temporal
Superior epigastric
Superior gluteal
Superior hemorrhoidal
Superior mesenteric
Superior ophthalmic
Superior palpebral
Superior phrenic
Superior thyroid
Superior vena cava
Supraorbital
Suprarenal
Testicular
Thoracoepigastric

Transverse cervical
Transverse facial
Transverse scapular
Ulnar
Urethral
Uterine
Uterovaginal
Vaginal
Vein of cochlear canal
Vertebral
Vesical
Vesicular
Volar digital
Volar metacarpal

SKELETAL ANATOMY

The skeletal framework of the body is made up of 206 separate bones which are distributed as follows:

Skull	22
Hyoid bone	1
Vertebral column	26
Ribs and sternum	25
Auditory ossicles (ear)	6
Lower extremities	62
Upper extremities	64
	206

The bones are joined at articulating points called joints. The articular ends of the bones are connected by bands of flexible connective tissue called ligaments. With the aid of muscles, the various parts of the body can be moved voluntarily. The muscles are attached to the bones by tendons. The ends of the muscles are further secured by aponeuroses and fasciae which also exert an influence on the direction of pull.

The bones, joints, ligaments and muscles are presented here to assist the secretary with the nomenclature of these structures.

BONES

CRANIAL BONES

Ethmoid
Frontal

Occipital
Parietal

CRANIAL BONES (Continued)

Sphenoid
Temporal
  mastoid
  petrous

squamous
styloid process
subperiosteal
tympanic

NECK

Hyoid

FACIAL BONES

Inferior turbinates
Lacrimal
Malar (zygomatic)
  zygomatic arch
Mandible (jaw bone)
  alveolar process
  condyloid process
  coronoid process
  ramus
Maxilla

alveolar process
frontal process
palatine process
Nasal
  ethmoid
  septum
    perpendicular plate
    cribriform process
Vomer

EAR BONES

Incus
Malleus

Stapes

BONES OF THE TRUNK

Ribs
Sternum
  manubrium
  gladiolus
  xiphoid (ensiform)
Vertebrae

cervical
thoracic
lumbar
sacral (sacrum)
coccygeal (coccyx)

SHOULDER GIRDLE

Clavicle (collar bone)

Scapula (shoulder blade)

UPPER LIMBS

Humerus
Radius & Ulna
Carpal Bones (wrist)
  capitate (os magnum)
  greater multangular (trapezium)
  lesser multangular (trapezoid)
  hamate (unciform)

lunate (semilunar)
navicular (scaphoid)
pisiform
triangular (cuneiform)
Metacarpals
Phalanges

PELVIC GIRDLE

Pelvis
  ilium

ischium
os pubis

LOWER LIMBS

Femur (thigh bone)
  condyle, lateral
  condyle, medial
  head
  neck
  shaft
  trochanter, greater
  trochanter, lesser
Tibia & Fibula
Patella (knee bone)
  medial meniscus

lateral meniscus
Tarsal Bones (ankle)
  calcaneus (os calcis)
  cuboid
  cuneiform, inner
  cuneiform, middle
  cuneiform, outer
  navicular (scaphoid)
  talus (astragalus)
Metatarsals (foot bones)
Phalanges (toe bones)

JOINTS AND LIGAMENTS

Joints are points at which the bones of the skeleton are joined to one another. They may be classified into three groups: the immovable, the slightly movable and the freely movable. An example of the immovable joint may be found in the articulations of the bones of the skull. Slightly movable joints may be found between the vertebral bodies. The joints most often referred to in orthopedic surgery are the freely movable, such as the elbow, wrist, hip, knee, etc. These bones are completely separated from one another permitting a wide range of motion. Their articular surfaces are covered with cartilage and a joint capsule and they are attached to one another by strong fibrous bands called ligaments. The ligaments actually form the joint.

The nomenclature for the ligaments and joints constitutes an important phase of surgical terminology and should be familiar to the secretary. Alphabetically arranged tables of these structures are presented in this section for reference and review purposes.

THE JOINTS

The movable joints and some of the slightly movable ones which are important to the surgeon are listed here.

Acromioclavicular . . . . shoulder
Atlantooccipital . . . . vertebral colume with cranium
Carpometacarpal . . . . wrist

126

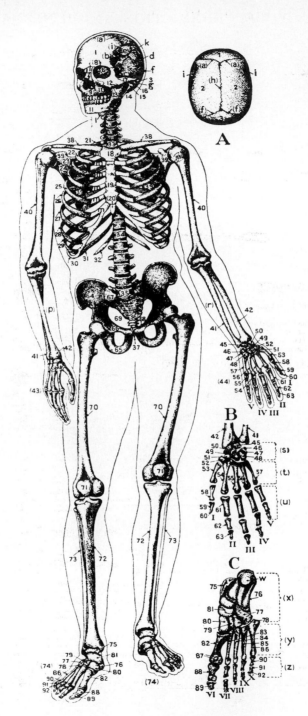

SKELETON OF ADULT MAN

HEAD OR SKULL
Bones of the Cranium
A Top of Skull showing Sutures
1 Frontal
2 Parietal (two in number)
3 Squamous Portion of Occipital
4 Greater Wing of Sphenoid
5 Squamous Portion of Temporal (two)
6 Ethmoid

Bones of the Face
7 Nasal (two)
8 Lachrymal (two)
9 Vomer
10 Maxilla or Superior Maxillary; (two)
11 Mandible or Inferior Maxillary
12 Zygomatic (two)
(The Palatine Bones (two), the Inferior Conchae or Inferior Turbinated Bones (two), the Ethmoid (two), the Lachrymal (two), the Vomer (one), and the Bones of the Ear — Malleus, Incus, Stapes in each ear — are not indicated)

Principal Features of the Bones of the Head
13 Coronoid Process of Mandible
14 Condyloid Process of Mandible
15 Styloid Process of Temporal
16 Mastoid Process
17 Zygomatic Arch
a Coronal Suture
b Sphenofrontal Suture
c Sphenosquamosal Suture
d Squamous Suture
e Sphenoparietal Suture
f Lambdoid Suture
g Occipitomastoid Suture
h Sagittal Suture
i Superior Temporal Line
k Inferior Temporal Line
l Hyoid Bone

THORAX OR CHEST
Bones of the Breast
18 First Bone of the Sternum, called also Manubrium, Presternum
19 Second Bone of the Sternum, called also Mesosternum
20 Xiphoid process

Sternal or True Ribs
21 to **27** First to Seventh Ribs inclusive (two of each)

Asternal or False Ribs
28 to **32** Eighth to Twelfth Ribs inclusive
(**31** and **32** are the Floating Ribs) (two pairs)
m. m. m. etc. Costal Cartilages

TRUNK
Spinal Column
33 First Thoracic Vertebra
34 Twelfth Thoracic Vertebra
35 Fifth Lumbar Vertebra
36 Fifth Sacral Vertebra (last bone of the Sacrum)
37 Coccyx

UPPER EXTREMITY
Shoulder
38 Clavicle or Collar Bone (two)
39 Scapula or Shoulder Blade (two)

Arm
40 Humerus (two)
41 Ulna (two)
42 Radius (two)
(p) Bones of Forearm in Prone Position
(r) Same in Supine Position

Bones of the Hand
(43) Bones of Right Hand (Dorsal, or Back, Surface)
(44) Bones of Left Hand (Volar, or Palm, Surface)
Diagram **B** Bones of the Left Hand (Dorsal Surface)
(s) Carpus, or Wrist
(t) Metacarpus, or Palm
(u) Phalanges of Thumb and Fingers

Bones of the Carpus
45 Lunatum (two)
46 Pisiform (two)
47 Triquetrum (two)
48 Hamatum (two)
49 Capitatum (two)
50 Navicular (two)
51 Multangulum minus (two)
52 Multangulum majus (two)

Bones of the Metacarpus
53 to **57** First to Fifth Metacarpal Bones (two of each)

Phalanges (28 in all)
58 and **59** First and Second Phalanx of Thumb (two of each)

60 Ungual Tuberosity
61 Proximal, or First, Phalanx of Index
62 Middle, or Second, Phalanx of Index
63 Distal, Terminal, Ungual, or Third, Phalanx of Index

LOWER EXTREMITY
Bones and Principal Parts of Pelvic Girdle
64 Ilium (two)
65 Ischium (two)
66 Pubis (two)
67 Sacrum
68 Brim of Pelvis
69 True Pelvis

Bones of Leg
70 Femur, or Thigh Bone (two)
71 Patella, or Kneepan (two)
72 Tibia, or Shin Bone (two)
73 Fibula (two)

Bones of the Feet
(74) View from Dorsal Surface
Diagram **C** Bones of Right Foot (Plantar, or Sole, Surface)
(x) Tarsus, or Ankle
(y) Metatarsus
(z) Phalanges of Toes

Bones of the Tarsus
75 Talus, Astragalus, or Ankle Bone (two)
76 Calcaneus, or Heel Bone (two)
w Tuberosity of Calcaneus
77 Cuboid (two)
78, 79, 80 Cuneiform Bones (six in all)
81 Navicular, or Scaphoid, Bone (two)

Bones of the Metatarsus
82 to **86** First to Fifth Metatarsal Bones (ten in all)
87 Sesamoid Bones
VI First Digit, Hallux, or Great Toe
VII to **IX** Second to Fourth Digits, or Toes
X Fifth Digit, or Little Toe

Phalanges (28 in all)
88 and **89** First and Second Phalanx of Hallux
90 to **92** First, Second, and Third Phalanx of Fifth Digit

JOINTS (Continued)

Costochondral .... ribs and cartilage
Costosternal .... ribs and sternum
Costotransverse .... ribs and transverse processes
Costovertebral .... ribs and vertebrae
Coxal .... hip
Cuboideonavicular .... ankle-foot
Cuneocuboid .... foot
Cuneonavicular .... foot
Hip .... trunk and leg
Humeral .... shoulder
Intercarpal .... wrist
Interchondral .... cartilages of ribs
Intercuneiform .... foot
Intermetacarpal .... hand
Intermetatarsal .... foot
Interphalangeal .... toes or fingers
Intertarsal .... ankle
Knee .... upper and lower leg
Lumbosacral .... trunk
Metacarpophalangeal .... hand and fingers
Metatarsophalangeal .... foot and toes
Midcarpal .... wrist
Midtarsal .... ankle
Radiocarpal .... wrist
Radioulnar .... wrist
Sacrococcygeal .... lower trunk
Sacroiliac .... lower trunk
Scapuloclavicular .... shoulder
Shoulder .... upper arm and trunk
Sternal .... upper trunk (sternum)
Sternoclavicular .... sternum and clavicle
Sternocostal .... sternum and ribs
Symphysis pubis .... lower trunk
Talocalcaneal .... intertarsal (ankle)
Talocalcaneonavicular .... intertarsal (ankle)
Talocrural .... ankle
Tarsal .... ankle
Tarsometatarsal .... ankle-foot
Temporomandibular .... mandible-temporal bone
Tibiofibular, distal .... ankle
Tibiofibular, superior .... knee
Tibiotarsal .... ankle

THE LIGAMENTS

In addition to connecting the articular ends of bones at the joint, the ligaments also serve to support viscera, muscles and fasciae. These structures are encountered in the surgery of almost all of the specialties. They have been listed here alphabetically to provide an expedient source of reference.

LIGAMENTS

Accessory
Acromioclavicular
Alar
Annular
Anococcygeal
Apical odontoid
Arantius'
Arcuate, lateral
Arcuate, medial
Auricularis
Axis (of malleus)
Bardinet's
Barkow's
Bellini's
Berry's
Bertin's
Bichat's
Bifurcated
Bigelow's
Botallo's
Bourgery's
Broad
Brodie's
Burns's
Calcaneocuboid
Calcaneofibular
Calcaneonavicular, external
Calcaneonavicular, lateral
Calcaneonavicular, plantar
Calcaneotibial
Caldani's
Campbell's suspensory
Camper's
Capsular
Cardinal
Caroticoclinoid
Carpal dorsal
Carpal palmar

Carpometacarpal, dorsal
Carpometacarpal, palmar
Caudal
Cervical
Check, lateral
Check, medial
Ciliary
Civinini's
Clado's
Collateral, fibular
Collateral, metatarsophalangeal
Collateral, radial
Collateral, tibial
Collateral, ulnar
Colles'
Conoid
Cooper's
Coraco-acromial
Coracoclavicular
Coracohumeral
Corniculopharyngeal
Coronary (of knee)
Coronary (of liver)
Costoclavicular
Costocolic
Costotransverse, anterior
Costotransverse, middle
Costotransverse, posterior
Costoxiphoid
Cotyloid
Cricoarytenoid posterior
Cricopharyngeal
Cricosantorinian
Cricothyroid
Cricotracheal
Crucial
Cruciate, of atlas of spine
Cruciate, of knee

LIGAMENTS (Continued)

Cruciate, of the leg
Cruciform
Cruveilhier's
Cubonavicular
Cuneocuboid
Cystoduodenal
Deltoid
Denonvillier's
Dental
Denticulate
Denuce's
Diaphragmatic (kidney)
Epihyal
External lateral (wrist)
Falciform
Falciform, of the liver
Fallopian
Ferrein's
Flood's
Fundiform (penis)
Gastrolienal
Gastrophrenic
Gastrosplenic
Gerdy's
Gillette's suspensory
Gimbernat's
Gingivodental
Glenoid
Glossoepiglottic
Gunz's
Helmholtz'
Henle's
Hensing's
Hepatocolic
Hepatoduodenal
Hepatogastric
Hepatorenal
Hesselbach's
Hey's
Holl's
Heuck's
Humphry's
Hunter's
Hyoepiglottic
Hypsiloid
Iliofemoral

Iliolumbar
Iliopectineal
Iliotrochanteric
Infundibulo-ovarian
Infundibulopelvic
Inguinal
Inguinal reflex
Intercarpal
Interchondral
Interclavicular
Interclinoid
Intercornual
Intercostal
Intercuneiform
Interfoveolar
Intermetacarpal
Intermetatarsal
Internal lateral (wrist)
Interspinous
Intertransverse
Intra-articular
Ischiofemoral
Jarjavay's
Jugal
Krause's median puboprostatic
Laciniate
Lacunar
Lannelongue's
Lateral (bladder)
Lauth's
Lienophrenic
Ligament teres of liver
Ligamenta flava (spine)
Ligamentum nuchae
Lisfranc's
Lockwood's
Longitudinal
Lumbocostal
Luschka's
Mackenrodt's
Malleolar
Mauchart's
Meckel's
Nuchal
Occipito-axial (Membrana tectoria)
Odontoid

LIGAMENTS (Continued)

Orbicular (radius)
Ovarian
Palpebral, lateral
Palpebral, medial
Pectinate (iris)
Pectineal
Perineal
Petit's
Phrenicocolic
Phrenicosplenic
Phrenogastric
Phrenosplenic
Pisiunciform
Pisohamate
Pisometacarpal
Plantar
Popliteal arcuate
Popliteal oblique
Poupart's
Pterygospinous
Pterygomandibular
Pubic
Pubocapsular
Pubofemoral
Puboprostatic
Pubovesical
Pulmonary
Quadrate
Radiate
Radiocarpal
Retzius'
Rhomboid
Robert's
Round
Sacrococcygeal
Sacroiliac, anterior
Sacroiliac, interosseous
Sacroiliac, posterior
Sacrosciatic
Sacrospinous
Sacrotuberous
Sappey's
Sheath
Soemmering's
Sphenomandibular
Spinoglenoid

Spiral of cochlea
Spring
Stanley's cervical
Stellate
Sternoclavicular
Sternocostal
Sternopericardial
Stylohyoid
Stylomandibular
Suprascapular
Supraspinous
Suspensory
Sutural
Synovial
Talocalcanean
Talofibular
Talonavicular
Talotibial
Tarsal
Tarsometatarsal
Tarsotibial
Temporomandibular
Teutleben's
Thyroepiglottic
Thyroepiglottidean
Thyrohyoid
Tibiofibular
Tibionavicular
Transverse
Trapezoid
Treitz's
Triangular
Umbilical
Uterosacral
Vaginal
Valsalva's
Ventricular
Vertebropelvic
Vesalius
Vesicouterine
Vesicoumbilical
Vestibular
Vocal
Von Helmholtz'
Weitbrecht's
Winslow's

LIGAMENTS (Continued)

Wrisberg's
Y-shaped
Yellow

Zaglas'
Zinn's

MUSCLES, FASCIA, APONEUROSES AND TENDONS

The muscles are organs of voluntary motion which, through contraction, effect movement of the various parts of the body. Muscle tissue is either smooth or striated (striped). It is either voluntary or involuntary. Smooth muscle, such as that of the intestine and the striated muscle of the heart are involuntary. The striated muscles, except for that of the heart, are voluntary because they can be controlled with conscious effort. When we refer to the muscles, we usually refer to the skeletal, striated, voluntary variety.

Other important musculoskeletal tissues include the fasciae, aponeuroses and tendons which take their names from the muscle with which they are identified.

The fasciae consist of fibrous connective tissues whose function it is to cover, separate and support the muscles, as well as other organs throughout the body. The entire fascial system is divided into three categories: the deep fascia, the subserous fascia, and the superficial fascia. The most extensive of the three types is the deep fascia, binding and enveloping the muscles. The subserous fascia lies within the body cavities. It covers and supports the viscera. It forms the fibrous layer of the serous membranes, such as the peritoneum, pericardium and pleura, and serves as an attachment for the parietal aspect of the serous membranes to the deep fascia situated on the inner surface of the body wall. The superficial fascia permits free movement of the skin by intervening between the deep fascia and the skin.

Another structure of the muscles is the aponeurosis which extends from the muscle as a flattened tendon. These tissues assist in the contraction of the muscle. The tendons also function in this capacity. They are strong flexible cords which connect the muscle to the bone or other structures. With the exception of their point of attachment, they are enveloped in a sheath of fine fibro-elastic connective tissue. These structures are often partially or completely severed in lacerations of the extremities.

An alphabetical table of thé muscles and a listing by regions follows.

NB: Although the tables listing anatomic structures throughout these pages show the first letter capitalized in every item listed, in context these terms would appear in the lower-case. Only the Latin B.N.A. names of muscles and those named after an individual are capitalized. The English versions of anatomic titles are used with the lower-case.

MUSCLES

NB: Capitalize first letter in names listed in this table. For authority see Gray's Anatomy.

Abductor digiti minimi manus
Abductor digiti minimi pedis
Abductor hallucis
Abductor pollicis brevis
Abductor pollicis longus
Accelerator urinae
Adductor brevis
Adductor hallucis
Adductor longus
Adductor magnus
Adductor minimus
Adductor obliquus hallucis
Adductor obliquus pollicis
Adductor pollicis
Adductor transversus hallucis
Anconaeus
Antitragicus
Arrectores pilorum
Articularis genu
Aryepiglotticus
Arytenoideus obliquus
Arytenoideus transversus
Aryvocalis
Attollens aurem
Attrahens aurem
Auricularis anterior
Auricularis posterior
Auricularis superior
Azygos uvulae
Biceps brachii
Biceps femoris
Biceps flexor cruris
Biventer mandibulae
Brachialis
Brachioradialis
Bronchooesophageus
Buccinator
Buccopharyngeus
Bulbocavernosus
Caninus
Cephalopharyngeus
Ceratocricoideus
Ceratopharyngeus
Cervicalis ascendens
Chondroglossus
Chondropharyngeus

Ciliaris
Cleidoepitrochlearis
Cleidomastoideus
Cleidooccipitalis
Coccygeus
Complexus
Complexus minor
Compressor naris
Compressor urethrae
Constrictor pharyngis inferior
Constrictor pharyngis medius
Constrictor pharyngis superior
Constrictor urethrae
Coracobrachialis
Corrugator cutis ani
Corrugator supercilii
Cremaster
Cricoarytenoideus lateralis
Cricoarytenoideus posterior
Cricopharyngeus
Cricothyreoideus
Crureus
Cucullarius
Deltoideus
Depressor angulioris
Depressor labii inferioris
Depressor septi
Depressor supercilii
Depressor urethrae
Detrusor urinae
Diaphragma
Digastricus (digastric)
Dilator naris
Dilatator pupillae
Ejaculator seminis
Epicranius
Epitrochleoanconeus
Erector clitoridis
Erector penis
Erector spinae
Extensor brevis digitorum
Extensor brevis pollicis
Extensor carpi radialis brevis
Extensor carpi radialis longus
Extensor carpi ulnaris
Extensor coccygis

MUSCLES (Continued)

Extensor communis digitorum
Extensor digiti minimi
Extensor digitorum
Extensor digitorum brevis
Extensor digitorum brevis manus
Extensor digitorum longus
Extensor hallucis brevis
Extensor hallucis longus
Extensor indicis
Extensor longus digitorum
Extensor longus pollicis
Extensor minimi digiti
Extensor ossis metacarpi pollicis
Extensor pollicis brevis
Extensor pollicis longus
Flexor accessorius digitorum
Flexor brevis digitorum
Flexor brevis hallucis
Flexor brevis minimi digiti
Flexor carpi radialis
Flexor carpi ulnaris
Flexor digiti minimi brevis
Flexor digiti minimi brevis
Flexor digitorum brevis
Flexor digitorum longus
Flexor digitorum profundus
Flexor digitorum superficialis
Flexor hallucis brevis
Flexor hallucis longus
Flexor longus digitorum
Flexor longus hallucis
Flexor longus pollicis
Flexor pollicis brevis
Flexor pollicis longus
Flexor profundus digitorum
Flexor sublimis digitorum
Frontalis
Gastrocnemius
Gemellus inferior
Gemellus superior
Genioglossus
Geniohyoideus
Glossopalatinus
Glossopharyngeus
Gluteus maximus
Gluteus medius

Gluteus minimus
Gracilis
Helicis major
Helicis minor
Hyoglossus
Hyopharyngeus
Iliacus
Iliacus minor
Iliocapsularis
Iliocostalis
Iliocostalis cervicis
Iliocostalis dorsi
Iliocostalis lumborum
Iliocostalis thoracis
Iliopsoas
Incisivus labii inferioris
Incisivus labii superioris
Incisurae helicis
Infracostalis
Infraspinatus
Intercostalis externus
Intercostalis internus
Intercostalis intimus
Interosseus dorsalis manus
Interosseus dorsalis pedis
Interosseus palmaris
Interosseus plantaris
Interosseus volaris
Interspinalis
Intertransversarius
Ischiocavernosus
Ischiococcygeus
Keratopharyngeus
Laryngopharyngeus
Latissimus dorsi
Levator alae nasi
Levator anguli oris
Levator anguli scapulae
Levator ani
Levator costae
Levator glandulae thyreoideae
Levator labii inferioris
Levator labii superioris
Levator labii superioris alaeque nasi
Levator palati
Levator palpebrae superioris

MUSCLES (Continued)

Levator prostatae
Levator scapulae
Levator veli palatini
Longissimus capitis
Longissimus cervicis
Longissimus thoracis
Longitudinalis dorsi
Longitudinalis inferior
Longitudinalis superior
Longus capitis
Longus colli
Lumbricalis manus
Lumbricalis pedis
Masseter
Mentalis
Multifidus
Mylohyoideus
Mylopharyngeus
Nasalis
Obliquus auriculae
Obliquus capitis inferior
Obliquus capitis superior
Obliquus externus abdominis
Obliquus inferior
Obliquus internus abdominis
Obliquus superior
Obturatorius externus
Obturatorius internus
Occipitalis
Occipitofrontalis
Omohyoideus
Opponens digiti minimi
Opponens digiti quinti
Opponens minimi digiti
Opponens pollicis
Orbicularis oculi
Orbicularis oris
Orbicularis palpebrarum
Orbitalis
Orbitopalpebralis
Palatoglossus
Palatopharyngeus
Palatosalpingeus
Palatostaphylinus
Palmaris brevis
Palmaris longus

Papillaris
Pectinatus
Pectineus
Pectoralis major
Pectoralis minor
Peroneocalcaneus
Peroneus brevis
Peroneus longus
Peroneus tertius
Petropharyngeus
Petrostaphylinus
Pharyngopalatinus
Piriformis
Plantaris
Platysma
Pleurooesophageus
Popliteus
Procerus
Pronator pedis
Pronator quadratus
Pronator teres
Prostaticus
Psoas major
Psoas minor
Pterygoideus externus
Pterygoideus internus
Pterygoideus lateralis
Pterygoideus medialis
Pterygopharyngeus
Pterygospinosus
Pubococcygeus
Puboprostaticus
Puborectalis
Pubovesicalis
Pyramidalis
Pyramidalis auriculae
Pyramidalis nasi
Pyriformis
Quadratus femoris
Quadratus labii inferioris
Quadratus labii superioris
Quadratus lumborum
Quadratus menti
Quadratus plantae
Quadriceps femoris
Rectococcygeus

MUSCLES (Continued)

Rectourethralis
Rectouterinus
Rectovesicalis
Rectus abdominis
Rectus capitis anterior
Rectus capitis anticus major
Rectus capitis lateralis
Rectus capitis posterior major
Rectus capitis posterior minor
Rectus externus
Rectus femoris
Rectus inferior
Rectus internus
Rectus lateralis
Rectus medialis
Rectus superior
Rectus thoracis
Retrahens aurem
Rhomboatloideus
Rhomboideus major
Rhomboideus minor
Risorius
Rotatores
Rotatores cervicis
Rotatores lumborum
Rotatores thoracis
Sacrococcygeus anterior
Sacrococcygeus dorsalis
Sacrococcygeus posterior
Sacrococcygeus ventralis
Sacrolumbalis
Sacrospinalis
Salpingopharyngeus
Sartorius
Scalenus anterior
Scalenus medius
Scalenus minimus
Scalenus posterior
Scansorius
Semimembranosus
Semispinalis capitis
Semispinalis cervicis
Semispinalis colli
Semispinalis dorsi
Semispinalis thoracis
Semitendinosus

Serratus anterior
Serratus magnus
Serratus inferior posterior
Serratus posterior superior
Soleus
Sphenosalpingostaphylinus
Sphincter ampullae
  hepatopancreaticae
Sphincter ani externus
Sphincter ani internus
Sphincter oris
Sphincter pupillae
Sphincter pylori
Sphincter urethrae
Sphincter urethrae membranaceae
Sphincter vaginae
Sphincter vesicae
Spinalis capitis
Spinalis cervicis
Spinalis colli
Spinalis dorsi
Spinalis thoracis
Splenius capitis
Splenius cervicis
Splenius colli
Stapedius
Staphylinus externus
Staphylinus internus
Staphylinus medius
Sternalis
Sternochondroscapularis
Sternoclavicularis
Sternocleidomastoideus
Sternofascialis
Sternohyoideus
Sternothyreoideus
Styloauricularis
Styloglossus
Stylohyoideus
Stylolaryngeus
Stylopharyngeus
Subclavius
Subcostalis
Subcrureus
Subscapularis
Supinator

MUSCLES (Continued)

Supinator longus
Supraclavicularis
Supraspinalis
Supraspinatus
Suspensorius duodeni
Tarsalis inferior
Tarsalis superior
Temporalis
Tensor fasciae latae
Tensor palati
Tensor tarsi
Tensor tympani
Tensor veli palatini
Teres major
Teres minor
Thyreoarytenoideus
Thyreoarytenoideus **externus**
  and internus
Thyreoepiglotticus
Thyreohyoideus
Thyreopharyngeus
Tibialis anterior
Tibialis gracilis
Tibialis posterior
Tibialis secundus
Tibiofascialis anterior
Trachealis
Tracheloclavicularis
Trachelomastoideus
Tragicus
Transversalis abdominis

Transversalis capitis
Transversalis cervicis
Transversalis nasi
Transversospinalis
Transversus abdominis
Transversus auriculae
Transversus linguae
Transversus menti
Transversus nuchae
Transversus perinei profundus
Transversus perinei superficialis
Transversus thoracis
Trapezius
Triangularis
Triangularis labii inferioris
Triangularis labii superioris
Triangularis sterni
Triceps brachii
Triceps surae
Triticeoglossus
Uvulae
Vastus externus
Vastus intermedius
Vastus internus
Vastus lateralis
Vastus medialis
Ventricularis
Verticalis linguae
Vocalis
Zygomaticus (major & minor)

MUSCLES OF
THE FACE AND HEAD

Auricularis anterior
Auricularis posterior
Auricularis superior
Buccinator
Caninus
Caput zygomaticum
Depressor septi nasi
Epicranius
Levator palpebrae superioris

Masseter
Mentalis
Nasalis, pars alaris
Nasalis, pars transversa
Obliquus inferior oculi
Obliquus superior oculi
Orbicularis oculi
Orbicularis oris
Platysma

Figs. 1 and 2. MUSCULAR SYSTEM OF MAN

Fig. 1, FRONTAL VIEW. Fig. 2, DORSAL VIEW.

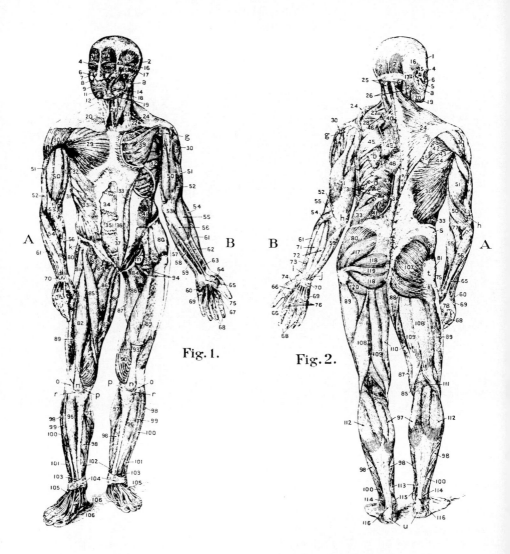

Fig. 1.   Fig. 2.

FIGS. 1 AND 2.   MUSCULAR SYSTEM OF MAN

FIG. 1, FRONTAL VIEW.   FIG. 2, DORSAL VIEW.

HEAD AND NECK

1 Frontalis (2)
2 Occipitalis (2)
3 Temporal (1)
4 Orbicularis Oculi
5 Zygomaticus
6 Zygomatic Head of the Quadratus Labii Superioris, or Zygomaticus Minor
7 Angular Head of the Quadratus Labii Superioris (1)
8 Nasalis (1)
9 Orbicularis Oris (1)
10 Triangularis Menti (1)
11 Quadratus Labii Inferioris (1)
12 Mentalis (1)
13 Masseter (1)
14 Buccinator (1)
15 Auricularis Anterior
16 Auricularis Superior
17 Auricularis Posterior
a Parotid Gland
18 Mylohyoid
19 Digastric
20 Platysma or Platysma Myoides
21 Sternocleidomastoid
22 Omohyoid (1)
23 Sternohyoid (1)
24 Trapezius (1)
25 Splenius Capitis (2)
26 Splenius Cervicis (2)
27 Levator Scapulae (2)
28 Supraspinatus (2)

TRUNK

29 Pectoralis Major (1)
30 Deltoid
31 Latissimus Dorsi
32 Serratus Anterior
33 External Oblique
34 Rectus Abdominis (1)
35 Umbilicus (1)
36 Abdominal Aponeurosis (1)
37 Linea Alba (1)
38 Subclavius (1)
39 Pectoralis Minor (1)
40 Serratus Posterior Superior (1)
41 Internal Oblique
42 Infraspinatus (2)
43 Teres Minor (2)
44 Teres Major (2)
45 Rhomboideus Major (2)

46 Rhomboideus Minor (2)
b Scapula (2)
c 9th Rib (2)
d 10th Rib (2)
e 11th Rib (2)
f 12th Rib (2)
47 Serratus Posterior Inferior (2)
48 Lumbodorsal Fascia (2)
49 Sacrospinalis (2)

UPPER EXTREMITY

50 Biceps Brachii
51 Triceps Brachii
52 Branchialis
53 Lacertus Fibrosus
54 Extensor Carpi Radialis Longus
55 Brachiorodialis
56 Flexor Carpi Radialis
57 Palmaris Longus (1)
58 Flexor Digitorum Sublimis (1)
59 Flexor Carpi Ulnaris
60 Palmaris Brevis
61 Extensor Carpi Radialis Brevis
62 Flexor Pollicis Longus (1)
63 Pronator Quadratus (1)
64 Flexor Pollicis Brevis (1)
65 Palmaris Longus (cut across in Fig. 1)
66 First Dorsal Interosseus
67 First Lumbricalis (1)
68 Fibrous Sheaths of the Tendons
69 Adductor of the Little Finger
70 Annular Ligament of the Carpus
g Head of Humerus (showing Bicipital Groove)
71 Extensor Digitorum Communis (1)
72 Extensor Carpi Ulnaris (2)
73 Extensor Pollicis Longus
h Medial Epicondyle of Humerus (2)
i Lower End of Radius (2)
j Lower End of Ulna (2)
74 Tendons of Extensor Pollicis Longus and Brevis (2)
75 Adductor Pollicis (2)
76 Tendons of the Extensors (2)
77 Pronator Teres (2)
78 Palmar Aponeurosis (2)

LOWER EXTREMITY

k Anterior Superior Spine of Ilium (1)
79 Iliacus (1)

80 Gluteus Medius
81 Tensor Fasciae Latae
82 Rectus Femoris (1)
83 Psoas Major (1)
84 Pectineus (1)
85 Sartorius
86 Adductor Longus (1)
87 Adductor Magnus
88 Gracilis
89 Vastus Lateralis
90 Vastus Medialis
91 Gluteus Minimus (1)
92 Superior Extremity of Rectus Femoris (1)
93 Inferior Extremity of Rectus Femoris (1)
m Head of Femur (1)
94 Inferior Extremities of Psoas and Iliacus (1)
95 Adductor Brevis (not shown)
n Patella (1)
o Head of Fibula (1)
p Medial Condyle of Femur (1)
r Tuberosity of Tibia (1)
96 Tibialis Anterior
97 Gastrocnemius, Medial Head (1)
98 Soleus
99 Extensor Digitorum Longus (1)
100 Peroneus Longus
101 Peroneus Brevis (1)
102 Flexor Digitorum Longus (1)
103 Extensor Hallucis Longus (1)
104 Ligamentum Cruciatum Cruris (1)
105 Extensor Digitorum Brevis (1)
106 Abductor Hallucis (1)
s Ilium
t Greater Trochanter
107 Gluteus Maximus (2)
108 Biceps Femoris (2)
109 Semitendinosus (2)
110 Semimembranosus (2)
111 Plantaris (2)
112 Gastrocnemius, Lateral Head (1)
113 Flexor Digitorum Longus (2)
114 Peroneus Tertius (2)
115 Tendon of Tibialis Posterior (2)
116 Achilles' Tendon (2)
117 Pyriformis (2)
118 Gemellus Superior and Gemellus Inferior (2)
119 Obturator Internus (2)
120 Quadratus Femoris (2)

MUSCLES OF THE FACE AND HEAD (Continued)

Procerus
Pterygoideus externus
Pterygoideus internus
Quadratus labii inferioris
Quadratus labii superioris
Rectus inferior oculi
Rectus lateralis oculi

Rectus medialis oculi
Rectus superior oculi
Risorius
Temporalis
Triangularis
Zygomaticus

MUSCLES OF THE NECK

Constrictor pharyngis inferior
Constrictor pharyngis medius
Constrictor pharyngis superior
Digastricus
Genioglossus
Geniohyoideus
Glossopalatinus
Hyoglossus
Intrinsic tongue muscles
Levator veli palatini
Longus capitis
Longus colli
Musculus uvulae
Mylohyoideus
Omohyoideus

Pharyngopalatine
Rectus capitis anterior
Rectus capitis lateralis
Scalenus anterior
Scalenus medius
Scalenus posterior
Sternocleidomastoideus
Sternohyoideus
Sternothyroideus
Styloglossus
Stylohyoideus
Stylopharyngeus
Tensor veli palatini
Thyrohyoideus

MUSCLES OF THE TRUNK

Cremaster
Iliocostalis
Intercostales externi
Intercostales interni
Interspinalis
Latissimus dorsi
Levatores costarum
Longissimus
Multifidus
Obliquus capitis inferior
Obliquus capitis superior
Obliquus externus abdominis
Obliquus internus abdominis
Pyramidalis

Quadratus lumborum
Rectus abdominis
Rectus capitis posterior major
Rectus capitis posterior minor
Rotatores
Sacrospinalis
Semispinalis
Serrati posteriores
Spinalis dorsi
Splenius
Transversus abdominis
Transversus thoracis
Trapezius

MUSCLES OF
THE FOREARM AND HAND

Abductor digiti quinti manus
Abductor pollicis brevis
Abductor pollicis longus
Abductor pollicis
Brachioradialis
Extensor carpi radialis brevis
Extensor carpi radialis longus
Extensor carpi ulnaris
Extensor digitorum communis
Extensor digiti quinti proprius
Extensor indicis proprius
Extensor pollicis brevis
Flexor carpi radialis
Flexor carpi ulnaris

Flexor digiti quinti brevis manus
Flexor digitorum profundus
Flexor digitorum sublimis
Flexor pollicis longus
Interossei dorsales manus
Interossei volares
Lumbricales manus
Opponens digiti quinti manus
Opponens pollicis
Palmaris brevis
Palmaris longus
Pronator quadratus
Pronator teres
Supinator

MUSCLES OF
THE HIP AND KNEE

Adductor brevis
Adductor longus
Adductor magnus
Biceps femoris
Gemellus inferior
Gemellus superior
Gluteus maximus
Gluteus medius
Gluteus minimus
Gracilis
Iliacus
Obturator externus
Obturator internus

Pectineus
Piriformis
Psoas major
Rectus femoris
Quadratus femoris
Sartorius
Semimembranosus
Semitendinosus
Tensor fasciae lata
Vastus intermedius
Vastus lateralis
Vastus medialis

MUSCLES OF
THE PERINEUM AND PELVIS

Bulbocavernosus
Coccygeus
Iliacus
Iliococcygeus
Ischiocavernosus
Levator ani
Obturator internus

Piriformis
Pubococcygeus
Sphincter ani, externus
Sphincter urethrae membranaceae
Transverse perinei superficialis
Transversus perinei profundus

MUSCLES OF
THE ARM AND SHOULDER

Anconeus
Biceps brachii
Brachialis
Deltoideus
Infraspinatus
Latissimus dorsi
Levator scapulae
Pectoralis major
Pectoralis minor

Rhomboideus major
Rhomboideus minor
Serratus anterior
Subscapularis
Supraspinatus
Teres major
Teres minor
Trapezius
Triceps brachii

MUSCLES OF
THE LEG AND FOOT

Abductor digiti quinti pedis
Abductor hallucis
Dorsal interossei dorsales pedis
Extensor digitorum longus pedis
Extensor hallucis longus
Flexor digiti quinti brevis pedis
Flexor digitorum brevis
Flexor digitorum longus
Flexor hallucis brevis
Flexor hallucis longus
Gastrocnemius

Interossei plantares
Lumbricales pedis
Peroneus brevis
Peroneus longus
Peroneus tertius
Plantaris
Popliteus
Quadratus plantae
Soleus
Tibialis anterior
Tibialis posterior

THE PERIPHERAL NERVOUS SYSTEM

Terminology referable to the peripheral nervous system is used more frequently in surgical dictations than is that of the central nervous system; however, in addition to developing a familiarity with the names of the nerves, the secretary should have an intelligent concept of the divisions of the nervous system as a whole.

Grossly, the nervous system is divided into the central nervous system (brain and spinal cord), and the peripheral nervous system (cranial and spinal nerves and end organs). The peripheral nervous system may be further divided into the cerebrospinal (voluntary) system and the visceral (autonomic or splanchnic) system.

The cerebrospinal system connects the central nervous system with the body wall, controls skeletal muscles and includes those parts of the brain governing consciousness and mental activities. The autonomic system innervates the viscera and involuntary tissues such as the heart, the glands and plain muscle tissue which cannot be consciously controlled.

The autonomic system may be further subdivided into the parasympathetic (craniosacral) and sympathetic (thoracolumbar) systems.

The fibers of the parasympathetic arise from the midbrain, the medulla oblongata and the sacral segment of the spinal cord. Stimulation of the parasympathetic system causes contraction of the smooth muscle of the stomach and intestine, constriction of the arterioles, bronchioles and pupils of the eyes. It also causes a slowing of the heart.

The sympathetic division runs parallel on either side of the vertebral colume and is connected to the spinal cord by thoracic and lumbar fibers. Its functions are opposite and antagonistic to those of the parasympathetic system. A balance exists between the two systems to maintain proper body function.

Some of the more important peripheral nerves are the cranial which are referred to by number (based on the order in which they emerge from the brain) as often as by name. Medical students use a rhyme to assist them in recalling the nerves in their proper order, where the first letter of each word coincides with the first letter in the name of each nerve—ON OLD OLYMPUS TOWERING TOPS, A FINN AND GERMAN VIEWED A HOPS.

The Cranial Nerves Are: (12 pairs)

I.	Olfactory	VI.	Abducent
II.	Optic	VII.	Facial
III.	Oculomotor	VIII.	Acoustic
IV.	Trochlear	IX.	Glossopharyngeal
V.	Trigeminal	X.	Vagus
	ophthalmic branch	XI.	Accessory
	maxillary branch	XII.	Hypoglossal
	mandibular branch		

The numbers are just as important as the names in identifying these nerves. The surgeon will often refer to the 5th nerve rather than to specify it as the trigeminal. He is just as apt to refer to a nerve branch by name and the nerve proper by number, as for example, the ophthalmic branch of the 5th nerve.

THE NERVES

The names in this table may be used in the lower case except where they are named after an individual.

Abdominal	Alveolar, superior
Abducens	Anococcygeal
Accessory	Aortic plexus
Acoustic	Auditory
Adrenal plexus	Auricular
Alveolar, inferior	Auricular, great

THE NERVES (Continued)

Auricular, posterior
Auriculotemporal
Axillary
Brachial, cutaneous
Bronchial
Buccal, of facial
Buccinator
Calcaneal, medial
Cardiac
Caroticotympanic
Carotid, of glossopharyngeal
Cavernous, of penis
Celiac, of vagus
Cervical
Chorda tympani
Ciliary, long
Ciliary, short
Circumflex, of clitoris
Clunical
Coccygeal
Cochlear
Crural, anterior
Cutaneous
Cutaneous surae lateralis
Deep branch of radial
Dental
Descending ramus of hypoglossal
Digastric
Digital
Dorsal, of penis
Dorsal scapular
Dural
Erigentes
Esophageal
Esophageal plexus
Ethmoidal, anterior
Ethmoidal, posterior
External nasal
Facial
Femoral
Frontal
Gastric
Gastroduodenal plexus
Genitofemoral
Glossopharyngeal

Gluteal, inferior
Gluteal, superior
Great auricular
Greater occipital
Hemorrhoidal
Hepatic branches of vagus
Hypogastric
Hypoglossal
Iliohypogastric
Ilioinguinal
Incisive
Inferior dental to infrahyoid
Infraorbital
Infrapatellar
Infratrochlear
Intercostal
Intercostobrachial
Intermedius, of Wrisberg
Intermesenteric plexus
Internal calcaneal
Interosseous, anterior
Interosseous, posterior
Jacobson's
Jugular
Labial, inferior
Lacrimal of Lancisi
Laryngeal, inferior
Laryngeal, recurrent
Laryngeal, superior
Laryngopharyngeal
Lesser splanchnic
Lingual
Long ciliary
Lowest splanchnic
Lumbar
Lumbo-inguinal
Mandibular
Masseteric
Maxillary
Median
Meningeal
Mental
Mesenteric plexus
Middle superior alveolar
Motor

THE NERVES (Continued)

Musculocutaneous
Mylohyoid
Nasal
Nasociliary
Nasopalatine
Obturator
Occipital
Oculomotor
Olfactory
Ophthalmic
Optic
Orbital
Ovarian
Palatine
Palpebral, inferior
Pelvic
Perineal
Peroneal, common
Peroneal, deep
Peroneal, superficial
Petrosal, greater superficial
Petrosal, lesser
Petrosal, lesser superficial
Pharyngeal
Phrenic
Phrenic plexus
Plantar
Popliteal
Posterior scrotal
Presacral
Pterygoid
Pterygopalatine
Pudendal
Pudendal plexus
Pudic, internal
Pulmonary
Pyloric
Radial
Recurrent laryngeal
Renal
Respiratory, of Bell
Saphenous
Scapular

Sciatic
Solar plexus
Spermatic
Sphenopalatine
Spinal accessory
Spinosus
Splanchnic
Splenic plexus
Stapedial
Stylohyoid
Stylopharyngeal
Subscapular
Supraclavicular
Supraorbital
Suprascapular
Supratrochlear
Sural
Temporal
Tensor tympani
Tensor veli palatini
Tentorial
Testicular
Thoracic, anterior
Thoracic, long
Thoracodorsal
Thyrohyoid
Tibial
Tibial, anterior
Tibial, posterior
Tonsillar
Trigeminal
Trochlear
Tympanic
Ulnar
Ureteric
Uterovaginal plexus
Vagus to vertebral artery
Vestibular
Vidian (of pterygoid canal)
Volar digital of Wrisberg
Zygomatic
Zygomaticofacial
Zygomaticotemporal

Section III - Regional Surgery

General Surgery	Chapter 7
ENT	Chapter 8
Eye	Chapter 9
Neurosurgery	Chapter 10
OB & Gyn	Chapter 11
Orthopedics	Chapter 12
Plastic Surgery	Chapter 13
Thoracic Surgery	Chapter 14
Urology	Chapter 15
Vascular Surgery	Chapter 16

7 { *General Surgery*

The field of general surgery encompasses a wide variety of operations and is not confined to particular organs or systems as are the surgical specialties. The modern, well trained general surgeon is qualified to perform many of the operations which we usually think of as specialty surgery with the exception of those procedures which require highly specialized knowledge and training. For example, the general surgeon might perform major ENT surgery such as a laryngectomy and yet not venture into delicate ear operations as, for instance, a stapedectomy or tympanoplasty.

We will confine our considerations of general surgery to those cases which do not encroach on the specialties presented elsewhere in this book. Representative cases, performed most frequently in the general hospital, have been selected to exemplify the work of the general surgeon. Other technical information has been included with these case presentations which should be of value to the secretary.

HERNIA (pl. herniae)

The term hernia is used to describe any bulging or rupture of organs through a weakness in the supporting structures, particularly of the abdominal wall.

VARIOUS TYPES OF HERNIA

Abdominal
Amniotic
Bladder (abdominal)
Diaphragmatic
Epigastric
Femoral
Incisional (ventral)
Inguinal
  congenital

direct
incarcerated
indirect (oblique)
interstitial
recurrent
sliding
strangulated
Internal

150

TYPES OF HERNIA (Continued)

Interstitial
  inguino-superficial (Kuster)
  interparietal
  properitoneal (Krönlein)
Ischiorectal
Linea alba (abdominal)
Littre-Richter's
Lumbar
Maydl's
Obturator (anterior iliac hernia;
  thyroidal; opeocele; hernia
  foraminis ovalis)
Omental
Pantaloon

Perineal
Richter's
Sciatic
Sliding (hernia en glissade)
  intraperitoneal—sliding hernia with
    complete sac
  paraperitoneal—sliding hernia with
    incomplete sac
  extraperitoneal—sliding hernia
    without a sac
Spigelian (abdominal)
Umbilical
Ventral
Voluminous

TECHNIQUES FOR
REPAIR OF INGUINAL HERNIA
(Herniorrhaphy)

Andrews Modification of Bassini
Anson-McVay
Babcock
Bassini
Bevans Right-Sliding
Bloodgood
Ferguson
Ferguson-Coley
Gallies
Graham Roscie Sliding Sigmoidal
Halsted Rectus Sheath Flap
Handley Darn & Staylace
Hey Grooves
Hotchkiss
Houget (Pantaloon Hernia)
Hunt's

Inlay
Keel
Mackid's (sliding)
Mair's Whole Skin Graft
Mayo
McVay
Mermingas
Nuttall
Ogilvie
Tanner Slide Operation
Turner
Wangensteen
Wise's Method
Wyllys Andrews Imbrication
Zieman Indirect Repair
Zimmerman (sliding)

ANATOMIC FEATURES
INVOLVED IN
INGUINAL REPAIRS

Aponeurosis of ext. oblique
Areolar tissues
Circumflex iliac superficial fascia
Conjoined tendon
Cooper's ligament
Cremaster fascia

Cremaster muscle
Deep epigastric vessels
Direct component
External oblique
External pudic vessels
Funiculus spermaticus

ANATOMIC FEATURES INVOLVED IN
INGUINAL REPAIRS (Continued)

Gimbernat's ligament
Hesselbach's triangle
Hypogastric branch of
  iliohypogastric nerve
Iliohypogastric nerve
Ilioinguinal nerve
Infundibuloform fascia
Inguinal ligament
Inguinal ring
Lacunar ligament
Leaf (leaves) of muscle
Ligamentum inguinale
Os pubis spine
Pampiniform plexus
Pillars, external and internal

Plexus pampiniformis
Poupart's ligament
Processus vaginalis
Properitoneal fat
Pubic bone
Pubic crest
Pudendal vessels
Rectus sheath
Sac
Scarpa's fascia
Shelving edge of Poupart's
Spermatic cord
Transversalis fascia
Vas deferens

McVay Inguinal Herniorrhaphy

After satisfactory general anesthesia, the patient's abdomen was prepared and draped in the usual manner.

A right groin incision was made and carried through the skin and subcutaneous tissues. Hemostasis was secured with clamps and individual ligatures. Sharp and blunt dissection was employed to free the entire inguinal ligament inferiorly and medially. The aponeurosis of the external oblique was sharply incised, opening the external ring. Sharp and blunt dissection was employed to free the round ligament and its contents. Prior to this, the ilioinguinal nerve was visualized, identified, isolated and retracted out of the way.

Rather extensive dissection in the operative area failed to reveal the presence of any hernial sac, even though the indirect area was dilated and loose in character. The round ligament was transected. A high ligation with transfixing suture was done. The internal ring was undisturbed. There was a mild weakness in the direct component. The inferior epigastric artery was identified, visualized and retracted inferiorly. Palpatation along the femoral canal revealed the presence of a defect about 1½ fingerbreadths in diameter. It was elected, therefore, to perform a herniorrhaphy of the McVay (Cooper's ligament) type repair.

Interrupted 00 dacron sutures were employed to coapt Cooper's ligament to the internal oblique aponeurosis and this was accomplished down to the level of the femoral artery and vein, where a transitional suture of the same material was placed, from the inguinal ligament, to Cooper's ligament, to the femoral sheath. This completely closed the defect. The aponeurosis of the external oblique was closed with a running suture of 000 chromic. Subcuticular closure with interrupted sutures of 000 chromic was done and a pull-out suture of 00 nylon was used to close the skin. Blood loss was negligible and none was replaced. Sponge count was correct on two occasions.

Bassini Operation for Inguinal Herniorrhaphy

Under general anesthesia, the patient was sterilely prepared and draped in the supine position.

An oblique incision was made about ½ inch above and parallel to Poupart's ligament, from a point opposite the anterior superior spinous process of the ilium, to the spine of the os pubis. The incision was deepened to expose the fascia of the external abdominal oblique muscle. The incision severed the superficial epigastric vessels, running at right angles to them. These were carefully ligated. The superficial external pudic vessels and the superficial circumflex vessels were also encountered.

Exposure and identification of the components of the external abdominal ring was accomplished. A Kocher was introduced through the external ring. The aponeurosis of the external abdominal oblique muscle was divided from the external ring, along the line of incision, for 2 or 3 inches. The edges of the aponeurotic flaps were retracted and the upper flap was separated inward. The lower flap was separated from Poupart's ligament. The index finger, covered with gauze, was used to strip and expose the lower leaf of the divided external oblique muscle from the underlying structures. The contents of the inguinal canal were exposed. The ilio-inguinal nerve was identified and avoided.

The conjoined tendon was identified. Full exposure was accomplished by retraction. The hernial sac and cord were raised en masse. By stripping and dissection, the sac was completely isolated from the spermatic cord as high as possible in relation to the internal ring. The sac was opened and its contents examined. The contents were returned to the abdominal cavity.

The conjoined tendon was retracted. The hernial sac was transfixed at its base, as high as possible, with chromic catgut. The deep epigastric vessels were avoided. The ligature was tied. The neck of the sac was encircled and the ligature tied once more. The redundant sac was removed. The stump of the sac retracted beyond the internal ring. A strip of tape was insinuated under the cord and it was retracted out of the way. Six # 2 catgut sutures were introduced beneath the cord, from before, backward and from within, outward. This united the conjoined tendon with the transversalis fascia, muscles and the lower fibers of the internal oblique muscle with Poupart's ligament. Sutures were tied and tissues approximated.

The cord was replaced on its new floor. The aponeurosis of the external oblique muscle was approximated with interrupted sutures of # 2 catgut. There was no constriction of the cord at its exit from the newly constructed external ring. This was verified by introduction of the little finger into the external opening. The skin was closed with interrupted silkworm-gut.

TYPES OF
FEMORAL HERNIORRHAPHY

Anson-McVay
Combined femoral-inguinal approach
Extra-peritoneal approach
Gallie's
Henry
High Operation (inguinal approach)

Lotheissen (high operation)
Lower Operation (femoral approach)
Marcy Purse-String Method
McEvedy
Ogilvie
Wyllys Andrews

FEMORAL
ANATOMIC STRUCTURES

Aponeurosis (pl. aponeuroses)
Conjoined tendon
Cooper's ligament
Cribriform fascia
Crural canal
External iliac vessels
Falciform process of fascia lata
Fascia lata of thigh
Femoral canal
Femoral sheath
Gimbernat's ligament
Hesselbach's triangle

Iliopectineal line
Lacunar ligament
Leaf (leaves) of aponeurosis
Pectineal fascia
Pectineal ligament
Pectineal line
Pectineus fascia
Peritoneum
Poupart's ligament
Properitoneal fat
Scarpa's triangle
Transversalis fascia

Femoral Herniorrhaphy

Under general anesthesia, the patient was placed in the supine position. An incision was made between the left corner of the pubic bone and the left anterior superior iliac spine. It was carried down to the fascia. The bleeders were clamped with Kelly clamps and tied with 000 chromic sutures.

The large hernial sac was visualized. It was opened and found to contain a large piece of omentum. The omentum was partially necrotic and was therefore excised. It was clamped with several hemostats, divided and the hemostats replaced with sutures of 000 chromic catgut. The sac was freed. The remaining omentum was replaced into the abdomen. The base of the sac was sutured with a 00 intestinal catgut, tied and the sac removed. The femoral vessels could easily be palpated.

Poupart's ligament was sutured to the fascia with interrupted 00 cotton sutures. A second layer of suture was placed approximating the aponeurosis of the external oblique to Cooper's ligament with 00 interrupted cotton sutures.

A small catheter drain was inserted into the wound because of oozing. It was brought out below the incision, through a small stab wound. The skin edges along with the subcutaneous tissues were approximated with interrupted mattress sutures of 00 cotton. Pressure dressing was applied to the wound.

Diaphragmatic Herniorrhaphy—Transthoracic approach for hiatal hernia

The patient was prepared and draped after being positioned on his right side. It was decided to enter the thoracic cavity through the 7th intercostal space. A skin incision was made coursing from the spine to the midaxillary line. The skin incision was deepened into the musculature for its entire length. A small section of the 7th and 8th ribs was removed to facilitate entry into the pleural cavity. The left phrenic nerve was crushed.

The abdominal contents were carefully examined and no incarceration was noted. There was no other pathology nor were there any marked adhesions. A few small adhesions were lysed and hemostasis secured. The intestinal contents were replaced in the abdomen after a gastrotomy had been performed and the stomach lining found to be normal. No ulcerations were noted. Adhesions were found binding the fundus of the stomach to the liver. These were freed by blunt and sharp dissection. The gastroesophageal junction was visualized and freed from adhesions. The defect was found and measured approximately 7 cm. in diameter and easily admitted three fingers.

By blunt and sharp dissection, the right and left crus of the diaphragm were freed and reapproximated with interrupted 00 silk. The hiatal hernia was then further diminished by approximating the crus anterior to the esophagus with one interrupted 0 silk stitch. The defect at the termination of the procedure measured approximately 2 cm. in diameter and admitted two fingers.

The peritoneum was then closed with interrupted 00 chromic and the fascia was reapproximated with interrupted figure-of-eight #30 wire. The subcutaneous tissue was closed with chromic and the skin edges brought together with interrupted cotton.

Umbilical Herniorrhaphy

Under general anesthesia the patient was placed in the supine position. A curved elliptical incision was made inferior to the umbilicus extending laterally for a distance of approximately $1\frac{1}{4}$ inches. The incision was made down through the subcutaneous tissues and down to the fascia proper. The underlying sac was freed from its entire circumference and carefully opened. Upon opening the sac, a small piece of omentum was found to be incarcerated. The omentum was then handled by division between curved Kelly clamps. The sac was freed. The peritoneal contents were in place. The peritoneum, itself, was freed from the surrounding edges.

An attempt was made to explore the abdominal cavity, but because of the fact that there were so many abdominal adhesions from previous surgery, the exploration was quite inadequate. After having excised the redundant peritoneum, the peritoneum was closed with a continuous atraumatic suture.

The rectus sheath had already been freed from the subcutaneous tissue. It was also freed from the underlying peritoneum to permit correction of the midline defect. Following this, an overlapping type of repair was performed by placing a series of mattress sutures which would imbricate the upper flap over the lower flap. The closure was further reinforced by again approximating the upper flap to the distal flap, to the lower flap with interrupted 000 cotton sutures.

After adequate bleeding control was achieved, closure was accomplished by first approximating the subcutaneous tissue with interrupted 000000 cotton sutures. The umbilicus was then sutured to the underlying fascia with one interrupted 000000 cotton suture. Closure of the skin was accomplished with interrupted 00000 dermalon sutures.

500 cc. of 5% glucose in water was used during the operation.

Left Radical Groin Dissection

An incision was made just above a previous hernial incision for the removal of a carcinomatous testicle. The incision was carried through the subcutaneous tissue, to the aponeurosis of the external oblique. It was then carried to the internal oblique muscle, following the extension of the incision through the internal oblique. A portion of the internal oblique muscle and transversalis were incised. Bleeders were clamped, cut and ligated with 000 chromic suture. Following incision through the muscles, the extraperitoneal tissue and preperitoneal fascia were encountered. The peritoneum was reflected medially. The cord, which had been ligated previously, was encountered. This was isolated between the muscle layers and was dissected further towards its origin. Clamps were applied and the vessels were ligated. Following the excision of the spermatic cord, dissection was carried out exposing the ureter. This was reflected medially. The iliac vessels and hypogastric vessels were all isolated and were entered. The internal and external iliacs were exposed. The peri-iliac glands were dissected out carefully. There were several pudendal glands. The nerve was oriented at this point and the obturator palpated. Dissection was carried along the common iliac to the aorta and this was palpated high towards the region of the kidney. All of the perivascular fatty tissue as well as the glands between the aorta, at the bifurcation of the iliac, and at the common, internal and external iliacs were exposed and dissected out. There were no unusual tumor masses palpable anywhere in the extraperitoneal area.

A drain was inserted into the pelvic cavity and brought out through the superior portion of the wound.

Repair was carried out using interrupted 000 and 00 dacron sutures for the various fascial and muscle layers. Partial covering of the internal oblique was accomplished with interrupted 000 dacron. The fascia of the external oblique was approximated with interrupted 00 dacron and the subcutaneous tissue with interrupted chromic. The skin was closed with subcuticular nylon.

A separate longitudinal incision was then made commencing just inferior to Poupart's ligament and extending down along the greater saphenous vein, exposing the femoral artery. There were several small glands encountered here. The artery and vein were carefully dissected out. Several branches of the greater saphenous were clamped, cut and ligated. The perivascular fatty tissue and glands were removed for a distance of about 5 inches. The tissues were approximated with 000 interrupted chromic suture and the skin with subcuticular nylon.

THE NAILS

Traumatic injuries to the fingernails or toenails and ingrown nails of the large toes constitute the principal reasons for surgery of these structures. These conditions often require radical excision of the nail rather than simple excision, and in such instances, the patient is admitted to surgery.

Some of the conditions which may be listed as the pre- or postoperative diagnosis have been listed here with structures commonly referred to in operative dictations of nail excisions.

NAIL STRUCTURES

Body
Cuticle
Cuticular fold
Dorsal plate
Eponychium

Lunula
Matrix
Nail bed
Nail fold
Root

DISEASES OF THE NAILS

Eggshell nails
Koilonychia
Leukonychia
Onychauxis
Onychia

Onychomycosis
Onychorrhexis
Paronychia
Polyunguia
Unguis incarnatus (ingrown)

Radical Excision of Toenails

The patient was admitted with recurrent ingrown toenails for which radical excision of the toenails was proposed.

Under general anesthesia, the patient was prepared and draped in the supine position.

Beginning with the right great toe, a tourniquet was applied to the base of the toe to create a bloodless field. A small incision was made in the soft tissue of the nail fold and eponychium, on a line with the incision, and extended back to the matrix. The nail was raised from its bed with scissors for its entire length. A loose piece of nail was grasped with forceps and by gradual traction and separation from the nail bed, it was removed in one piece.

Using a small curet, the matrix and nail bed were curetted to prevent recurrent nail growth. The same procedure was carried out on the left great toe.

INCISION AND DRAINAGE OF ABSCESS (EXTERNAL)
INSTRUMENTS

Backhaus towel clamp
Crile forceps
Grooved director
Kelly forceps

Mayo Hegar needle holder
Mayo Pean forceps
Mayo scissors
Thumb forceps

Incision and Drainage of Abscess on Buttocks

Under spinal anesthesia the patient was sterilely prepared and draped in the usual manner.

There was an abscess about the size of a small egg on the left buttocks which was incised and drained. The area of the abscess was dissected free and loculations were broken up.

The incision was cross-hatched over the surface of the abscess. A small Penrose drain was inserted. Culture was taken for bacteriologic identification and sensitivity studies.

Incision and Drainage, Dorsum of Hand

With the patient under general anesthesia, the hand was prepared and draped in the usual manner.

The abscess which presented on the dorsum of the hand, over the hypothenar surface, was incised in a stellate fashion and probed. It was then drained and cleaned of all purulent material.

The abscess cavity was packed with Iodoform gauze and the hand bandaged over a gauze compress and wad of mechanic's waste.

The patient tolerated the procedure well and was returned to the room in good condition.

Excision of Pilonidal Cyst

After satisfactory spinal anesthesia was obtained, the patient was placed in the prone flexed position. Sterile preparation and draping was carried out.

An elliptical incision was made after methylene blue injection of the sinus and it was excised en bloc. Hemostasis was secured with clamps and individual ligatures.

Interrupted 000 chromic catgut sutures were employed to coapt the deeper layers employing the fascia of the coccyx also. A maneuver of vertical mattress sutures of 00 cotton was done to coapt the edges entirely. A running subcuticular pull-out type 00 nylon suture was employed to close the skin. Sponge and needle counts on two occasions were correct.

THE BREASTS

The breasts, otherwise known as the mammae or mammary glands, give rise to a variety of surgical lesions which are usually treated by the general surgeon. It is argued in some quarters that surgery of the breasts belongs in the specialty of gynecology; however, this classification is not universally accepted. For this reason, we will consider the breasts in the category of general surgery. Operations designed to augment or reduce the size of the breasts belong in the category of plastic surgery.

One of the most common conditions involving the breast in the male is gynecomastia (excessive enlargement of the male breasts). Frequently seen surgical lesions in the female breast include abscesses, fibrocystic disease, blue dome cysts, cystic mastitis, fibroadenomas and other benign neoplasms. The breasts are also common sites of adenocarcinoma. Breast masses are usually biopsied to rule out carcinoma. The biopsy, generally, is followed with a frozen section examination by the pathologist. Discovery of malignancy is reported back to the surgeon immediately, while the patient is still on the operating table, following which, the patient is redraped and prepared for a radical mastectomy (removal of the breast and axillary lymph nodes). Post-mastectomy patients sometimes develop edema of the arm which is caused by a block in the venous system or in the deep and superficial lymphatics of the axilla. This condition is treated by the Kondoleon operation or the Beck operation designed to promote lymphatic drainage.

ANATOMIC FEATURES OF
THE BREAST and AXILLA

Acromiothoracic artery	Lactating breasts
Alar thoracic artery	Mammary gland
Alar thoracic vein	Nerve of Bell
Areola	Nipple
Areolar glands	Papilla
Cooper's ligament	Parenchyma
Ducts	Pectoralis major
Fascia of recti muscles	Pectoralis minor
Glands of Montgomery	Space of Mohrenheim
Internal mammary artery	Sulcus

ARTERIAL SUPPLY

Acromial	Internal mammary
Acromiothoracic	Long thoracic
Alar thoracic	Subscapular artery
Intercostals	Thoracic branch of axillary

MASTECTOMY INCISIONS

Elsberg	Meyer
Halsted	Rodman
Handley	Stewart
Jackson	Thomas-Warren

Right Breast Biopsy—Frozen Section—Right Radical Mastectomy

After satisfactory general endotracheal anesthesia, the patient's right breast was prepared and draped in the usual manner.

An areolar incision was made and, by sharp dissection, an excisional biopsy of the right breast was carried out. This mass was approximately 4 cm. in diameter and was immediately sent to the pathologist for frozen section examination. The wound in the areolar area was closed over a gauze pack with a continuous 000 nylon suture. Frozen section report of the excisional biopsy was malignant. A radical mastectomy was elected.

An elliptical incision was made from the middle of the clavicle down to about the end of the thoracic cage and the skin flaps developed. Sharp dissection was employed to develop fairly thin flaps on the medial aspect. These tapered out to relatively thick flaps at the base of the flap, per se. Hemostasis was secured with clamps and electrocautery. Sharp dissection was employed to find the distal attachment of the Pectoralis major. This was doubly cross clamped, divided and then suture ligated. Continuous sharp and blunt dissection was employed to identify the head of the Pectoralis minor. This was also transected between clamps and suture ligated. The entire axillary vein was then cleaned of all its inferior branches and surrounding fat. The axilla was likewise cleaned of its fat and lymphatic node content. The long thoracic nerve was visualized.

By sharp dissection, the Pectoralis major, Pectoralis minor and over-lying breast were removed. Hemostasis was secured with clamps and individual ligatures or electrocautery. The Serratus anterior was left intact.

The entire operative area was then inspected for hemostasis and it was found to be secure. Large Penrose drains were placed for drainage purposes and a French catheter for irrigation-suction purposes. The wound was irrigated with Clorpactin solution.

The skin was closed in one layer with vertical mattress type sutures. There was no area of discoloration of the skin and the flaps appeared to be viable. Blood loss sustained during the course of the operation was replaced in the operating room. Sponge counts taken on several occasions were found to be correct. The patient tolerated the operation well and was returned to the recovery room in satisfactory condition.

SURGERY OF THE SPLEEN

The spleen has several known functions, serving as a reservoir for the destruction of red blood corpuscles and the preparation of new hemoglobin from the iron thus produced; however, all of the functions of this lymph gland are not yet known. It is regarded as an organ which is not essential to life. Its removal (splenectomy) is not followed by any significant or permanent dysfunction.

Location of this organ in the left hypochondriac region, just beneath the diaphragm, and behind the stomach, predisposes it to rupture in cases of severe trauma to the abdominal wall. It is a very vascular organ, being supplied by the splenic (lienal) artery, a branch of the celiac.

IMPORTANT ANATOMIC
FEATURES OF THE SPLEEN

Accessory spleens (supernumerary)	Phrenic surface
Capsule	Phrenicocolic ligament
Celiac axis	Phrenicolienal ligament
Colic surface	Phrenicosplenic ligament
Diaphragm	Portal vein
Ectopic tissue	Posterior parietal peritoneum
Gastric surface	Presplenic fold
Gastroepiploic branch of lienal artery	Renal surface
Gastrolienal ligament	Short gastric br.-lienal artery
Gastrosplenic omentum	Splenic artery
Greater omentum	Splenic pulp
Hilum	Splenic vein
Lienal artery	Splenocolic ligament
Lienal vein	Splenomegaly
Lienorenal ligament	Splenunculi
Malpighian bodies	Tunica albuginea
Mesogastrium	Tunica serosa
Pancreaticosplenic ligament	Visceral surface
Pedicle of spleen	

TECHNIQUES
OF SPLENECTOMY

Carter thoracicoabdominal	Henry
Three clamp method of Federoff	Rives

Splenectomy

Under general anesthesia, after the patient had been sterilely prepared and draped, a left Kocher incision was made and the rectus muscle was divided and ligated. The peritoneal cavity was entered. There was

162

splenomegaly which descended to the costal margins.

By means of sharp dissection, the short gastric vessels in the gastro-splenic ligaments were isolated, clamped, divided and ligated with cotton. The splenic artery was identified running over the superior border of the pancreas. By means of a ligature carrier, the artery was isolated at a short segment and tied with 00 chromic just distally and proximally and then divided between ligatures. A second suture of 000 cotton was used to transfix the artery proximally; it was ligated for further safety. The artery and veins of the pedicle were clamped, divided and ligated close to the spleen, avoiding the pancreas. The colon and stomach were re-tracted out of the way to avoid injury. The splenocolic and splenorenal ligaments were clamped, divided and ligated. There were firm adhesions of the diaphragmatic attachments onto the posterior aspect of the spleen. These were lysed by blunt dissection. The spleen was removed. Further hemostasis was achieved with interrupted cotton stitches until the field was entirely dry. A medium size Penrose drain was placed beneath the diaphragm in the left side and brought out through a separate stab wound in the flank.

There were no accessory spleens palpable and the pelvic organs were felt to be entirely normal as was the remaining G.I. tract. The appendix could not be reached through this incision.

The peritoneum and posterior sheath were closed with a continuous locking 00 chromic suture. The fascia was approximated in layers with interrupted figure-of-eight 000 cotton. The subcutaneous tissue was closed with chromic sutures. The skin edges were approximated with a sliding dermalon. The drain was transfixed to the skin with a suture and safety pin. Dressing applied.

THE SALIVARY GLANDS

There are three pairs of salivary glands which communicate with the mouth, and pour their secretions into its cavity. They are the *parotid, submaxillary,* and *sublingual.* The secretions of these glands combine with those of the small buccal glands of the mouth to form saliva.

Parotid Gland

The parotid gland is the largest of the three, situated at the side of the face, below and in front of the external ear. The parotid duct

(Stensen's duct) opens upon the inner surface of the cheek opposite the second upper molar tooth. The gland is invested in a capsule continuous with the deep cervical fascia. A portion of the fascia, attached to the styloid process and the angle of the mandible, is somewhat thickened and forms the stylomandibular ligament which courses between the parotid and submaxillary glands.

Structures adjacent to the parotid and other salivary glands are important considerations in surgery of this area and therefore will be reviewed here to provide the secretary with an anatomic reference.

The main body of the parotid is situated between the mastoid process and Sternocleidomastoideus posteriorly and the ramus of the mandible anteriorly. The anterior surface is covered by the Pterygoideus internus and the Masseter. It slopes for a short distance between the two Pterygoid muscles. The outer lip of the gland extends over the superficial surface of the Masseter. There is a detached portion just below the zygomatic arch called the accessory part. The superficial surface of the gland is covered by superficial fascia containing the facial branches of the great auricular nerve. The posterior surface of the gland borders against the external acoustic meatus, the mastoid process, and the anterior edge of the Sternocleidomastoideus muscle. The deep surface of the parotid extends into the deep tissues with two processes, one of which is located in front of the styloid process, contacting the internal jugular vein, internal and external carotid arteries, and the glossopharyngeal and vagus nerves; the other is situated on the styloid group of muscles, styloid process and Digastricus muscle. It projects under the mastoid process and Sternocleidomastoideus.

The parotid duct (Stensen's duct) emerges in several branches from the anterior aspect of the gland, crosses the Masseter muscle, where it receives the duct of the accessory part of the parotid gland, continues through the corpus adiposum of the cheek and Buccinator muscle and finally opens upon the inside of the cheek, just opposite the second upper molar tooth.

STRUCTURES OF
THE PAROTID GLAND

Accessory duct	Great auricular nerve
Accessory part of gland	Masseter muscle
Apophysis	Parotid duct
Auriculotemporal nerve	Spinal accessory nerve
Deep cervical fascia	Stensen's duct
Facial nerve	Stylomandibular ligament

VESSELS OF
THE PAROTID GLAND

Common facial vein

External carotid artery

   int. maxillary branch

   posterior auricular branch

   superficial temporal branch

External jugular vein

Internal maxillary vein

Posterior auricular vein

Posterior facial vein

Superficial temporal vein

Temporal artery

Transverse facial artery

Parotidectomy (Aveline Gutierrez Technic—preservation of lower maxilla)

Using 0.5% Novocain, the auriculotemporal, auricular and anterior branches of the facial nerve were blocked. The facial nerve was likewise blocked.

Beginning at the malar arch, an incision was made parallel to the zygomatic arch, toward the tragus, under the anterior portion of the ear lobe, following the contour of the ear. The incision was carried further along the auriculomastoid line, toward the base of the mastoid apophysis. It was then carried downward toward the vertex, proceeding toward the anterior border of the sternocleidomastoid muscle, and then curving in the direction of the hyoid bone. The skin and underlying tissues were reflected.

The external jugular vein was ligated and divided at the level of the border of the maxilla. The sternocleidomastoid along with the mastoid apophysis were identified after deep dissection. The digastric muscle was further identified at the point where it meets the sternocleidomastoid. Further identification of structures was carried out to include the external branch of the spinal accessory nerve which courses in front of the transverse apophysis to the atlas. This was isolated. We also identified the great hypoglossal nerve, the internal jugular vein and the external carotid artery. The external carotid was dissected free and ligated with silk, the ligature passing from within, outward. The artery was divided between these ligatures.

By careful dissection, the parotid gland was divided from the pavilion of the ear and auditory canal. The temporal artery and sternocleidomastoid artery, coursing in front of the tragus, were ligated and divided. By placing forward traction on the parotid, we were able to expose the facial nerve.

An incision was then made for the purpose of removing the skin overlying the lesion of the parotid which extends, from the mid-portion of the zygomatic arch, toward the angle of the mandible. By mobilizing the anterior flap we were able to expose the anterior border of the parotid. This maneuver exposed the transverse facial artery and Stensen's duct. These structures were ligated and divided. The gland was then freed from the Masseter muscle. Bleeding was controlled.

By backward traction on the gland, we were able to expose the internal maxillary veins which were ligated and divided. The pharyngeal portion of the gland was isolated with a Kocher director. The dead space remaining after removal of the gland was obliterated by use of contiguous skin flaps which were mobilized and sutured in place. Horsehair sutures were used to approximate the skin edges. A drain was left in the lower portion of the wound. The specimen was sent to the pathologist for histopathologic examination.

Radical Neck Dissection, left

With the patient in the supine position and the head turned to the right, the left cheek, neck and upper chest were prepared and draped.

A routine double "Y" incision was made in the usual manner. Marked bleeding was encountered due to Cobalt therapy and old surgery in the area. Bleeders were controlled by clamping and ligating and/or electrocoagulation. After the flaps had been adequately elevated in all directions, the sternomastoid muscle was isolated anteriorly and its two heads of attachment sharply divided. The carotid sheath was entered. The internal jugular vein was isolated and doubly ligated, one of which was a suture ligature. The dissection was carried posteriorly to the scalene fat pad which was included in the specimen and carried down to the level of the fascia overlying the brachial plexus and scalene muscles. The phrenic nerve was tentatively identified and preserved. The dissection was carried posteriorly to the anterior border of the Trapezius and upward, including the spinal accessory nerve and its accompanying nodes. The sternomastoid was divided superiorly from the mastoid process. Beneath this, the digastric muscle was identified and retracted anteriorly to expose the upper end of the internal jugular vein. Anterior to this, a portion of the tail of the parotid gland was included as was the submaxillary gland. One additional involved node was noted just anterior to the bifurcation of the common carotid artery and was included with its surrounding fat and nodes in the specimen.

Considerable time was expended in controlling the bleeding. This was accomplished as stated above and the neck flaps reapproximated with a few interrupted 000 chromic catgut sutures.

Hemovac drainage tubes were inserted through two stab wounds and attached to the Hemovac units. The skin was then closed with interrupted simple and vertical mattress 00000 nylon sutures. A light dressing was applied.

Blood loss was approximated at about 1800 cc. During the operative procedure, the patient received 1000 cc. of whole blood and an additional 500 cc. in the recovery room.

Submaxillary Gland

The submaxillary gland is situated under the posterior tongue, largely in the submaxillary triangle, extending backward to the stylomandibular ligament and forward to the anterior belly of the Digastricus. Below, it usually overlaps the intermediate tendon of the Digastricus and the insertion of the Stylohyoideus.

The submaxillary duct (Wharton's duct) extends in branches from the deep surface of the gland and courses between the Genioglossus, Hypoglossus, Mylohyoideus and sublingual gland and opens at the side of the frenulum linguae.

SUBMAXILLARY GLAND STRUCTURES

Deep cervical fascia
Deep process
Facial nerve
Hypoglossal nerve
Lingual nerve
Mylohyoid nerve

Platysma muscle
Submaxillary ganglion
Submaxillary lymph nodes
Superficial fascia
Wharton's duct

SUBMAXILLARY GLAND CIRCULATION

Anterior facial vein
External carotid artery
External maxillary artery
Facial artery
Facial vein
Glandular br. of ext. maxillary

Hypoglossal vein
Jugular vein
Lingual artery
Mylohyoid vessels
Submental vessels

Sublingual Gland

The sublingual gland is the smallest of the salivary glands. It is located under the tongue, in the floor of the mouth, at the side of the frenulum linguae.

SUBLINGUAL
GLAND STRUCTURES

Duct of Bartholin
Ducts of Rivinus
Plica sublingualis

Sublingual depression
Sublingual ducts
Submaxillary duct

SUBLINGUAL CIRCULATION

Sublingual arteries

Submental arteries

OPERATIONS ON THE STOMACH
AND INTESTINES

The most frequently performed operation on the stomach is probably the gastrectomy (excision of all or a portion of the stomach), indicated in certain cases of gastric and duodenal ulcer and other surgical lesions of the stomach and duodenum. A partial or subtotal resection is performed more often than a complete or total excision. These resections are usually followed by either a gastroduodenostomy (anastomosis of the stomach and duodenum) or a gastrojejunostomy (anastomosis between the stomach and jejunum).

A number of techniques have been proposed for gastrectomy, all based upon the principles of the Billroth methods. They are, in essence, modifications of the Billroth I and II operations.

BILLROTH I   Resection of a portion of the stomach with an end-to-end anastomosis between the stomach and the duodenum.

BILLROTH II   An anastomosis following gastric resection, closing the end of the stomach and duodenum and attaching a loop of jejunum to a new opening in the stomach.

Other popular gastrectomy techniques include:

Schoemaker Modification of Billroth I

Billroth I except that the cut end of the stomach on the lesser curvature side is closed with a row of continuous chromic catgut and a row of interrupted silk resulting in a stoma of about 2 inches for anastomosis with the duodenum.

Anterior Polya

Resection of a portion of the stomach with end-to-end anastomosis between the stomach and jejunum, anterior to the transverse colon.

Posterior Polya

Removal of a portion of the stomach with end-to-end anastomosis between the stomach and jejunum, posterior to the transverse colon.

Hofmeister Modification of Polya

The stomach is partially resected and the lesser curvature of the remaining stomach is closed leaving a 2 inch opening on the side of the greater curvature. The stoma is anastomosed to the jejunum.

GASTRECTOMY TECHNIQUES

Aquirre
Balfour
Bancroft-Plenk
Billroth I
Billroth II
Braun and Jaboulay
Connell's Tube Operation
  (partial fundusectomy)
Deloyers reverse gastrectomy
Finsterer
Finochietto-Billroth I
Hofmeister
Hofmeister-Billroth II antecolic
Horsley
Krönlein
Lahey
Mayo

McKittricks two stage partial
Mikulicz
Moore
Moynihan
Nissen
Pauchet
Polya, anterior
Polya, posterior
Reichel
Roux-Y (Also: Roux-en-Y)
Schoemaker
Schoemaker-Billroth II
Stevenson
von Eiselsberg
von Haberer
von Haberer-Finney
Warren

GASTRECTOMY INSTRUMENTS

Allis forceps
Babcock forceps
Balfour retractor
Deaver retractor
Doyen clamps
Doyen cross-action forceps
Dunhill hemostats
Eastman clamp
Friedrich-Petz clamp
Furniss clamp

Halsted hemostats
Harrington forceps
Kelly clamps
Kocher clamps
Kocher forceps
Lane clamps
Lockwood clamps
Maingot hemostats
Martin needle
Mayo needle

GASTRECTOMY INSTRUMENTS (Continued)

Mayo scissors
Mayo-Ochsner box-joint forceps
Mosquito clamps
Moynihan clamps
Ochsner clamp
O'Sullivan-O'Connor retractor
Parker-Kerr forceps

Payr clamp
Rankin clamp
Roosevelt clamp
Spencer Wells forceps
Stevenson clamps
von Petz clamp

ANATOMIC
STRUCTURES ENCOUNTERED
IN GASTRECTOMY

Anterior rectus sheath
Azygos vein
Cardiac orifice
Celiac axis
Crus of diaphragm
Duodenum
Fundus of stomach
Gastric artery
Gastrocolic ligament
Gastroepiploic artery
Gastrohepatic ligament
Gastrohepatic omentum
Gastrolienal ligament
Gastrophrenic ligament
Greater curvature
Greater omentum
Hepatic artery
Hepatogastric ligament
Incisura angularis
Incisura cardiaca

Jejunum
Leaf of mesocolon
Lesser curvature
Ligament of Treitz
Muscularis
Posterior rectus sheath
Pyloric antrum
Pyloric orifice
Pyloric valve
Pyloric vestibule
Pylorus
Recti muscles
Rugae of stomach
Rugal folds
Seromuscular layer
Serosa
Stoma
Suspensory ligament of liver
Transverse colon
Vasa brevia

Gastrectomy and Gastroduodenostomy (Billroth I)

Under spinal anesthesia an incision was made approximately 1½ inches above the umbilicus to approximately 1 inch below the xiphoid. The incision extended through the superficial tissues, down to the linea alba. The linea alba was opened and the peritoneum incised.

Exploration revealed the liver, kidneys and gallbladder to be normal. There was no evidence of duodenal ulcer. Examination of the stomach did not reveal any gross evidence of an ulcer. In view of the difficulty in palpation for an ulcer, a longitudinal incision was made in an avascular area in the anterior wall of the stomach. 000 chromic intestinal sutures were placed. The stomach wall was incised. Upon examining the lumen of the stomach, a posterior penetrating ulcer measuring approximately $1\frac{1}{2}$ cm. in diameter was found. Grossly, it appeared to be benign. In view of this, the opening in the anterior wall of the stomach was closed with continuous running 00 chromic suture.

The gastrocolic omentum was freed by ligating and clamping the vessels. The duodenum, along its inferior border, was freed for a distance of about $1\frac{1}{2}$ inches. The right gastric artery and vein were doubly clamped, cut and ligated with dacron and chromic 0 sutures. The superior portion of the duodenum was freed. The left gastric vessels were doubly clamped, cut and ligated. Following this, the clamp was placed on the duodenum and the prepyloric area, and the stomach was divided. Approximately 65-70% of the stomach was resected.

The lesser curvature of the stomach was closed with three layers. First, the layer beneath the clamp was closed with an overlying 00 chromic suture and a running 000 cotton suture. The stoma of the opening in the stomach was then brought to the duodenum and approximated with it using interrupted 000 dacron sutures for the posterior seromuscular layer. Following the approximation of the posterior layer, through-and-through 00 chromic sutures were used for a posterior approximation of the mucous membrane. This was utilized as a Connell suture anteriorly with a reinforcing row of 000 dacron. Several sutures were placed along the inferior superior border of the duodenum and the stomach to remove any tension between the stomach and duodenal anastomosis. Following the anastomosis, inspection revealed no evidence of any further bleeding anywhere.

The peritoneum was closed with a continuous 00 chromic closure suture. The fascia was approximated with figure-of-eight 00 dacron suture and the skin with 00 nylon suture.

Subtotal Gastrectomy and Gastrojejunostomy (Billroth II)

Under spinal anesthesia the patient was placed in the supine position, prepared and draped in routine fashion.

A midline supraumbilical incision measuring 3 inches in length was made. The incision was carried down to the subcutaneous tissues and down through the anterior rectus sheath. This was incised vertically. The right and left recti muscles were retracted laterally. The posterior rectus sheath and peritoneum were grasped and opened.

Upon entering the abdominal cavity, palpatory exploration of the abdominal organs and contents was carried out. The examination was within normal limits except for the duodenum which contained both an anterior and posterior duodenal scar. On the anterior wall there was a very definite area of erythema and dimpling as well as an extensive area of scarring. By palpation with a finger in the foramen of Winslow, it was felt that the ulcer did not involve the common duct. It was decided that a resection would be the procedure of choice.

Attention was then turned to the stomach, where, under adequate visualization, the gastrocolic and gastrolienal ligaments were divided between curved Kelly clamps and ligated with sutures of 0 chromic catgut. After adequate mobilization of the duodenum and greater curvature, the index finger was placed through the gastrohepatic ligament in an avascular plane and the vessels and ligaments to the lesser curvature of the stomach were divided between curved Kelly clamps and ligated in a similar manner. The duodenum was then ready for division. The clamp was placed just proximal to the pylorus and the duodenum was divided just below this clamp. With the stump of the duodenum open, one could see that there was some posterior scarring. Bile was seen to flow freely from the duodenal stump.

The duodenal stump was closed with a three layer closure using 00 chromic catgut suture which was reinforced with interrupted 000 dacron sutures. The body of the stump was further mobilized by clamping and dividing further the gastrocolic and gastrohepatic ligaments for a distance involving approximately 70% of the stomach. The stomach was then ready for division.

Two long intestinal clamps were placed across two-thirds of the stomach in a transverse manner. The stomach was partially divided. A second set of clamps was placed across the lesser curvature portion of the stomach in 45 degree angles and the stomach divided. A continuous atraumatic chromic catgut suture was placed upon the lesser curvature clamp which was removed and the suture drawn taut. An additional chromic catgut suture was then run back and tied. A third layer of a continuous 000 cotton suture completed the closure of the lesser curvature aspect of the stomach.

The ligament of Treitz was found by grasping the transverse colon, maintaining general traction and bringing up a loop of jejunum, 14 to 18 cm. from the ligament of Treitz, to be anastomosed to the stomach in an antecolic fashion. The anastomosis was closed with a two layer closure using continuous 000 chromic catgut suture which was reinforced with interrupted 000 dacron sutures.

After adequate hemostasis had been attained, the anastomotic site and duodenal stump were checked for bleeding and leakage. None were found and therefore closure of the wound was begun by approximating the peritoneum with 00 general closure suture. The fascia was closed with interrupted 00 dacron figure-of-eight sutures. A medium size Penrose drain was inserted into the subcutaneous tissues and brought out through a separate stab wound incision, inferior to the primary incision. Subcutaneous tissues were then approximated with interrupted 000 chromic catgut sutures and the skin with 00 dermalon in a continuous subcuticular suture.

During the operation the patient received 500 cc. of 5% glucose in water and 500 cc. of whole blood.

GASTROSCOPY

The interior of the esophagus and stomach can be examined without recourse to surgery by means of endoscopic procedures called esophagoscopy and gastroscopy. A scope is introduced by way of the mouth and passed into the esophagus and stomach. With the aid of a light and a lens system, the interior of these organs may be visualized and even biopsied. Aspirations can also be collected by this method for Papanicolaou smears and cytologic studies.

Gastroscopy is an adjunct to roentgenologic studies. Any instrumentation is usually preceded by x-ray examinations of the esophagus, stomach and mediastinum to rule out the presence of conditions which would contraindicate such a procedure.

These examinations are performed by specially trained endoscopists who may be internists or surgeons. The otolaryngologist performs endoscopic examinations of the esophagus but does not, as a rule, carry his examination into the stomach.

GASTROSCOPES

ACMI	Ellsner
Benedict Operating	Herman Taylor
Bernstein modification	Housset-Debray
Chevalier Jackson	Janeway
Eder	Kelling
Eder-Chamberlin	Peroral Chevalier Jackson
Eder-Hufford	Schindler
Eder-Palmer	Wolf-Schindler

ESOPHAGOSCOPES

Ballooning	Chevalier Jackson
Boros	Haslinger

ESOPHAGOSCOPES (Continued)

Holinger
Jackson full lumen
Jesberg
Lell
Mosher
Moure

Roberts folding
Sam Roberts
Schindler optical
Tucker
Yankauer

Gastroscopy

Sodium amytal I.M. and atropine grains 1/150 were administered while the patient was on call to the OR. In the operating room, the buccal, oral and pharyngeal mucosa were sprayed with 1% Xylocaine with epinephrine. There were no untoward results. 100 mgm. of Demerol was given intravenously and the patient turned on her left side.

An Eder-Hufford gastroscope was introduced with minimal difficulty. The scope was passed to depth I. The incisura was readily identified. On the anterior and greater curvature wall of the stomach, just proximal to the incisura, there were noted six separate 3 to 5 mm. polyps, none of which were ulcerative. There was no evidence of surrounding infiltration. On the anterior wall, proximal to the polyps described, there was a linear fold which was a pseudopolyp. This was hemorrhagic, but without ulceration. The venous pattern could be readily seen throughout the stomach indicating an atrophic gastritis. The lesser curvature was normal.

The scope was gently withdrawn and the patient returned to the ward in satisfactory condition.

Esophagogastroscopy

The patient was given Sodium amytal grains 2 prior to coming to the operating room and atropine grains 1/100 on call to the OR. In the operating room, the buccal, oral and pharyngeal mucosa were sprayed with 1% Xylocaine and epinephrine. The patient was given 50 mgm. of Demerol and turned on his left side.

A flexible Eder-Hufford esophagoscope was introduced without difficulty. The epiglottis was visualized as was the pyriform sinus. The lumen of the esophagus was kept in constant view. The scope was gently urged through the Cricopharyngeus muscle as the patient swallowed. A definite hiatal hernia was noted measuring about 2-3 cm. The mucosa of the stomach and distal esophagus were markedly edematous. No true varices were seen. No evidence of esophagitis was noted. The scope was gently withdrawn.

An Eder-Chamberlin gastroscope was introduced to depth I. The pylorus was readily seen, unusually so, in all quadrants and appeared normal throughout. The scope was then withdrawn and reinserted into the body of the stomach and greater curvature. At the junction of the posterior wall there was a large fold, abnormal in color, with two pinpoint ulcerations on its surface measuring about 1-2 cm. and very highly suspicious of malignancy. The mucosa proximal to this area was markedly atrophic with a definite venous pattern. The scope was removed.

Esophagoscopy

The patient was given Sodium amytal grs. 2 I.M. and atropine grains 1/100 on the ward. In the OR, the buccal, oral and pharyngeal mucosa were sprayed with 1% Xylocaine and epinephrine with no untoward results. The patient was given 75 mgm. of Demerol intravenously. He was turned on his left side. The esophagoscope obturator was passed without difficulty. The cardioesophageal junction was identified.

There was no evidence of hiatal hernia, varicosities, ulcerations, tumefactions or areas of inflammation. As the scope was slowly removed, the mucosa was inspected. There were no lesions noted. No hyperemia of the mucosa was seen. The scope was removed and the patient returned to the ward in good condition.

GASTROSTOMY

The purpose of all gastrostomy procedures is to establish a fistulous communication between the stomach and the surface of the abdominal wall in order that the patient might be fed. A permanent fistula is formed in cases of inoperable stricture of the larynx, pharynx or esophagus. A temporary and palliative gastrostomy is formed in those cases where the disease process is obstructing and the patient does not have much longer to live or as an expedient measure in conditions which are being corrected.

GASTROSTOMY TECHNIQUES

Beck-Jianu
DePage-Janeway
Kader
Marwedel

Spivack
Stamm
Witzel

Gastrostomy

The patient's abdomen was sterilely prepared and draped. Using ½% Xylocaine as a local anesthetic, an area in the left upper quadrant of the abdomen was infiltrated through the skin and muscle.

A transverse incision was made midway between the umbilicus and xiphoid. The lateral fibers of the rectus muscle were clamped, divided and ligated. The posterior sheath was then infiltrated with Xylocaine and it was entered. The stomach was reached and brought out through the wound with gentle traction. A purse-string of 00 chromic was then used on the greater curvature near the vascular supply.

A stab wound was made in the stomach and a #30 mushroom catheter was inserted. The purse-string was then tied and the catheter was rein-serted into the stomach with two other circumferential purse-strings of chromic. This provided a secure gastrostomy. The stomach serosa was then tacked to the anterior peritoneal wall circumferentially with interrupted chromic stitches. The wound was closed in layers.

PYLOROPLASTY AND GASTRODUODENOSTOMY

The pylorus is the distal aperture of the stomach which opens into the duodenum. It is the site of frequent obstructing stenosis necessitating pyloroplasty. Surgery on the pylorus is also indicated to relieve gastric stasis and promote emptying of the stomach which loses its tone following vagotomy. The Heinecke-Mikulicz pyloroplasty is the most widely prac-ticed technique today for facilitating gastric drainage by enlarging the gastric opening.

PYLOROPLASTY TECHNIQUES

Finney	Judd
Heinecke-Mikulicz	Ramstedt
Horsley	Weinberg's Modification
Jaboulay	of Heinecke-Mikulicz

ANATOMIC FEATURES

Duodenum (duodenal)	Pyloric antrum
Gastrocolic omentum	Pyloric sphincter
Gastrohepatic omentum	Pyloric valve
Gastrolienal ligament	Pyloric vestibule
Greater and lesser curvature	Sulcus intermedius
Greater omentum	

Ramstedt Pyloromyotomy

Using ether anesthesia administered by drop and open mask method, a vertical 1½ inch rectus muscle splitting incision was made high in the epigastrium. It was carried through the posterior sheath to the peritoneum which was carefully picked up and incised.

The liver was carefully retracted upwards and the pyloric region of the stomach was brought into the wound. A longitudinal incision was then made in the hypertrophied area. A 1 inch incision was begun just proximal to the pyloric vein of Mayo at the gastroduodenal junction. It was carried through the peritoneal and superficial muscular layers over the pyloric lesion and then slightly beyond into the antrum of the stomach. The muscle fibers were bluntly separated with a knife handle for the length of the incision. The dissection continued until the mucous membrane gaped widely in the incision. Constricting fibers were released and patency of the pylorus assured. The duodenum was checked and found to be intact.

The stomach was replaced in the abdomen and the wound closed in layers with two continuous sutures of 000 chromic catgut. The skin edges were approximated with interrupted vertical mattress sutures of fine Deknatel.

Abdominal Vagotomy

In certain cases of duodenal ulcer, where the nervous phase of gastric secretion is found to be abnormally great, complete division of the vagus nerves to the stomach is indicated. This operation is called a gastric vagotomy and is usually performed in conjunction with a gastrojejunostomy or pyloroplasty.

Technique: (using transabdominal approach)

Under general anesthesia the patient was prepared and sterilely draped in the supine position.

A left paramedian incision was made extending from the xiphoid to 2 cm. below the umbilicus. The incision was carried through the anatomic layers of the abdomen. The peritoneum was picked up and incised.

The abdominal viscera were carefully examined and palpated. There was no pathology noted. The left lobe of the liver was pulled down into the operative field disclosed the coronary ligament which was divided with scissors. The left lobe of the liver was retracted to the right, exposing the lower esophagus and upper stomach. A 1 cm. transverse incision was then made about 1 cm. above the esophageal hiatus. This aperture was enlarged by blunt finger dissection. Using gentle finger dissection, the lower portion of the esophagus was separated from its areolar tissue. The esophagus was drawn downward, bringing into view the left (anterior) vagus nerve. It was seen to course along the front of the esophagus in the direction of the lesser curvature of the stomach. The right (posterior) vagus nerve was felt on the posterior aspect of the esophagus. By blunt finger dissection, the right vagus was separated from the esophageal wall. It was brought out on the left where it was ligated and divided between silk sutures, after it had been clamped superiorly. A 5 cm. segment of the nerve was resected. The left vagus was similarly treated, also being divided 7 cm. above its entrance into the stomach on the lesser curvature aspect.

The esophagus was drawn down further to facilitate investigation for additional vagus branches. None were found and the esophagus was therefore permitted to retract into the mediastinum. A few interrupted catgut sutures were used to close the opening in the diaphragm. The left lobe of the liver was returned to its former position without resuturing the coronary ligament.

A posterior gastroenterostomy was then performed with the anastomosis situated about 5 cm. from the pylorus. A satisfactory stoma was obtained.

SURGERY OF THE SMALL BOWEL

The small bowel begins at the duodenum with its sphincter of Oddi and papilla of Vater, followed by the jejunum, ileum and ileocecal valve. The gastrointestinal tract beyond this point is regarded as the colon or large intestine. Resection of the small bowel is referred to generally as an enterectomy whereas resection of the large bowel is termed colectomy. The same is true of anastomosis of the small bowel which is referred to as enterostomy or enteroenterostomy. The terms colostomy, colocolostomy, etc., are applied only to anastomoses of the large bowel.

An anastomosis may assume any of the following combinations:

ENTEROENTEROSTOMY
(small bowel to small bowel)

Duodenoduodenostomy	Jejunojejunostomy
Duodenojejunostomy	Jejuno-ileostomy
Duodeno-ileostomy	Ileoileostomy

ENTEROCOLOSTOMY
(small bowel to large bowel)

Jejuno-ileostomy
Jejunocolostomy
Ileocecostomy

Ileocolostomy
Ileosigmoidostomy

COLOCOLOSTOMY
(large bowel to large bowel)

Cecocolostomy
Cecosigmoidostomy
Colocolostomy

Colosigmoidostomy
Coloproctostomy
Sigmoidoproctostomy

A variety of methods have been devised to provide anastomosis between sections of the bowel following resection. The end-to-end method probably affords the most satisfactory anatomic continuity when the caliber of both segments of the bowel to be joined is alike. A number of factors dictate the surgeon's choice of techniques, some of which have been listed below.

CLOSED METHODS
OF ANASTOMOSIS

Basting stitch method
Bulkhead method
Dennis two-clamp & one layer silk
Furniss clamp method
Moskowitz & Rankin
  three-bladed clamp
O'Hara two-clamp method

Parker & Kerr basting stitch method
Parlavecchio & Halsted
  bulkhead method
Perret & Babcock one-clamp method
Schoemaker & Wangensteen
  modified two-clamp

OPEN METHODS
OF ANASTOMOSIS

End-to-end
Side-to-side

End-to-side
Side-to-end

Gastrojejunostomy

Gastrojejunostomy is a short-circuiting operation in which the pylorus leading into the duodenum is occluded and a new opening created between the stomach and the jejunum. The digestive route thereafter moves from the stomach to the jejunum rather than through the normal route of stomach, duodenum and jejunum. One of the most common indications for this operation is chronic duodenal ulcer. The operation is often utilized alone in the elderly, debilitated patient with a chronic duodenal ulcer or obstruction. In most instances, gastrojejunostomy is preceded by a vagotomy.

GASTROJEJUNOSTOMY
TECHNICS

Antecolic
Anterior
Antiperistaltic
Brenner
Isoperistaltic
Kocher

Lahey anterior
Mayo
Moynihan
No-Loop
Posterior

ANATOMIC
STRUCTURES ENCOUNTERED

Antral stoma
Duodenojejunal flexure
Gastrocolic ligament
Gastrocolic omentum
Gastroenteric stoma
Greater curvature
Incisura angularis
Jejunal loop

Ligament of Treitz
Mesocolon
Middle colic artery
Omentum
Proximal jejunum
Pylorus
Stoma
Vascular epiploic arch

Anterior Gastrojejunostomy

Anterior or antecolic gastrojejunostomy is sometimes indicated in cases of inoperable cancer involving the antrum of the stomach and pylorus, particularly when there is associated obstruction. The anterior gastrojejunostomy is performed more commonly than the posterior.

Technique:

Under spinal anesthesia, a semilunar incision was made approximately 1½ inches below the xiphoid. The incision extended directly over both recti. The anterior rectus sheath was dissected and transected transversely. The posterior rectus sheath and peritoneum were entered.

Upon entering the peritoneal cavity, there was a large tumor mass involving the prepyloric area, the pylorus and the first portion of the duodenum. The mass measured 14-15 cm. in diameter. It was hard and indurated. There was edema of the remaining portion of the stomach. The liver contained several hard nodules on the right, at the midportion. The tumor mass appeared to involve the hepatoduodenal ligament as well as the head of the pancreas and the hepatic triad. The entire hepatic triad was hard and firm upon examination through the foramen of Winslow. The tumor was also kissing into the pancreas. In view of these findings, resection of the stomach seemed advisable.

The jejunum was identified with the ligament of Treitz and brought anterior to the stomach. The stomach was brought into the operative field, toward the midportion, and an anastomosis accomplished anterior to the transverse colon using 000 cotton suture for the posterior seromuscular layer. The stomach and the jejunum were then incised for the anterior gastrojejunostomy.

A through-and-through 000 chromic suture was used for the posterior layer utilizing this as a continental anterior leaf. A second row of seromuscular sutures was placed. The stoma measured approximately 5-6 cm. in diameter.

The peritoneal cavity was closed with a continuous 00 chromic suture. The fascia was closed with 000 suture and the skin with subcuticular nylon suture.

Jejunostomy

In certain cases of gastric malignancy, a jejunostomy operation is indicated for feeding purposes. An opening is made in the abdominal wall and in a loop of jejunum which is anchored to the abdominal wall. A catheter is introduced through the opening and sutured in place. The feeding tube is usually fixed in the opening in such a way that it cannot be removed. The procedure serves the purpose of maintaining nourishment in far advanced, inoperable cases of cancer of the stomach where survival is not expected to exceed four to five months.

JEJUNOSTOMY TECHNIQUES

Marwedel	Travel
Mayo-Robson	Witzel

Marwedel Jejunostomy

The patient is prepared and draped sterilely in a routine manner. Under general anesthesia, a vertical 2 inch incision is made just below the tip of the ninth costal cartilage on the left. The incision is carried through the anatomic layers of the abdomen following which, the peritoneum is picked up and incised.

A loop of jejunum about 10 inches from the duodenojejunal flexure is selected for the jejunostomy. A 2 inch incision is carried down to the mucosa on the antemesenteric border of the loop of jejunum. The seromuscular layer is dissected from the mucosa on either side of the incision forming the trough in which the catheter will be implanted. Careful identification of the distal portion of the bowel is ascertained and a purse-string of 00 chromic catgut is placed. An opening made in the center of the bowel with a bistoury for insertion of the catheter. A # 14 French catheter is introduced for a distance of 11 cm., following which, suction is applied. The purse-string is drawn closed and tied with the ends being left long.

The seromuscular layer is closed over the catheter using interrupted fine silk sutures, the ends of which are also left long. A stab wound is then made through which the catheter and long ends of the purse-string are brought up, positioning the jejunum adjacent to the peritoneum. The long ends of the catgut used in the purse-string are fixed to the fascia. The seromuscular sutures are threaded on a free needle and sutured to the adjacent peritoneum. The jejunum is anchored to the abdominal wall for a distance of 3 inches to reduce the likelihood of angulation. The catheter is fixed permanently in place and sutured to the skin.

SURGERY OF THE COLON

The large bowel or colon extends beyond the ileocecal valve for about five or six feet. It consists of the cecum, ascending colon, transverse colon, descending colon, sigmoid and rectum, which have a noticeably larger caliber than the preceding small intestine. The average diameter of the large bowel is approximately two and one-half inches, diminishing somewhat toward the end of the tract.

Resection of any portion of the colon is termed a colectomy; however, excision of the cecum, sigmoid and rectum may be more specifically designated as cecectomy, sigmoidectomy and proctectomy, respectively. Total colectomy includes removal of the entire large bowel from its beginning at the cecum to its termination with the rectum.

Some other operations performed on the colon include *cecostomy*, performed for rupture of the cecum or colonic obstruction with severe distention; *loop colostomy*, for decompression and defunctioning of the bowel; and, *primary resection and anastomosis of the colon* for resectable lesions.

Malignant growths of the colon which cannot be resected in their entirety often require a palliative type procedure. Resection of the primary lesion and a short-circuiting operation such as an ileocolostomy or lateral colocolostomy, etc., are usually performed in cases where there is hope of extending survival for three or more years. In such cases, where the parent lesion cannot be removed, palliation may be afforded by a short-circuiting operation such as a lateral ileocolostomy.

In a colostomy procedure, an artificial opening is surgically formed, bringing the colon up to an opening in the abdominal wall. A single opening may be made in the colon or a double opening known as a double-barrel colostomy. Bowel contents are ejected through this newly formed opening into a pouch worn by the patient. A colostomy may be temporary for the purpose of defunctioning the bowel in preparation for a later resection, or may be a permanent opening. Regardless of which form it assumes, it is essentially a short-circuiting operation.

ANATOMIC FEATURES IN COLON SURGERY

Anastomotic site
Appendices epiploicae
Ascending colon
Cecum
Colic flexure
Colic valve
Descending colon
Duodenocolic ligament
Frenula of the valve
Gastrocolic omentum
Gastrosplenic omentum
Hepatic flexure
Houston's valves
Ileocecal junction
Ileocecal valve
Ileocolic junction
Ileum
Iliac colon
Iliacus
Lumen

Mesentery
Mesocolon
Omentum
Phrenicocolic ligament
Psoas major
Quadratus lumborum
Rectal ampulla
Rectosigmoid
Sigmoid colon
Sigmoid flexure
Sigmoid mesocolon
Splenic flexure
Stoma
Stump
Superior aperture of lesser pelvis
Taenia
Terminal ileal segment
Transverse colon
Transverse mesocolon
Vermiform process

ARTERIAL SUPPLY IN COLON SURGERY

Anterior cecal
Appendicular
External iliac
Ileal
Ileocolic
Inferior hemorrhoidal
Inferior mesenteric
Left colic
Marginal

Middle colic
Middle hemorrhoidal
Piriformis
Posterior cecal
Right colic
Sigmoidal br. of inf. mesenteric
Spermatic
Superior hemorrhoidal
Superior mesenteric

Left Segmental Colectomy

Under spinal anesthesia, the patient was placed in the supine position, prepared and draped in the usual manner.

An infraumbilical midline incision, measuring approximately 3 inches in length, was made. The incision was taken down through the subcutaneous tissues and down to the anterior rectus sheath, which was incised transversely. The left and right recti muscles were retracted laterally and the peritoneum was grasped and entered.

Upon entering the abdominal cavity, palpatory examination of the abdominal contents was carried out. A small 3 x 3 cm. lesion in the rectosigmoid about 2 inches above the peritoneal reflection was discovered. The lesion was freely movable. It was not adherent. No lymph nodes were palpable although there were some areas of pericolonic induration. Examination of the liver failed to disclose any metastatic implants. The remaining abdominal organs were found to be within normal limits. There were some adhesions in the right upper quadrant from previous gallbladder surgery.

The lateral attachment of the colon to the parietal peritoneum was divided from below the brim of the pelvis, up to and just above the sigmoid colon. As the colon was mobilized medially, the spermatic vessels came into view. The left ureter, close to the spermatic vessels, was identified and carefully reflected. After complete and adequate mobilization, the rectosigmoid was divided about 1.5 cm. below the lesion. Kocher clamps were also placed across the colon in antemesenteric fashion at the elected sites of resection, just at the level of the sigmoid colon. The adjacent tissues were carefully protected with laparotomy pads. The colon was divided and the specimen removed.

An anterior anastomosis was then performed using a two layer closure. Following this, the defect in the mesentery was closed by using a continuous 000 chromic catgut suture. Again, after rechecking the anastomotic sites and obtaining hemostasis, closure of the wound was begun. Closure was carried out by approximating the peritoneum with 00 general closure, the fascia with interrupted figure-of-eight 00 dacron sutures, the subcutaneous tissues with interrupted 000 chromic catgut sutures and the skin with 00 continuous dermalon suture.

500 cc. of 5% glucose in water and 500 cc. of whole blood were used during the operation.

Surgery of the Vermiform Appendix

The appendix is a worm-like projection of the cecum. It is a blind sac subject to inflammation, abscess, gangrene, perforation and tumors. The operation for removal of the appendix is called an appendectomy.

TERMS USED
IN APPENDECTOMY REPORTS

Appendiceal
Appendicular artery
Caput caeci
Cecum
Diffuse inflammation
Exudate
Fecalith
Fecopurulent
Friable tissue
Gangrenous
Intramural artery

Invaginated stump
Meckel's diverticulum
Meso-appendix
Oxyuriasis vermicularis (pin worms)
Peritonitis
Retrocecal
Seromuscular coat
Sheath of rectus muscle
Stump of appendix
Vermiform process

APPENDECTOMY INCISIONS

Battle's pararectal
Fowler-Weir
Kocher's Modified McBurney
McBurney's gridiron
Median

Paramedian
Rectus muscle splitting
Suprapubic
Transverse

Appendectomy

Under spinal anesthesia the patient was prepared and draped in a sterile manner.

A right lower quadrant McBurney incision was made and carried through the skin and anterior sheath, transversalis, posterior sheath and peritoneum.

The appendix was located in a retrocecal position. It was noted to be acutely inflamed. The meso-appendix was clamped and ligated with a 000 cotton suture. A purse-string suture of 000 cotton was applied around the base of the appendix; the appendix was excised and the base treated with phenol and alcohol. The base was inverted and the purse-string drawn taut and tied. Further inversion was accomplished with a Z-suture.

The cecum was examined and no Meckel's diverticulum was found. The peritoneum was closed with 000 intestinal. The transversalis, internal oblique and external oblique were closed with interrupted 000 chromic. The skin was closed with subcuticular nylon.

THE RECTUM AND ANUS

The colon ends in a 5 inch segment below the sigmoid colon which is called the rectum. The distal end of the rectum, which consists of the external aperture, is called the anus. The opening to the outside of the body is guarded by an internal and external sphincter which remains closed except to permit passage of feces during defecation.

The entire length of the rectum and anus is only 6½ inches but this short terminal segment of the gastrointestinal tract is susceptible to certain pathologic conditions. Internal and external hemorrhoids probably constitute the most common pathology of this area. Other common anorectal conditions include anal fissure, anal fistula and ischiorectal abscess. Adenocarcinoma is the most frequently encountered malignancy in this region.

ANORECTAL STRUCTURES

Anal canal
Anal orifice
Anal valves
Anococcygeal body
Anus
Columns of Morgagni
External sphincter
Houston's valves
Internal sphincter
Lateral ligaments
Levator ani
Mucocutaneous junction

Mucous membrane
Pelvic colon (sigmoid)
Rectal ampulla
Rectal columns
Rectal sinuses
Rectococcygeal muscles
Rectosigmoid
Sigmoid (pelvic colon)
Rugae
Sphincter ani
Transverse rectal folds

ANORECTAL CIRCULATION

Hemorrhoidal plexus
Hypogastric artery
Inferior hemorrhoidal artery
Inferior rectal vein
Internal iliac vein
Internal pudendal artery

Left colic vein
Middle hemorrhoidal artery
Middle hemorrhoidal vein
Superior hemorrhoidal branch
    of inferior mesenteric artery
Superior rectal veins

Incision and Drainage of Ischiorectal Abscess

Under spinal anesthesia the patient was prepared and draped. An ischiorectal abscess of the right buttocks was then drained in the following manner. A sinus was probed on the lateral middle surface of the abscess. It was approximately 1½ inches from the rectal surface. Following the probing, a crypt was made in the posterior one half of the anus.

Sims retractors were then placed in the rectum. Using a knife, the skin and subcutaneous tissue along with the rectal sphincter were transected. The redundant portion of the sinus tract was dissected free with blunt and sharp dissection using Metzenbaum scissors. The area was packed with Iodoform gauze. Bleeders were clamped and ligated with 000 chromic suture.

Sigmoidoscopy With Rectal Polypectomy

Under spinal anesthesia, the patient was placed in the prone jack-knife position, prepared and draped in the usual manner.

A sigmoidoscope was introduced into the anus and passed to a level of about 13 cm. without difficulty. At this level, a small broad sessile type polyp, somewhat necrotic in appearance and bleeding moderately, was noted. The lesion was irregular in size and shape and had an extremely broad base. It measured 2 cm. in its greatest diameter. It was initially believed to be malignant and a biopsy was therefore taken. Bleeding was minimal and required no cautery or coagulation.

The scope was passed a little further and another small polyp was seen at approximately 15 cm. This polyp was also sessile but only measured 3 mm. in diameter. This was also removed. Without any further manipulation, the scope was removed. The specimens were sent to the laboratory for histopathologic examination.

Hemorrhoidectomy

Under spinal anesthesia the patient was placed in the prone jack-knife position, prepared and draped in routine fashion.

Examination of the rectum and anus revealed that there were hemorrhoids located in the usual positions, right anterior and posterior and left lateral. With the Fansler anoscope in place, internal and external hemorrhoid tags were noted in the right anterior position. A 00 chromic catgut suture was placed through the apex of the internal hemorrhoidal tag, pulled taut and tied. The hemorrhoidal tissue was excised. Excision was carried down to the external sphincter. Distally, excision extended to the level of the mucocutaneous junction.

Hemostasis was obtained by approximating the mucous membrane with a continuous 00 chromic catgut suture. Bleeding was minimal and controlled with hemostats and ligatures, as necessary.

The hemorrhoidal tags and tissue located at the other positions were treated in a similar manner. After adequate hemostasis, a rubber glove filled with Pontocainal ointment was placed in the rectum for comfort and dilatation.

Anal Sphincterotomy and Excision of Hemorrhoidal Tags

Under spinal anesthesia, the patient was placed in the prone position and the buttocks retracted. Manual dilatation of the anal canal revealed some external hemorrhoidal tags at the 12, 3 and 6 o'clock positions. There were also a few internal hemorrhoids present.

The hemorrhoidal vessels were ligated with 000 chromic catgut suture. A partial dissection of the external and internal hemorrhoids was carried out. The sphincter was completely dissected, posteriorly. A partial sphincterotomy was done. Following resection of the mucus membrane of the internal and external hemorrhoids, the mucous membrane was anastomosed to the skin with 0000 chromic intestinal suture.

Abdominal-Perineal Resection—**Proctosigmoidectomy (Miles Operation)**

The patient is placed in the Trendelenburg position, prepared and draped. The abdominal cavity is entered through a right paramedian incision which begins at the crest of the pubis and is carried upward to a point 2 inches above the umbilicus. The skin margins are protected and a self-retaining retractor is introduced for the abdominal portion of the operation.

Exploration of the abdominal and pelvic cavity is carried out. There is no evidence of peritoneal implants. The liver is normal. The colon is thoroughly examined and no other area of pathology noted. The gallbladder is within normal limits with no evidence of stones. There are no palpable nodes along the inferior mesenteric vessels.

The intestines are packed away out of the operative field and the pelvic colon is drawn up through the wound. Scissors are used to lyse the adhesions which attach the sigmoid loop to the lateral wall of the pelvis. This lysis is carried out on the outer side of the pelvic mesocolon to facilitate delivery of the colon out of the abdominal cavity. The stem of the inferior mesenteric artery is ligated close to the aorta. The inferior mesenteric vein is then isolated and ligated as high up as is possible. The lateral peritoneal leaf of the mesosigmoid is then divided and the incision carried down into the pelvis, along the rectum, across the base of the bladder and then upward on to the other side of the mesentery. This provides better mobilization of the sigmoid and rectum. The pelvic mesocolon is completely divided, followed by the peritoneum, as far as the promontory of the sacrum. Care is taken to avoid injury to the ureter. Following division of the peritoneum on both sides, the fingers of the operator's left hand are introduced into the cellular space between the terminal pelvic mesocolon and anterior surface of the sacrum. The terminal pelvic colon and rectum are stripped from their attachments as far down as the sacrococcygeal articulation. Adhesive bands, extending from the sacrum to the fascia propria, are lysed with scissors. With the operator's left hand in the presacral space, the rectum is pressed upward and forward. The pelvic peritoneum, elevated in this process, is divided on either side following the brim of the true pelvis to the base of the bladder. The ureters are carefully identified and kept out of the way. The incisions in the peritoneum are extended until they come together anteriorly behind the base of the bladder. Separation of the rectum from the base of the bladder and from the vesiculae seminales is carried out. The separation of the rectum anteriorly is extended as far as the upper limits of the prostate gland. The lateral ligaments, attaching the rectum, are completely divided down to the upper surfaces of the levator ani muscles. The middle hemorrhoidal artery is divided and ligated.

Using three deMartel clamps, the pelvic colon is crushed approximately 3 inches from the end of the descending colon. The middle clamp is removed and a cautery used to burn through the colon between the two remaining clamps. The divided ends of the bowel are wrapped in waterproof sheeting which is securely tied to avoid spillage. The peritoneum is then mobilized for reconstruction of the floor of the pelvis. The edges of the defect in the peritoneum are approximated posteriorly, in front of the promontory of the sacrum and are then sutured to the stump of the pelvic mesocolon. Peritoneum is brought up from the base and lateral aspects of the bladder to cover the remaining defect. The newly constructed pelvic floor is sutured securely.

A permanent colostomy is created by bringing the proximal pelvic colon, which was severed, up through a circular opening (2 inches in diameter) in the abdominal wall. Silk sutures are used to fix the stump into position. The stump is allowed to protrude for about 3 inches beyond the skin level. A few interrupted catgut sutures are placed between the lateral wall of the pelvis and the cut edge of the pelvic mesocolon. Packs and swabs are removed and the incision is sutured in layers. The wound is dressed and the patient repositioned in the Sims' position on his left side for the perineal procedure.

The anus is closed with a purse-string suture. A transverse incision, about four inches in length, is made at the level of the sacrococcygeal articulation. From the center of this, a longitudinal incision is made in the internatal furrow and extended to a point one inch from the posterior margin of the anus. Radiating from the inferior extremity, incisions are made to the left and to the right of the anus in a horseshoe-shaped fashion, and the extremities of these are joined by a transverse cut. As a precaution against recurrence, the incision is made to embrace a wide area of perianal skin.

The coccyx is exposed by reflecting and retracting the gluteal skin flaps. An opening is made in the sacrococcygeal joint and the coccyx dissected out. The incisions around the anus are deepened to include as much of the ischiorectal fat as possible. A small transverse incision is made in the connective tissue below the sacrum. The index finger is then introduced into the space containing the isolated bowel. A transverse incision is made through the Coccygeus muscle on either side and carried to the sacrosciatic ligaments. The isolated bowel is drawn down through this opening. Traction is made on the bowel with the left hand causing the Levatores ani to come into view. The anterior wall of the anal canal is then dissected away from the central aspect of the perineum. The rectum and isolated portion of the pelvic colon are removed.

The skin incision is closed with sutures and the wounds dressed. The deMartel clamp on the proximal end of the pelvic colon is removed and the open end of the bowel wrapped in a protective covering and a pad of gauze. A Foley type bag-catheter is inserted into the dead space and brought out of the most dependent anterior portion of the wound.

THE GALLBLADDER

There are several operations which are commonly performed on the gallbladder because of the tendency for calculi to form in this organ (cholelithiasis). These stones often occlude the common bile duct (choledocholithiasis) making it necessary to explore this region as well as the gallbladder proper.

Some of the operations performed on the gallbladder include:

CHOLECYSTECTOMY	Excision of the gallbladder.
CHOLECYSTOTOMY	Incision into the gallbladder.
CHOLECYSTOSTOMY	Incision and drainage of the gallbladder.
CHOLECYSTOLITHOTOMY	Incision into the gallbladder with removal of calculus.
CHOLEDOCHOLITHOTOMY	Incision into the common bile duct with removal of calculus (calculi).

ANATOMIC STRUCTURES
ENCOUNTERED IN
GALLBLADDER SURGERY

Ampulla of Vater
Bile duct
Common duct
Cystic artery
Cystic duct
Ductus choledochus
Ductus hepaticus
Foramen of Winslow
Fossa in the liver

Fundus of gallbladder
Gallbladder bed
Hartmann's pouch
Heister, spiral valve of
Hepatic artery
Hepatic duct
Hepatic fossa
Liver bed

Cholecystectomy

Under spinal anesthesia the patient was prepared and draped in the supine position.

A right subcostal Kocher incision was made. The skin was incised and the incision carried down through the anterior rectus sheath, rectus muscle, posterior sheath and peritoneum. Bleeders were clamped and ligated with 000 chromic suture.

The gallbladder was found to be markedly edematous, thickened and hyperemic. It measured approximately 15 cm. in length and 4 cm. in diameter. There were numerous adhesions around the gallbladder which were lysed by blunt dissection.

Exploration of the abdominal contents was normal. The finger could be inserted into the foramen of Winslow. The common duct was free of stones.

The gallbladder was removed by using Carmel clamps to grasp the fundus and Hartmann's pouch. The cystic duct was then clamped, divided and doubly ligated with 000 cotton. The cystic artery was likewise clamped, divided and ligated with 00 cotton and the gallbladder removed. The gallbladder bed was oversewn with a continuous locking 00 chromic. A medium sized Penrose drain was placed into the foramen of Winslow and brought out through a separate stab wound in the abdomen.

The peritoneum was closed along with the posterior sheath using chromic. The fascia was closed in layers with cotton, the subcutaneous tissue with chromic and the skin edges were approximated with dermalon.

Transduodenal Excision of Common Duct Stone; Sphincterotomy of Oddi

The patient had sustained a cholecystectomy 18 months previously. She has had repeated episodes of right upper quadrant intermittent abdominal pain associated with nausea and vomiting since. I.V. cholangiograms revealed a large calculus within the common duct with dilation of the duct.

Under spinal anesthesia, an incision was made through a previous scar and extended through the anterior rectus sheath, posterior rectus sheath and peritoneum. Multiple dense adhesions were encountered. The adhesions were lysed from the peritoneum. The renal vessels were visualized. Small bleeders were ligated. The duodenum and the common duct were identified.

The ampulla was palpated by inserting two fingers in the foramen of Winslow and getting the duodenum and pancreas in front of the fingers. A calculus measuring 1½ cm. was felt within the second portion of the duodenum near the sphincter of Oddi. It appeared to be firmly stuck at this point.

A longitudinal incision was made in an avascular area. The incision extended down through the sphincter. A calculus measuring 1½ cm. was extracted from the ampulla of Vater. The sphincter was cut in removing the stone. Bile was expressed very easily following removal of the stone. It appeared to be clear.

The duodenum was closed with a Connell 0000 continuous chromic suture and an interrupted three layer of cotton suture. All bleeding points were ligated. A through-and-through # 30 wire suture was used to approximate the various layers. A drain was inserted in the gallbladder bed and brought out through a separate stab wound.

PANCREATODUODENECTOMY

Resectable growths of the head of the pancreas and of the ampullary region are treated by radical pancreatoduodenectomy. This is not a commonly performed procedure because only the early and favorable cases are selected for resection. During the exploration which precedes and determines resectability, the surgeon examines the liver for neoplastic studding, the portal fissure for malignant nodes and the peritoneum, pelvic shelf, omentum and mesentery for malignant seedlings. The surgeon further determines whether or not there is any extension or invasion of the vena cava, portal vein or superior mesenteric vessels which would contraindicate surgery.

A description of the Whipple operation follows to illustrate the terminology encountered in descriptions of this operation.

PANCREATODUODENECTOMY
TECHNIQUES

Brunschwig	Two-Stage
Cattell	Warren
Child's	Watson
One-Stage	Waugh
Poth	Whipple

Whipple Operation (Pancreatoduodenectomy)

Under general and spinal anesthesia, the patient was prepared and draped in the usual manner.

An epigastric transverse incision was made subcostally, approximately 14 to 16 inches in length. The anterior rectus sheath was incised, rectus muscle transected on the right and the posterior sheath and peritoneum opened.

It was noted on exploration that the area of the pancreas was somewhat enlarged and the head of the pancreas was quite hard in consistency. Upon palpation of the ampulla of Vater, a small nodule was detected. The liver was free of implants. There was no evidence, on inspection and palpation, of metastases or involvement of the great vessels. Resection was decided upon.

The peritoneal reflection of the duodenum was incised and a Kocher's maneuver used to reflect the peritoneum laterally. The common duct was dissected free. It was noted that the common duct and the gallbladder were also greatly enlarged, the duct being approximately a half inch in diameter.

The greater curvature of the stomach was dissected free and bleeders were clamped and ligated with 0 chromic suture. The lesser curvature was isolated in a similar fashion. The stomach was then transected and approximately 40% of it was removed. A clamp was left in the proximal segment distally with the common duct being transected approximately 2 inches from its terminal portion. With blunt and sharp dissection, the duodenum was dissected free. In the area of the ligament of Treitz, dissection was performed. Bleeders were clamped and ligated with 000 intestinal. The mesentery was then dissected from the jejunum to the superior mesenteric artery. With blunt and sharp dissection, the duodenum was carried, in a retrograde fashion, behind the superior mesentery and brought out anteriorly. It was noted that the head of the pancreas was then easily dissectible. Dissection was therefore carried out in a blunt and sharp manner. There was no invasion in the area of the superior mesentery or celiac axis. There were two nodes present in the area of the common duct which were removed with the dissection. On pathologic examination they were reported as possibly malignant.

On transection of the head of the pancreas, it was noted that the ducts of Wirsung and Santorini were greatly dilated. A stem of a # 14 rubber catheter was placed in the duct of Wirsung. Santorini's duct was ligated. With a through-and-through suture, the rest of the pancreas was ligated so that no evidence of any leakage was present at this point. This completed the dissection of the duodenum, the first portion of the jejunum, and the head of the pancreas along with part of the common duct. The terminal portion of the jejunum was placed over the duct of Wirsung with an interrupted row of 000 cotton sutures. Another row was used for further inversion in a circumferential fashion. The common duct was tied with two 00 cotton sutures and the fundus of the gallbladder was then anastomosed to the jejunum with a posterior row of 000 cotton sutures. A musculomucosal row of 000 chromic intestinal posteriorly, locked anteriorly, was Connelled to anastomose the gallbladder and the jejunum. Further inversion was performed with 000 cotton, anteriorly.

The jejunum was grasped and brought up the proper length to the stomach. A Polya anastomosis was then accomplished posteriorly with 000 cotton. A musculomucosal row of 000 continuous chromic posteriorly, locked anteriorly, Connell type suture was placed. Further inversion was accomplished with 000 cotton. Upon completion of this procedure, a drain was placed in the area of the duodenum and the head of the pancreas, brought out through a separate stab wound incision and tied in place with an interrupted row of 000 cotton. There was no evidence of bleeding.

The posterior sheath and peritoneum were closed with 00 chromic general type closure anteriorly. The anterior rectus sheath and external oblique were closed with # 32 wire. The skin was closed with interrupted 000 silk suture.

The patient tolerated the procedure well. During the operation, 1000 cc. of 5% glucose in water and 1000 cc. of whole blood were administered. The patient left the operating room in satisfactory condition.

THE THYROID GLAND

The thyroid gland consists of two lobes situated at the front and sides of the neck, on either side of the trachea. The right and left lobes are joined across the midline by a narrow isthmus.

The thyroid is one of the ductless endocrine glands, the others being; the parathyroids, the pituitary and the adrenals (suprarenals). These glands do not possess ducts and therefore pour their secretions (hormones) into the blood stream.

Benign adenomas and thyroid goiters provide the most frequent indications for surgery of this gland. Subtotal resections are performed more commonly than total thyroidectomy.

THYROID AND ASSOCIATED STRUCTURES

Accessory thyroid glands
Colloid goiter
Cricothyroid
Deep fascia
Hyoid bone
Isthmus
Levator glandulae thyreoideae
Omohyoid muscle
Parathyroids
Platysma muscle
Pyramidal lobe
Recurrent nerves

Ribbon muscles of the neck
Sternal notch
Sternocleidomastoid muscle
Sternohyoid muscle
Sternothyroid muscle
Strap muscles of the neck
Superficial fascia
Thyroid capsule
Thyroid cartilage
Thyroidea ima
Thyroid notch

THYROID CIRCULATION

Anastomotic branch of artery
Brachiocephalic vein
Common carotid artery
Inferior thyroid artery
Inferior thyroid vein

Internal jugular vein
Middle thyroid vein
Subclavian artery
Superior thyroid artery
Superior thyroid vein

THYROID UPTAKE
(Radioisotopes)

Medotopes
Radiocaps

Sodium Radio-Iodide (I^{131})

Subtotal Thyroidectomy—with resection of pyramidal lobe

Under general endotracheal anesthesia, the patient was sterilely prepared and draped in the usual fashion.

An orbicular incision, two fingerbreadths above the sternoclavicular notch, was made. The skin was incised as was the Platysma which was dissected free to the thyroid notch. Dissection was carried inferiorly to the retrosternal space of Burns with sharp dissection. Bleeders encountered were clamped and ligated with 000 intestinal suture. Upon completion of this procedure, a vertical incision was made in the midline between the two prethyroid muscle bundles. This incision was extended from the thyroid notch to the level of the sternal notch. The incision was carried to the sternothyroid and sternohyoid muscles. These were retracted and the surgical capsule of the thyroid gland was incised.

On inspection, the thyroid was noted to be approximately 2 to 3 times larger than normal size and there were diffuse, nodular areas throughout the entire thyroid substance.

Dissection was continued by grasping the superior lobe of the thyroid and using blunt and sharp dissection, the superior thyroid vessels were dissected free. These were clamped and ligated with 00 cotton suture. The middle thyroid vein and inferior thyroid vessels were similarly treated. In the area of the inferior thyroid, blunt and sharp dissection were used to dissect free the recurrent laryngeal nerve. After identification and under good visualization, the inferior thyroid vessels were cut, ligated with 000 cotton suture and checked for hemostasis. At this time, the hemostats were used to transect the base of the thyroid in subcapsular fashion, leaving some thyroid tissue present. Upon completion of the transection to the isthmus of the thyroid, the thyroid was dissected from the trachea using both sharp and blunt dissection. The pyramidal lobe was noted superiorly. This was dissected using blunt and sharp dissection. Bleeders were clamped and ligated with 000 cotton suture. Upon removal of the right lobe, the left lobe was similarly removed. Persistent bleeders were clamped and ligated with 000 cotton suture or 000000 cotton.

Two drains were placed into the thyroid fossa and brought out laterally through the sternocleidomastoid muscle. The midline was closed with interrupted # 60 cotton and the subcutaneous tissue and Platysma with 0000 chromic. The skin was closed with a mattress cotton suture.

The patient tolerated the procedure well and was transferred to the recovery room in good condition.

8 } *Otolaryngology (E.N.T.)*

EAR—NOSE—THROAT

Otolaryngology, also referred to as E.N.T. (Ear, Nose and Throat) or otorhinolaryngology, is a surgical specialty which concerns itself with inflammatory and surgical lesions of the ears, nose and throat. These conditions are treated medically as well as surgically with antibiotics providing important therapeutic support.

The introduction of antibiotics has probably not influenced any surgical specialty to the extent that it has otolaryngology. Many of the conditions which were formerly common occurences in the practice of the otolaryngologist are seldom seen today as a result of early antibiotic intervention. Antibiotics have also produced many ear, nose and throat conditions which were uncommon before their use.

Advances in modes of treatment have been attended by dramatic new developments in surgical techniques which enable the modern otolaryngologist to successfully manage conditions for which, only a few years ago, no help was available.

In the field of otology (ear), some of the most spectacular progress has been made. There is possibly no more exacting and sensitive operation in any branch of surgery than the *stapedectomy*, performed for clinical otosclerosis.

In the field of rhinology (nose), pyogenic infections are better controlled; however, surgical conditions such as deviated nasal septum, nasal polyps, sinus defects and nasal fractures are no less common.

The otolaryngologist, skilled in modern surgical techniques, is equipped to care for almost all conditions of the neck with the possible exception of thyroidectomy operations. He does not routinely perform thyroidectomies unless the thyroid must be sacrificed in the course of a radical neck operation.

One of the more recent developments in laryngology (throat) is an

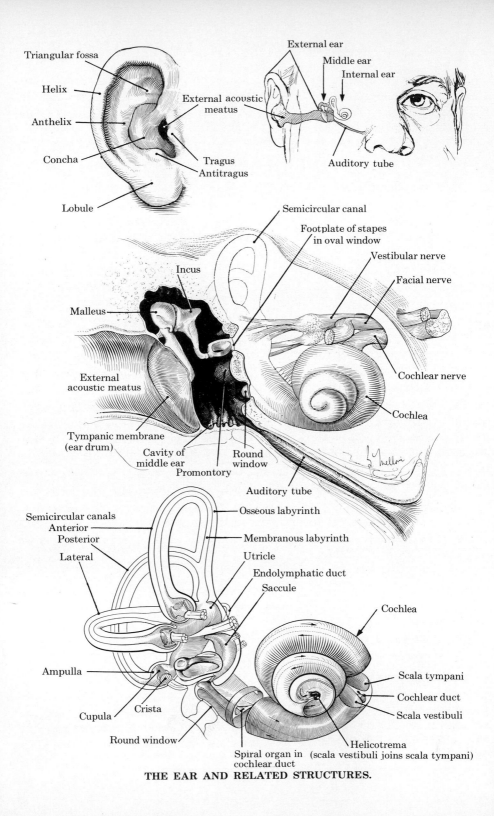

THE EAR AND RELATED STRUCTURES.

operation known as an *arytenoidectomy* which provides a more adequate airway to relieve respiratory obstruction in the throat. A description of this procedure has been included in this chapter under the section dealing with operations on the throat.

THE MIDDLE EAR

The ear is anatomically divided into the external ear, the middle ear and the internal ear. The internal ear is surgically inaccessible for all practical purposes. The middle ear is more important in the specialty of otolaryngology than is the external ear, the latter often being managed by the plastic surgeon. We will confine our considerations of the ear in this chapter to the middle ear.

The tympanic cavity, otherwise known as the middle ear, is a minute air cavity in the petrous portion of the temporal bone. It contains an ossicular chain of three small bones designated as the *malleus, incus,* and *stapes* which transmit vibrations of sound across the middle ear cavity to the internal ear.

The middle ear contains five openings which include: one into the external auditory canal (separated by the tympanic membrane), one into the auditory (eustachian) tube, one into the mastoid sinuses, and two into the internal ear. The latter two openings or windows are called the *fenestra rotunda* (also: fenestra cochleae or round window) and the *fenestra ovalis* (also: fenestra vestibuli or oval window).

The anatomic structures of the external ear are listed in Chapter 13. Important surgical features of the middle ear and associated structures are listed below.

ANATOMIC FEATURES OF THE MIDDLE EAR AND RELATED STRUCTURES

Aditus
Annular ligament
Annulus tympanicus
Anterior ligament of the malleus
Anterior process
Anterior wall
Articular capsule
Attic
Auditory canal
Auditory tube (eustachian)
Axis ligament
Base of the stapes
Capitulum of the stapes

Carotid canal
Cartilaginous portion
Chorda tympani nerve
Cochlea (pl. cochleae)
Cog-tooth of malleus
Columella
Crura
Crus
Deep petrosal nerve
Drumhead (tympanic membrane)
Endaural
Epitympanic recess
Epitympanum

ANATOMIC FEATURES OF THE MIDDLE
EAR AND RELATED STRUCTURES (Continued)

Eustachian canal
Eustachian tube
External acoustic meatus
External ligament of the malleus
Fenestra cochleae (round window)
Fenestra ovalis (oval window)
Fenestra rotunda (round window)
Fenestra vestibuli (oval window)
Foot-plate
Fossa incudis
Fundus tympani
Glaserian fissure
Head of the malleus
Horizontal canal
Hyaline cartilage
Incudomalleolar joint
Incudostapedial joint
Incus
Isthmus
Iter chordae, anterior, posterior
Jugular wall or floor
Labyrinthic wall
Lateral ligament of the malleus
Lateral process of the malleus
Lenticular process of the incus
Long crus
Long process of the incus
Malleo-incudal joint
Malleolar folds
Malleus
Manubrium of the malleus
Mastoid
Mastoid antrum
Mastoid air cells
Mastoid wall
Medial wall
Membranous (lateral) wall
Meniscus
Notch of Rivinus
Osseous portion
Ossicles
Oval window

Oval window niche
Oval window reflex
Paries jugularis
Paries tegmentalis
Pars flassida
Petrotympanic fissure
Postauricular area
Posterior ligament of the incus
Posterior wall
Prominence of the facial canal
Promontory
Pyramidal eminence
Round window
Round window reflex
Secondary tympanic membrane
Semicanal for Tensor tympani
Semicircular canal
Septum canalis musculotubarii
Short crus of the incus
Sigmoid sinus
Sino-dural
Sinus tympanicus
Spine of Henle
Spur of the malleus
Stapedius muscle
Stapedius tendon
Stapes
Superior ligament of the incus
Tegmen tympani
Tegmental wall roof
Temporalis muscle
Tensor tympani muscle
Torus tubarius
Trautmann's triangle
Tympanic antrum
Tympanic cavity
Tympanic membrane (drumhead)
Tympanic orifice
Tympanic sulcus
Tympanomeatal
Umbo
Vestibule

Endolymphatic-Subarachnoid Shunt

After injection with 1% Xylocaine with epinephrine, a routine post-auricular incision was made. The subcutaneous tissue and periosteum were divided by sharp dissection. Bleeders were clamped and electro-coagulated. The periosteum was incised and retracted. This exposed the mastoid cavity. The cortex was entered with a cutting bur at the spine of Henle. The entire operation was performed using the operating micro-scope.

After drilling away a few superficial cells, the antrum was reached. The anterior prominence of the lateral sinus was identified as was the semicircular canal. Trautmann's triangle was now completely exenterated with cutting burs. The posterior semicircular canal was roughly skele-tonized. From this point on, the Diamond bur and continuous irrigation with Ringer's solution were used. The posterior semicircular canal was thinned down but not to a point where blue line was visible.

The dural plate overlying the posterior cranial fossa was removed partly with a Diamond bur and partly with small curettes. The endo-lymphatic sac was identified. Its outer layer was then incised through the dura with a House tympanoplastic knife. Care was taken to avoid opening any of the large veins in the dura.

The medial wall of the endolymphatic sac was incised and the incision continued into the subarachnoid space. A small amount of cerebrospinal fluid escaped. A Teflon endolymphatic shunt tube was inserted into the incision.

From the postauricular incision, the muscle and fascia graft was ob-tained by sharp dissection. The entire exposed posterior fossa region was covered with this as a free graft. The mastoid cavity was packed with Gelfoam soaked in Chloromycetin. The postauricular incision was closed with interrupted 0000 dermalon mattress sutures. A gauze wick smeared with Achromycin-Hydrocortisone Ointment was inserted into the external auditory canal. A routine mastoid dressing was applied.

Labyrinthotomy, Left Transmeatal

Under general anesthesia, the left ear was prepared and draped. After injection with 1% Xylocaine with epinephrine and using the operating microscope throughout the procedure, an incision was made in the bony external auditory canal from 6 to 12 o'clock. The tympanomeatal flap was elevated. The tympanic membrane was lifted out of its sulcus and the middle ear was exposed. Some bone was curetted away from the posterior superior annulus to expose the stapes well. The chorda tympani was displaced in a downward direction. The incudostapedial joint was cut along with the Stapedius and the stapes was removed in toto.

Suction was applied through the oval window into the vestibule of the inner ear. Immediately, as soon as suction was withdrawn, a large amount of what appeared to be spinal fluid flowed out of the oval window to fill the middle and external auditory canal. This could not be controlled well with suction but it was finally brought under control. Working with two hands, the inferior margin of the oval window was widened by curettage. The curet was used to destroy the accessible parts of the inner ear. The inner ear was packed as well as possible with Gelfoam. The tympanomeatal flap was replaced. The external auditory canal was packed with a strip of gauze smeared with Achromycin-Hydrocortisone Ophthalmic Ointment and a mastoid dressing was applied.

TYMPANOPLASTY

The middle ear is separated from the external auditory canal by the tympanic membrane (drumhead). This membrane is connected to the internal ear by a series of three small bones or ossicles known as the *malleus, incus* and *stapes.*

As a result of trauma or infection, the tympanic membrane is often ruptured. When such a perforation exists in the presence of a normal ossicular chain (malleus, incus and stapes) it may be repaired with an operation called a *myringoplasty* (same as tympanoplasty I). When the damage exceeds perforation, a *tympanoplasty* is performed in those cases amenable to surgery. Descriptions of the various types of tympanoplasty have been included here to provide the secretary with an understanding of the differences between these procedures and the criteria which dictate selection of the procedure.

Types of Tympanoplasty

TYPE I   This operation is essentially a myringoplasty with repair of the perforated tympanic membrane by means of a graft. It is done in those cases which present a perforated tympanic membrane with a normal ossicular chain.

TYPE II   In this operation the malleus and complete tympanic membrane are replaced by a graft in contact with the incus or remainder of the malleus. This procedure is elected in those cases which present erosion of the malleus in addition to perforation of the tympanic membrane.

TYPE III A graft is used to replace the tympanic membrane. It is placed in contact with the stapes and also affords protection for the round window. This type of reconstruction is performed when the tympanic membrane is destroyed along with the incus and malleus, leaving only the stapes mobile and intact.

TYPE IV   A graft is attached to the promontory, extending over the tympanic orifice of the eustachian tube with attachment to the outer inferior margin of the middle ear space. A small air-containing cavity is thus developed between the round window and graft affording protection for the round window. The mobile foot-plate remains exposed. This operation is done when there is a functioning oval window membrane and mobile foot-plate even though the head, neck and crura of the stapes have been destroyed.

TYPE V   A window (fenestra) is created in the horizontal canal and is covered by a rather extensive skin graft which also forms a small tympanic cavity. The middle ear is sealed off by the skin graft thus providing sound protection for the round window. This operation is performed in cases of non-functioning oval window and fixed foot-plate.

Tympanoplasty   *Type I* — **Right Myringoplasty With Skin Graft Donor Site: External Auditory Canal**

Preliminary exposure of the middle ear was accomplished through an ear speculum with a magnifying loupe. After exposure, the Zeiss operating microscope was used for greater magnification.

Under high power magnification, using small picks and tympanoplastic knives, the remnants of the tympanic membrane were denuded of their epithelial layers.

After complete elevation of the epithelium, a longitudinal incision was made with a House knife in the bony auditory canal at 5 and 8 o'clock, respectively. Both incisions were connected about 5 mm. external to the annulus. This portion of the canal skin was elevated completely and freed. It was then shifted over the denuded portions of the tympanic membrane and external auditory canal, taking the utmost care to evert the edges of the graft.

Prior to this manipulation, the middle ear was filled with Hydrocortisone-Achromycin Ointment. The outer portions of the canal were loosely packed with a gauze strip smeared with the same ointment.

Tympanoplasty Type II — With Exploratory Meatoantrotomy

The left ear was prepared and sterilely draped. Local anesthesia was accomplished by injecting 2% Xylocaine with epinephrine in the usual manner at the entrance of the external canal. The entire operation was carried out using the Zeiss operating microscope under 6, 10 and 16 power magnification.

A Heerman endaural incision was made splitting the membranous canal at 12 o'clock and carrying the incision out parallel to the crus of the helix. Two self-retaining Wullstein retractors were inserted crosswise thus exposing the entire bony wall canal including the superior canal wall.

The usual meatal incisions for an exploratory tympanotomy were made and a tympanomeatal flap was elevated. The tympanic membrane which appeared quite thickened was elevated out of the tympanic sulcus together with the annular ligament without perforation. There were adhesions in the middle ear. These were dissected free under high power magnification. They mainly involved the long process of the incus and the tympanic membrane as well as the posterior annular region.

The mucous membrane of the middle ear appeared to be slightly thickened but there was no evidence of cholesteatoma or of irreversible pathology. The attic was explored by removing the posterior superior aspect of the annular region and thus, the lateral wall of the attic. There was no evidence of cholesteatoma. A few more adhesions around the ossicular chain were found and freed. Using a Diamond bur, a meatoantrotomy was performed, turning the bone over the aditus away and exposing the mastoid antrum. There was no evidence of cholesteatoma.

The entire middle ear and exposed part of the mastoid were thoroughly irrigated with Ringer's solution. A Teflon sheet was then placed over the areas where the adhesions were sectioned. The middle ear and mastoid antrum were filled with Achromycin-Hydrocortisone Ointment.

The tympanomeatal flap was replaced in its original position covering the defect in the bone wall. The endaural incision was closed with interrupted 00000 dermalon sutures. The external auditory canal was packed with gauze smeared with Achromycin-Hydrocortisone Ointment. A mastoid dressing was applied.

Tympanoplasty Type III

The left ear was sterilely prepared and draped in the usual manner. A postauricular approach was used making an incision precisely in the postauricular fold. These subcutaneous tissues were dissected down to the periosteum and the periosteum was divided sharply and retracted.

Bleeders were controlled by electrocoagulation. The mastoid cortex was entered at the spine of Henle with a cutting bur and as the cells were reached, they were found to be filled with mucoid fluid. Granulations were also noted in the mastoid. The antrum was reached. Exenteration of all of the mastoid cells was done with a cutting bur. The tip cells were removed. The sino-dural angle was cleaned. A small dural exposure occurred there. Trautmann's triangle was cleaned and the posterior bony canal wall was thinned down. All cells showed evidence of inflammation of a rather active degree with granulation. There was no evidence of cholesteatoma.

The aditus region was widened until the thickened lining of the incus came into view. This was not disturbed. The entire mastoidectomy was performed using the operating microscope to assure good exenteration of all cells. Under high power magnification, the posterior superior and superior lining of the bony external auditory meatus was now elevated. The tympanic membrane together with the annular ligament were lifted out of the annulus and the middle ear was thus opened. It was immediately apparent that there was an adhesion between the head of the stapes and the tympanic membrane. There had been a necrosis of the long process of the incus. There was no connection between the long process of the incus and the head and neck of the stapes. The stapes appeared to be mobile and intact. Gentle rocking movements were applied and a good round window reflex could be seen.

Working in the middle ear was considerably hindered by intense capillary bleeding. The chorda tympani was now elevated in a downward direction and could be placed in such a position that it filled the gap between the head of the stapes and the remaining long process of the incus. Prior to this, the tympanic membrane was carefully dissected free from the capitulum of the stapes. A small tear in the tympanic membrane from this dissection was repaired by using a free fascia graft obtained by sharp dissection through a postauricular incision.

After proper realignment of the ossicular chain, a small piece of Teflon sheeting was placed over the long process of the incus to prevent adhesions between it and the inner surface of the tympanic membrane. Achromycin-Hydrocortisone Ophthalmic Ointment was injected into the middle ear cavity. The tympanomeatal flap was replaced. The external auditory canal was cleaned and inspected.

A myringotomy incision was made in the tympanic membrane and a Shea polyethylene drainage tube was inserted through the incision to provide adequate drainage. The mastoid cavity was filled with Achromycin-Hydrocortisone Ointment. A small polyethylene drain was inserted into the mastoid cavity and brought out through a postauricular incision.

The incision was closed with 0000 dermalon sutures. A routine mastoid dressing was applied.

206

Revision of Type III Tympanoplasty with Insertion of 4.5 x 0.6 mm. Stainless Steel Malleal Foot-plate Piston

With the patient in the supine position and the head turned to the right, the left ear was sterilely prepared, draped and injected with 1% Xylocaine with adrenalin.

A vein was taken from the left antecubital area which was closed in the usual manner.

A Lempert endaural incision was made and hemostasis obtained by clamping and ligating or electrocoagulation. As the graft cholesteatoma appeared to extend outward on the posterior canal wall, a canal wall flap was not made. The cholesteatomatous portion of the old graft was outlined by sharp incision and this was carefully dissected from the drum and ossicles as well as the attic area. The drum inferiorly was noted to be normally intact and on removing the graft, it was found that the fibrous middle layer and the mucosal layer left gave an intact drum. However, there was a skin pocket in the attic which extended inferiorly behind the body of the incus. It was later noted that this pocket which contained some cholesteatoma debris had destroyed the greater portion of the incus leaving only a portion of the long process and a small portion of the ossicular surface with the malleus. The skin pocket was then dissected from behind the ossicles and a small amount of skin was removed from behind the head of the malleus. However, this area was felt to be skin free prior to grafting. The middle ear space was entered by a standard tympanomeatal flap and the chorda tympani nerve was sacrificed. The distal portion of the incus was thin and fibrotic and did not transmit motion of the incus to the stapes.

The incudostapedial joint was therefore divided as was the malleoincudal joint and the remnant of the incus was then removed. This was insufficient for a columella and was discarded.

The stapes appeared to be fully intact and the mucosal layer over the mid-portion of the malleal handle was incised and elevated from the malleus.

A 4.5 x 0.6 mm. stainless steel piston which was angled posteriorly and inferiorly was then inserted to contact the stapes foot-plate and was crimped over the malleus. Motion was transmitted well through this columella.

A small amount of bone was taken down from the atticotomy posteriorly; however, only slightly swollen mucosa was noted in this area and further mastoid work was not done. The atticotomy was obliterated with Gelfoam and soft tissue and two strips of vein were laid in to cover the raw outer surface of the upper one half of the tympanic membrane as well as the attic space.

The usual packing of rayon strips and Cortisporin soaked cotton was inserted after which the endaural incision was closed in the usual manner.

The patient tolerated the procedure well and left the operating room in good condition, after a head dressing had been applied.

Tympanoplasty Type IV — Using Fascia, Skin Grafts and Teflon Prosthesis

After surgical preparation and draping, the left mastoid cavity was exposed through a Lempert's endaural incision. A previous musculo-plasty had been done and the muscle, as expected, had been replaced by dense connective tissue which served to fill in the mastoid cavity. The skin was carefully peeled off this mass and the middle ear was exposed.

The middle ear was filled with granulation tissue and scar tissue. This was carefully removed to peel the back from the medial wall of the tym-panic cavity. The eustachian tube was probed and found to be patent. The foot-plate of the stapes remained and this was mobile. A Teflon umbrella prosthesis was fitted onto the foot-plate and held in place by packing around it with Gelfoam soaked in Achromycin-Hydrocortisone Ointment.

A very thin portion of skin graft from along the posterior wall of the external auditory canal was cut out. A graft obtained from the left arm was used to replace it. The fascia obtained from the left Temporalis muscle was placed over the Teflon umbrella prosthesis and fitted under-neath the previous existing graft in the tympanic cavity. Skin was placed over this fascia. The skin graft and fascia graft were held in place with Gelfoam packing reinforced with Iodoform gauze packing.

All incisions were closed with white nylon subcutaneously and 00000 dermalon for the skin. A mastoid bandage was applied. At the conclusion of surgery, when the patient reacted, it was noted that the facial nerve function was normal.

Tympanoplasty Type V — Fenestration from Vestibule and Insertion of Stainless Steel Wire Prosthesis

The left ear was sterilely prepared and draped in the usual manner. After injection of 1% Xylocaine with epinephrine at the usual points, a Heerman incision was made following the outline of the old incision.

A small eye retractor was inserted splitting the external auditory canal in its membranous portion. A tympanomeatal flap was outlined with the usual incisions and elevated. The tympanic membrane was lifted out of its sulcus together with the annular ligament. A flap was reflected forward and the middle ear was exposed. It was immediately apparent that the previously placed wire had slipped off the long process of the incus and was not in contact with the incus or oval window region any more. It was attached by adhesions to the undersurface of the tympanic membrane. It was carefully removed by sharp dissection using high power magnification. Following this, the oval window region was reinspected. There was still a small puncture opening. Proceeding from this area, a wide opening was made into the vestibule of the inner ear. This was technically difficult because thick bone had to be removed piecemeal with small foot-plate hooks. No drill was used in order to avoid injury to the inner ear structure. The facial nerve was clearly visualized and appeared to be completely exposed in its course through the middle ear. There was a very marked overhang of the facial nerve.

An attempt was made to place a wire piston prosthesis into the newly created opening into the vestibule. This proved impossible because of the continuous contact of the piston with the exposed facial nerve. Therefore a House wire of suitable size was selected and placed on the long process of the incus with its proximal end into the open vestibule. It was crimped in place tightly. The excess opening was covered up with compressed Gelfoam. The middle ear was now filled with Achromycin-Hydrocortisone Ointment.

The tympanomeatal flap was reflected into its original position where it was gently packed in place with a gauze strip smeared with the same ointment. The endaural incision was closed with interrupted 00000 dermalon sutures. A mastoid dressing was applied.

Myringotomy With Insertion of Polyethylene Collar Buttons, Bilaterally

The Zeiss operating microscope was brought into position and the tympanic membrane was well visualized.

An incision was made in the posterior inferior quadrant of the tympanic membrane. The middle ear was aspirated. Following this, a polyethylene collar button was inserted with a tympanoplastic alligator forceps and a pick through the myringotomy incision. The same procedure was carried out on the opposite ear.

Musculoplasty With Skin Grafting

After surgical preparation and draping, the left mastoid was exposed through a Lempert endaural incision.

The mastoid cavity was found to be filled with granulation tissue. There were two or three areas of definite cholesteatoma. These were all removed. The mastoid cavity had been operated on previously but many pockets of bone and overhangs remained. These were drilled out completely.

Musculoplasty was performed by rotating a free muscle pedicle graft from the left Temporalis muscle into the mastoid cavity. A postauricular skin graft was obtained and sutured in place. The skin was also held in place by packing which consisted of Gelfoam and Iodoform gauze.

Modified Radical Mastoidectomy

Under general anesthesia employing an endotracheal tube, the area of the right ear was prepared with pHisoHex and draped sterilely.

A Lempert endaural incision was made and carried down to the periosteum of the mastoid process. The periosteum was reflected anteriorly and posteriorly with a periosteal elevator after fashioning a conchal flap. A self-retaining endaural retractor was inserted. Using a Jordan-Day drill and cutting bur, the mastoid antrum was approached using Henle's spine as a landmark.

Upon approaching the mastoid antrum it became evident that a considerable amount of granulation tissue filled the antrum and extended posteriorly and inferiorly towards the mastoid tip. The granulation tissue was removed. The mastoid was quite sclerotic. The mastoid was not well pneumatized and the mastoid cells were few. The dura was quite low and the sigmoid sinus was situated quite far anteriorly. After removing the granulation tissue from what few mastoid cells there were, the dissection was carried anteriorly.

The lateral wall of the epitympanum was then removed and the bony bridge was also removed. At this point it became evident that the entire attic was filled with cholesteatoma. This was meticulously removed. The cholesteatoma had imbedded in the incus and head of the malleus and had extended into the sinus tympanicus. It was therefore necessary to remove the incus and to amputate the head of the malleus following which, the cholesteatoma matrix was carefully removed from the remaining portion of the malleus and undersurface of the tympanic membrane. It was also removed from the sinus tympanicus. The middle ear appeared normal, otherwise.

At one point the dura was exposed; however, the dura was not penetrated. The meatal flap was laid over the facial ridge which had previously been taken down. All of the diseased tissue appeared to have been removed.

Sulfadiazine powder was sprinkled into the cavity. The cavity was then packed with vaseline gauze. Additional Sulfadiazine powder was then placed externally into the meatus.

The postauricular incision was sutured in two layers using 0000 plain and 00000 dermalon sutures for the skin. A small Penrose drain was left in the inferior aspect of the posterior auricular incision and a mastoid type dressing was applied. The facial nerve function was normal at the conclusion of the procedure.

THE STAPES

The stapes is one of the three small bones of the middle ear. It is shaped like a stirrup and can be replaced by a prosthesis to restore continuity to the ossicular chain. Commonly used techniques are listed as follows:

STAPEDECTOMY TECHNICS:

Guilford   Schuknecht
Hough   Shea
House

Left Stapedectomy With Piston Prosthesis

The left ear was sterilely prepared and draped in the usual manner. Local anesthesia was obtained by injection of 2% Xylocaine with adrenalin.

A Heerman incision was made splitting the membranous portion of the external auditory canal at 12 o'clock. A semicircular incision was now made about 4 to 5 mm. external to the annulus tympanicus around the posterior circumference of the bony external auditory canal. The tympanomeatal flap was elevated. The tympanic membrane was lifted out of its sulcus together with the annular ligament without perforation. The tympanomeatal flap was reflected anteriorly, thus exposing the middle ear. A fair amount of bone was curetted away from the posterior superior aspect of the annulus, thus exposing the long process of the incus, stapes and oval window niche.

The stapes showed whitish otosclerotic bone anteriorly and a complete anterior fixation. The posterior portion of the foot-plate was blue. The niche was very deep with an overhanging facial nerve.

A small hole was made in the blue portion of the foot-plate with a fine stapes pick. Following this, the incudostapedial joint was separated sharply. The Stapedius tendon was cut, the crura fractured and the superstructure of the stapes removed. Using fine stapes hooks, the posterior part of the foot-plate was now removed.

The wire piston prosthesis was manipulated over the long process of the incus and hooked onto its long process with the piston part of the wire prosthesis protruding into the opening in the oval window. The wire was crimped down to assure a good fit. The hearing of the patient improved immediately on the operating table.

The tympanomeatal flap was replaced in its original position. The external canal was filled with Achromycin-Hydrocortisone Ointment and a small gauze wick with the same ointment was inserted.

The Heerman incision was closed with interrupted 00000 dermalon sutures and a routine mastoid dressing was applied.

Stapedectomy With Stainless Steel Prosthesis and Gelfoam

After surgical preparation and draping, 1% Xylocaine with adrenalin was infiltrated into the external auditory canal.

An incision was made in the posterior wall of the external auditory canal about 5 mm. external to the tympanic membrane. The tympanomeatal flap was elevated. The posterior portion of the bony annulus was removed extensively with a curet. The stapes was found to be fixed. The incudostapedial joint was dislocated. The stapedial tendon was cut and the superstructure of the stapes was removed. A very thick foot-plate was removed with some difficulty using picks and fistula hooks.

Gelfoam was placed over the open oval window and a 4½ mm. preformed House stainless steel prosthesis was fitted. The proximal end laid on the Gelfoam and oval window. The distal end was crimped around the long process of the incus. A good round window reflex was obtained and the patient's response to gross testing was satisfactory.

The middle ear was cleansed of blood. Achromycin-Hydrocortisone Ointment was instilled. The tip of the meatal flap was replaced. The entire ear canal was filled with Achromycin-Hydrocortisone Ointment.

Fenestration of Right Lateral Semicircular Canal

The right ear was sterilely prepared and draped in the usual manner. A Shambaugh endaural incision for fenestration was made. The anterior portion of the conchal cartilage was removed in a semilunar fashion and the subcutaneous tissue was excised. The entire operation was performed using a Zeiss operating microscope.

The canal incisions were made in the usual fashion at about 12 and 6 o'clock, respectively. The membranous canal was dissected free in its posterior circumference. For a short distance, the bony canal was separated from its periosteal membranous lining. Using cutting burs, the bony part of the canal was widened. A few superficial mastoid cells were drilled away and the exenteration of mastoid air cells was continued to the antrum. Following this, the middle ear was explored under high power magnification. There were no new findings. There was no evidence of any oval window reflex present. The facial nerve was identified superiorly, above the oval window. The lateral wall of the attic was now removed, partly with Diamond burs, partly with curets and partly with cutting burs. This exposed the short process of the incus and the body of the incus, as well as the long process of the incus. The incus was malformed and was fused to the head of the malleus. The head of the malleus and the incus were now removed. The surgical dome of the vestibule, consisting of the anterior part of the lateral semicircular canal, was now clearly in view as was the facial nerve.

The middle ear was again inspected and a round window niche was visualized, but we could not be certain that there was a round window membrane. The cavity was smoothed out. All bleeding was controlled with a Diamond bur. A flap was then fashioned until a perfect fit had been obtained and the flap fitted well over the surgical dome of the lateral ends of the semicircular canal. Following this, the entire cavity was thoroughly irrigated and all bone dust removed. Bleeders were again carefully and meticulously controlled.

The next step consisted of the creation of a fenestra into the lateral semicircular canal. This was done with a Diamond bur under continuous irrigation with Ringer's solution. The surgical dome of the semicircular canal was first encumberalized after the blue line was visualized. The remainder of the fenestra was completed by a cupula technique. An opening in the labyrinth was made after the cupula had been completed with a small pick. The bone was completely removed from the fenestra. A good, clean fenestra was obtained under high power magnification. The membranous part of the semicircular canal was clearly visible.

No remarkable bleeding occurred during this procedure. There was no large accumulation of blood in the vestibule. The tympanomeatal flap was now placed over the broken fenestra and secured with a cotton pack smeared with Achromycin-Hydrocortisone Ointment. The flap was then packed in place with gauze smeared with the same ointment. The outer part of the cavity was packed with the same material. The upper portion of the endaural incision was approximated with a 00000 dermalon suture and a routine mastoid dressing was applied.

The patient moved the right side of his face indicating that the facial nerve was unimpaired.

THE LARYNX

The larynx is a musculocartilaginous structure which has the shape of an inverted triangle. This pyramidal tube, situated above the trachea in the neck, is regarded chiefly as the organ of speech. When excision of the larynx (*laryngectomy*) becomes necessary due to carcinoma or other grave condition, the patient is fitted with an artificial larynx and rehabilitated until he can communicate distinctly enough to be understood.

Examination and biopsy of the larynx is performed endoscopically by a procedure called a *laryngoscopy*, using an instrument called a *laryngoscope*. Some of the other commonly used laryngeal instruments have been listed here to further familiarize the secretary with the armamentarium of the otolaryngologist.

ANATOMIC FEATURES OF THE LARYNX

Anterior commissure
Arch
Articular capsule
Aryepiglottic fold
Arytenoid cartilage
Cartilages of Santorini
Cartilages of Wrisberg
Conus elasticus
Cords
Corniculate cartilage (Santorini)
Cornu
Cornua
Cricoarytenoid ligament
Cricoid cartilage
Cricotracheal ligament
Crista arcuata
Cuneiform cartilage (Wrisberg)
Cuneiform tubercle
Esophageal introitus
Epiglottis
False cords
Foveae

Fusiform fossa
Glossoepiglottic folds
Hyoepiglottic ligament
Hyothyroid ligament
Hyothyroid membrane
Inferior laryngeal nerve
Intrathyroid cartilage
Lamina
Laryngeal prominence (Adam's apple)
Mucous membrane
Pyriform sinus
Rima glottidis
Superior laryngeal nerve
Thyroid cartilage
Thyroid notch
Thyroepiglottic ligament
True cords
Valleculae
Ventricular bands
Vestibule
Vocal cords
Vocal process

MUSCLES OF THE LARYNX

Arytenoideus (interarytenoid)
Cricoarytenoideus
Cricothyroid
Interarytenoid (Arytenoideus)

Internal thyro-arytenoid
Lateral crico-arytenoid
Posterior crico-arytenoid
Thyroarytenoideus

LARYNGEAL INSTRUMENTS

Abraham laryngeal cannula
Abraham laryngeal syringe
Andrews chest support
Artificial larynx
Carabelli mirror cannula
Cordes-New laryngeal punch
Dean laryngeal applicator
Erich laryngeal biopsy forceps
Fauvel forceps
Ferguson-Metzenbaum scissors
Fraenkel forceps
Haslinger head rest
Holinger cannula
Holinger laryngeal dissector
Jackson core mold
Jesberg laryngectomy clamp

Jurasz laryngeal forceps
Killian suspension gallows
Krause laryngeal snare
LeJuene laryngofissure scissors
Lewy laryngoscope holder
Lukens laryngeal syringe
Lynch knife
McKenzie laryngeal forceps
Myerson laryngectomy saw
New's speaking tube
Record laryngeal syringe
Roberts vocal cord fixer
Sawtell laryngeal applicator
Tobold-Fauvel forceps
Vasconcelos-Barretto clamp
Yankauer-Little tube forceps

LARYNGEAL TUBES

Chevalier Jackson
Clerf
Holinger

Lewis
Martin
Schell

LARYNGOSCOPES

Adult reverse bevel
Albert Andrews modified Jackson
Anterior commissure
Atkins-Tucker shadow free
Bizzarri-Giuffrida
Broyles anterior commissure
Broyles optical
Broyles wasp waist
Chevalier Jackson
Clerf
Dual distal lighted
E.S.I.
Fink
Flagg
Foregger
Guedel
Haslinger
Holinger anterior commissure
   hour-glass
Holinger anterior commissure
   slotted

Holinger modified Jackson
Hook-on folding
Jackson
Lewy
Lundy
Lynch suspension
McIntosh
Miller
Multipurpose
Polio
Roberts self-retaining
Rotating
Sam Roberts
Sanders intubation
Siker mirror
Standard
Tucker anterior commissure
Welch-Allyn
Wis-Foregger
Wis-Hipple
Yankauer

Direct Laryngoscopy With Stripping of Cord

Under general anesthesia, using an endotracheal tube in the posterior commissure, a Jackson anterior commissure laryngoscope was inserted and held in the operative position with a Luer retractor.

There was a marked irregularity of the left and right vocal cord, particularly at the anterior third. Numerous biopsies were taken from both cords. The mucosal lining was stripped from the right cord. No other areas of tumefaction, ulceration or bleeding were noted. The scope was withdrawn and the biopsy specimens submitted to the pathologist for histopathologic examination.

Total Laryngectomy — with radical neck dissection

General anesthesia was administered via endotracheal tube. The right neck and part of the chest were prepared and draped in a sterile manner.

A double Y-incision was made and the upper limb of the incision extended from the symphysis of the mandible anteriorly, to the mastoid process posteriorly. This was joined by the vertical limb which extended into the inferior limb, stretching from the suprasternal notch to the posterior triangle of the neck. Skin flaps were dissected by blunt and sharp dissection and a radical neck dissection was carried out.

Following the neck dissection, the hyoid bone was freed from the suprahyoid musculature which was detached by sharp dissection. Midline dissection was then continued and the thyroid cartilage was identified. The thyroid isthmus was ligated.

Attention was then turned to the right upper area of dissection and the superior cornu of the hyoid bone was retracted. The thyrohyoid membrane was identified. Superior laryngeal vessels consisting of the superior laryngeal artery, vein and laryngeal nerve were ligated. The superior thyroid artery was previously ligated during the neck dissection. A similar procedure was repeated on the left side. The superior laryngeal blood vessels and nerves on the left were also sectioned. The dissection was continued downward. The left lobe of the thyroid gland was left intact. The attachments of the inferior constrictor muscles to the thyroid cartilage were sectioned and the ribbon muscles were sectioned inferiorly. The larynx became quite mobile and was retracted with ease to the right side. The trachea was then sectioned at the level between the second and third tracheal rings. The endotracheal tube was then removed and a new tube was placed in the tracheal stump. The dissection continued from the lower aspect of the trachea. The superior stump of the trachea and larynx were separated from the esophagus, bluntly. The superior cornu of the right thyroid cartilage was then identified and the pharynx was entered at this area.

There was a large lesion involving the right pyriform sinus, right side of the epiglottis and base of the tongue. The pharyngeal mucosa was then cut approximately 2 cm. away from the lesion obtaining free healthy margins. The specimen consisting of the right sternocleidomastoid muscle, jugular vein, submandibular gland, thyroid gland, larynx and hyoid bone was removed in toto. This necessitated a ligation of the inferior thyroid arteries on both sides. Bleeding was minimal.

The pharynx was closed with 0000 continuous catgut sutures and closed over with 000 silk sutures. The closure was quite adequate. A feeding tube was inserted prior to the closure. The tracheal stump was then mobilized and a button hole was made in the suprasternal notch. The tracheal stump was brought to the outer surface and sutured to the skin with 000 silk sutures. Anesthesia was then administered via the tracheal stump. The skin flaps were attached to the underlying tissues by catgut sutures and the skin was closed with interrupted 0000 dermalon. Pressure dressing was applied. Only 500 cc. of whole blood was given during the operation.

Laryngoplasty With Insertion of Teflon Mold and

Right Arytenoidectomy; Tracheotomy

The neck was sterilely prepared and draped in the usual manner. The tracheotomy was performed under local anesthesia, using 1% Xylocaine. An incision was made in the old tracheotomy scar which was dissected away. A longitudinal incision was made in the trachea at the level of the previous tracheotomy and a #8 tracheotomy tube was inserted. An anesthetist's endotracheal tube was then inserted into the tracheotomy tube and general anesthesia was administered.

The neck was entered through a previous arytenoidectomy incision on the right side. Dissection was carried through heavy scar tissue to the site of the previously removed thyroid cartilage. Dissection was carried deeper in order to find the arytenoid cartilage. It was located but it was noted that there was very extensive cicatrization of the endolarynx.

The incision was widened and the upper portion of the trachea and the entire larynx in its right lateral aspect were freed. It was now apparent that this was an extensive crushing injury of the larynx with much scar tissue formation and that this was the cause of the patient's airway obstruction, rather than the recurrent laryngeal nerve paralysis.

The arytenoid cartilage was freed by sharp dissection with much difficulty through heavy scar tissue and lateral pull was again exerted on it while the larynx was inspected through an anterior commissure laryngoscope. The lateral pull did not give an adequate airway and it was therefore decided to split the larynx, excise the scar tissue and do an arytenoidectomy. It was further decided to split the anterior larynx with an endolaryngeal mold in order to assure a good airway later.

A vertical midline incision was then made from the tracheotomy incision to the hyoid region. The strap muscles were divided in the midline and the framework of the larynx was exposed. The thyroid cartilage was split in the midline. The endolaryngeal tissues were divided by sharp dissection, a short distance right of the anterior commissure, in order not to injure the anterior commissure. The lumen of the larynx was thus entered.

The entire dissection had to be carried through very heavy scar tissue. Arytenoidectomy was completed with removal of the right arytenoid cartilage. Endolaryngeal scar tissue was dissected free and removed.

Teflon sheeting was now used and a suitable sized triangular shape mold was made. This was inserted into the laryngeal lumen extending from the cricoid region in a superior direction, to about the arytenoid region. The laryngeal mold was sutured in place with #30 wire sutures being brought out on both sides of the neck lateral to the midline incision. One #30 wire suture was then used to reapproximate the thyroid cartilage. The muscle and fascial layers were closed with interrupted 0000 chromic catgut and the skin was closed with interrupted 0000 white nylons and 00000 dermalon.

The lateral incision was closed in a similar fashion and a small Penrose drain was inserted deep into the incision. A pressure dressing was applied to the neck.

Bleeding was quite heavy during the operation and very hard to control; however, this was done by clamping and electrocoagulation. The patient received 50 cc.'s of whole blood in addition to 1000 cc.'s of 5% glucose in water intravenously.

THE TRACHEA

The trachea (windpipe) is a membranocartilaginous tube-like structure which extends for about $4\frac{1}{2}$ inches from the larynx down into the thorax where it bifurcates into the right and left bronchus. The tracheal tube consists of a series of segments composed of semicircular rings which do not close on the back surface of the tube. Their continuity is provided by muscle fibers and fibrous tissue. By placing the fingers to the throat, one can feel these ring-like segments.

Incision into the trachea (*tracheotomy*) is often employed as a life saving measure to establish an airway. This is usually followed by introduction of a tube to maintain an open airway.

TRACHEA INSTRUMENTS

Bernay tracheal retractor
Brewster retractor
Flexible shaft retractor
Jackson laryngofissure retractor
Jackson perichondrial elevator
Jackson tracheal bistoury
Jackson tracheal scalpel
Jackson tracheal scissors
Jackson tracheal tenaculum
Jackson-Trousseau dilator

Laborde tracheal dilator
Lukens thymus retractor
Moore tracheostomy buttons
Rockey cannula
Rockey trachea forceps
Rockey mediastinal cannula
Rockey fenestration scope
Rockey vascular clamp
Salvatore-Maloney tracheotome

TRACHEA TUBES

Atkins-Cannard
Chevalier Jackson
Gabriel Tucker
Holinger
Jackson
Jackson cane-shaped
Jackson extra long
Jackson short length
Kistner plastic

Lepley-Ernst
Lore-Lawrence
Luer
Martin
Mosher life-saving
Pilling
Pilling duralite
Polisar-Lyons
Tucker suction

Tracheotomy

Under local anesthesia, a skin incision was made 2 fingerbreadths above the sternoclavicular junction. The Platysma was incised. Bleeders were clamped and ligated with 000 intestinal sutures. The midline between the strap muscles was grasped and the fascia was incised. Using blunt and sharp dissection, the trachea was exposed. An orbicular ring was cut from the anterior surface. A #8 tracheostomy tube was placed. Interrupted 000 chromic sutures were used to close the subcutaneous tissue and cotton was used to close the skin.

Tonsillectomy and Adenoidectomy (T & A)

The patient was taken to the operating room where general anesthesia was administered employing an intratracheal tube. A Jennings mouth gag was inserted.

The tonsils were removed by sharp dissection and a tonsil snare. It was necessary to insert one 00 chromic suture in the superior pole of both tonsillar fossae to secure hemostasis.

The adenoids were removed with adenoid curettes and St. Clair-Thompson forceps. The fossa of Rosenmuller was cleaned with St. Clair-Thompson forceps and a Meltzer punch.

After the procedure was completed, both tonsillar fossae were injected with a mixture of Depo-Medrol, Depo-Cer-O-Cillin and 2% Xylocaine.

Tonsillectomy

Under local anesthesia, the patient was prepared and draped in a re-clining position.

A retractor was applied to the hypertrophied tonsil and the anterior pillar was pulled forward. The entire mass of the tonsil was grasped with a forceps and the handles were closed. A curved elevator was used to lift the anterior pillar away from the tonsil after being inserted at the upper attachment of the pillar. The snare wire was drawn into the cannula, removing the tonsil. As the stylet of the snare impinged upon the ton-sillar tissue, the handle of the instrument was directed outward.

The remaining defect was packed with a sponge to control bleeding. The mouth and throat were suctioned. After a few minutes, the sponge was removed. Further bleeding was controlled with 00 double catgut sutures.

THE NOSE AND PARANASAL SINUSES

Surgery on the inner nose and paranasal sinuses is performed by the otolaryngologist. This phase of ENT surgery is called *rhinology* and should not be confused with plastic surgery although these specialties overlap in this area. The plastic surgeon often performs a submucous resection, Weir operation, turbinate crushing, etc. in the course of a rhinoplasty.

Examples of operative procedures performed on the nose, other than those listed in Chapter 13 are presented here with descriptions of pro-cedures performed on the accessory sinuses.

ANATOMIC STRUCTURES OF THE NOSE AND PARANASAL SINUSES

Ala (pl. alae)
Alanasi
Alar cartilages
Aponeurosis
Atrium
Bridge
Bulla ethmoidalis
Cartilaginous septum
Cartilaginous vault
Choana (pl. choanae)
Clinoid process
Columella
Columna
Concha (pl. conchae)
Cribriform plate of ethmoid
Crista galli
Crura
Crus laterale
Crus mediale
Dorsum nasi
Ethmoidal air cells
Frontal processes of maxillae
Greater alar cartilage
Hamular process
Hiatus semilunaris
Hypophyseal fossa
Inferior meatus
Infundibulum
Kiesselbach's plexus
Lateral crus
Lateral wall
Lesser alar cartilage

Medial crus
Middle meatus
Mucoperichondrium
Mucous membrane
Nares
Nasal bones
Nasal conchae
Nasal crest
Nasal spine
Nasion
Nasolabial junction
Nasopalatine recess
Nostrils
Ostium maxillare
Palatine bone
Perpendicular plate of ethmoid
Piriform opening
Plica nasi
Rostrum of sphenoid
Septum
Septum mobile nasi
Sesamoid cartilages
Sinus groove
Spheno-ethmoidal recess
Sphenoidal process
Superior meatus
Turbinates
Uncinate process
Vestibule
Vomer
Vomeronasal cartilage
Vomeronasal organ of Jacobson

PARANASAL SINUSES

Ethmoidal
Frontal

Maxillary
Sphenoidal

ARTERIES OF THE NOSE

Alar br. of ext. maxillary
Alveolar br. of int. maxillary
Ant. ethmoidal br. of ophthalmic
Dorsal nasal br. of ophthalmic
Infraorbital br. of int. maxillary

Pharyngeal br. of int. maxillary
Post. ethmoidal br. of ophthalmic
Septal br. of ext. maxillary
Septal br. of superior labial
Sphenopalatine br. of int. maxillary

NERVES OF THE NOSE

Ant. alveolar br. of maxillary

Anterior ethmoidal

Anterior palatine

External nasal

Facial

Infraorbital of maxillary

Infratrochlear br. of ophthalmic

Nasal br. of sphenopalatine ganglion

Nasociliary br. of ophthalmic

Nasopalatine

Nerve of pterygoid canal

Olfactory

Nasal Polypectomy and Caldwell-Luc

The right side of the nose was packed with 10% cocaine. The area over the canine fossa on the right side was injected with 1% Xylocaine and epinephrine.

A ½ inch horizontal incision was made over the fossa, through the mucosa and submucosal tissues and periosteum. An elevator was used to fracture the lateral wall of the right antrum. Bone biting forceps were used to enlarge the opening.

The mucosa of the antrum was very edematous and polypoid. The antrum was scraped clean and bleeding was minimal. The ostium appeared to be markedly enlarged.

The pack was removed from the nose and some small polypi were removed from the middle meatus. A large polyp remained and this had to be removed from behind the soft palate, through the mouth. The ostium was further enlarged. When bleeding was controlled the antrum was packed with two Cod liver oil soaked strips. The two ends of the strips were brought out into the nasal cavity. The incision was closed with two 000 silk sutures. There was no evidence of bleeding in the posterior nasopharynx.

Submucous Resection   (Also: Septectomy or SMR)

Under local anesthesia, a curvilinear incision was made on the convex side of the septum with a Freer knife. Particular care was taken not to enter the mucous membrane or perichondrium. The mucoperichondrium and mucoperiosteum were raised intact. The mucoperichondrium and cartilage of the opposite side were separated utilizing an elevator. The cartilage was exposed and the mucous membrane retracted on each side of the nasal septum. The cartilage was trimmed with a Ballenger swivel knife and removed as a single piece with forceps.

Using a Foster-Ballenger forceps, we grasped the portion of the perpendicular plate of the ethmoid to be removed and snipped it away piecemeal. Hurd's reversible septal ridge forceps were introduced into the incision and the deflected portion of the vomer was bitten away. Hajek's chisel was further utilized in this procedure. All bleeding was controlled. The wound was left open to permit drainage.

Bilateral Intranasal Ethmoidectomy, Transnasal Sphenoidotomy and Caldwell-Luc

An infraorbital block was accomplished with 1% Xylocaine with epinephrine. The septum and anterior ethmoid region were infiltrated. Using cocaine flakes on applicators, a bilateral sphenopalatine block and anterior ethmoid block were carried out.

There was a marked spur of the anterior septum on the right. An incision was made in the right mucocutaneous junction. Bilateral mucoperiosteal elevation was carried out. The spur was removed using a chisel and mallet.

A thorough exenteration of all accessible ethmoid cells was carried out through the nose under direct vision. Much polypoid tissue was also noted in both sphenoid sinuses. The sphenoid sinuses were also exenterated. The sphenoid and ethmoid sinuses on both sides were packed off with Tincture of Benzoin gauze.

An incision was made in the right canine fossa and carried through submucosal tissue and periosteum. The periosteum was elevated and the right maxillary sinus was entered through the canine fossa. It was noted to be completely filled with polypoid tissue and polypoid degeneration of the lining. The entire lining of the maxillary sinus was removed. A large window was made at the level of the inferior nasal meatus. An inferior pedicle mucosal flap was developed from the nasal mucosa of the inferior meatus and folded into the maxillary sinus. The maxillary sinus was then packed with Compound Tincture of Benzoin gauze. This was repeated on the opposite side. The incision was closed with interrupted 0000 chromic catgut sutures. The nose was packed with finger cots smeared with Achromycin-Hydrocortisone Ointment after closing the septal incision with 0000 chromic catgut sutures.

Blood loss was estimated at 500 cc.'s because of copious bleeding during the operation. Transfusion was not deemed necessary.

9 } *Ophthalmology*

Ophthalmology is the surgical specialty concerned with diseases of the eye and its associated structures to include the eyelids, ocular muscles and lacrimal apparatus. Surgery of the eyelids is not confined exclusively to ophthalmology since lid surgery is also performed by the plastic surgeon. Eye surgery is otherwise the exclusive domain of the ophthalmologist.

ANATOMY OF THE EYE AND ACCESSORY STRUCTURES

The eyes are spherical shaped organs with an anterior rounded projection which bulges from the globe proper. This is the portion of the eye which can be seen when the eyelids are open. The major part of the eye is housed in the cavity of the orbit which is lined by fat to afford further protection to the eyeball. The actual socket in which the eyeball moves consists of a thin membranous sac, the *fascia bulbi* (Tenon's capsule) which extends from the optic nerve at the back of the eyeball to the ciliary region toward the front of the eyeball.

The eyeball, per se, consists of three tunics or coverings which include:

(1) a fibrous tunic (sclera behind and cornea in front)
(2) a vascular, pigmented tunic (choroid, ciliary body and iris)
(3) a nervous tunic (retina)

The sclera (white of the eye) is the outermost tough layer which gives the eyeball its shape. It covers the entire eyeball as the sclera on the back and sides and continues as the transparent cornea over the front of the eye. The point at which the sclera continues as the cornea is called the sclerocorneal junction.

The middle (vascular) tunic contains an abundance of pigment and blood vessels. The posterior five-sixths of the middle layer consists of the choroid, while the anterior portion is comprised of the ciliary body, suspensory ligament and iris. The iris is that portion of the eye around the pupil which we refer to when we speak of the color of the eyes.

The innermost tunic of the eye, consisting of the retina, does not cover the entire eyeball. It extends from the optic nerve at the back of the eyeball as far forward, toward the front of the eyeball, as the ciliary body where it terminates in the ora serrata. Beyond this point it extends only as a non-nervous, pigmented membrane over the back of the ciliary processes and iris.

The eyegrounds (fundus of the eye) may be examined by the physician with an instrument called an ophthalmoscope. This is a fundoscopic examination of the eyes which permits the physician to see through the cornea, pupil, lens and eye fluids into the retina. The optic disc is also visible in this examination, representing the point at which the optic nerve enters the retina.

The eyeball is not a solid organ. It actually contains a large hollow interior consisting of the anterior and posterior cavities. The posterior cavity is the greater of the two, consisting of all of the area behind the lens. It contains a gelatinous substance, the vitreous humor, which provides intraocular pressure and helps to support the layers of the eyeball.

The anterior cavity, situated in front of the lens, consists of an anterior and posterior chamber. A clear fluid called the aqueous humor fills the entire anterior cavity.

The muscles of the eye are extrinsic and intrinsic in type. The intrinsic muscles consist of the ciliary muscles and iris and are involuntary. The extrinsic muscles are voluntary muscles which control the movements of the eye. They are the inferior, superior, lateral and medial rectus and the inferior and superior oblique muscles.

ACCESSORY STRUCTURES OF THE EYE

The accessory structures of the eye consist of the eyelids, eyebrows, cilia (eyelashes) and lacrimal apparatus.

The opening between the eyelids through which the eye can be seen is known as the *palpebral fissure*. The point at which the upper and lower lids come together, closest to the upper nose, is the *inner canthus*. The outer corner of the lids is the *outer canthus*. The thickened margin of the eyelids is called the *tarsal plate*.

An important accessory structure of the eye is the lacrimal apparatus consisting of the lacrimal gland which secretes tears, lacrimal ducts (lacrimal canals), lacrimal sac and the nasolacrimal duct through which the secretions are carried into the nasal cavity.

These passages sometimes become occluded to the point where surgery is indicated. The operation for drainage of the lacrimal sac is called a dacryocystostomy. When a channel must be established between the lacrimal sac and the nasal cavity an operation called a dacryocystorhinostomy is performed.

SECTION THROUGH RIGHT EYE.

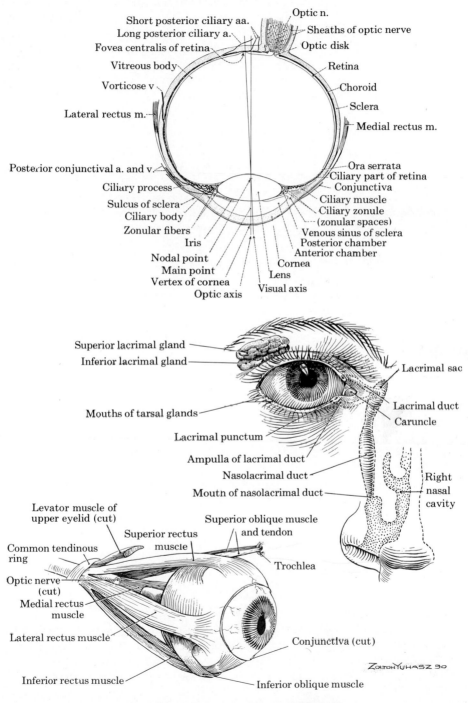

Optic n.
Short posterior ciliary aa.
Long posterior ciliary a.
Fovea centralis of retina
Vitreous body
Vorticose v
Lateral rectus m.

Sheaths of optic nerve
Optic disk
Retina
Choroid
Sclera
Medial rectus m.

Posterior conjunctival a. and v.
Ciliary process
Sulcus of sclera
Ciliary body
Zonular fibers
Iris
Nodal point
Main point
Vertex of cornea
Optic axis

Ora serrata
Ciliary part of retina
Conjunctiva
Ciliary muscle
Ciliary zonule
(zonular spaces)
Venous sinus of sclera
Posterior chamber
Anterior chamber
Cornea
Lens
Visual axis

Superior lacrimal gland
Inferior lacrimal gland

Lacrimal sac

Mouths of tarsal glands

Lacrimal duct
Caruncle

Lacrimal punctum
Ampulla of lacrimal duct
Nasolacrimal duct
Mouth of nasolacrimal duct

Right nasal cavity

Levator muscle of upper eyelid (cut)
Superior rectus muscle
Superior oblique muscle and tendon
Common tendinous ring
Optic nerve (cut)
Medial rectus muscle
Lateral rectus muscle
Trochlea
Conjunctiva (cut)

ZOLTAN YUHASZ 90

Inferior rectus muscle
Inferior oblique muscle

THE EYE AND RELATED STRUCTURES

ANATOMIC FEATURES OF THE EYE AND ACCESSORY STRUCTURES

Ampulla (pl. ampullae)
Annular plexus
Anterior chamber
Aqueous humor
Bowman's membrane
Canal of Schlemm
Canthus
Capsula lentis
Capsule of the lens
Capsule of Tenon
Caruncle
Choroid
Cilia (eyelashes)
Ciliaris muscle
Ciliary body
Ciliary processes
Ciliary veins
Conjunctiva
Cornea
Crystalline humor
Crystalline lens
Cul-de-sac
Descemet's membrane
Eyeball
Fascia bulbi (capsule of Tenon)
Fovea centralis
Hyaloid canal
Hyaloid membrane
Inferior fornix
Infratrochlear nerve
Intraepithelial plexus
Iris
Jacob's membrane (rods & cones)
Lacrimal duct
Lacrimal gland
Lacrimal papilla
Lacrimal sac
Lacus lacrimalis
Lamina basalis
Lamina choriocapillaris
Lamina cribrosa sclerae
Lamina suprachoroidea
Lamina vasculosa
Lens
Ligament of Zinn

Limbus
Macula lutea
Meibomian glands (tarsal)
Membrane of Demours
Membrane of Descemet
Muscles of the eye
    Levator palpebrae superi
    Obliquus inferior
    Obliquus superior
    Rectus inferior
    Rectus lateralis
    Rectus medialis
    Rectus superior
Nasolacrimal duct
Optic disk
Optic nerve
Ora serrata of retina
Orbicularis ciliaris
Orbicularis oculi
Palpebral commissure
Palpebral fissure
Pars ciliaris retinae
Pars iridica retinae
Pars optica retinae
Pectinate ligament of the iris
Pectinate villi
Periscleral space
Plica semilunaris
Posterior chamber
Punctum lacrimale
Pupil
Retina (tunica interna)
Sclera
Scleral spur
Sclerocorneal junction
Sinus venosus sclerae
Space of Tenon
Spaces of Fontana
Spatia zonularia (canal of Petit)
Sphincter pupillae
Stratum intermedium
Subepithelial plexus
Substantia propria
Superior tendon of Lockwood
Suspensory ligament of lens

ANATOMIC FEATURES OF THE EYE
AND ACCESSORY STRUCTURES (Continued)

Tapetum	Uvea
Tarsal plates (tarsi)	Vaginae bulbi (Tenon's capsule)
Tarsus	Vascular tunic
Tendon of Lockwood	Venae vorticosae
Tendon of Zinn	Vitreous body
Tenon's capsule	Vitreous humor
Trochlea	Zonula ciliaris
Tunica vasculosa	Zonule of Zinn

EYE ABBREVIATIONS

O.D. — right eye (oculus dexter)   O.U. — both eyes (oculi unitas)
O.S. — left eye (oculus sinister)

SOME MEDICATIONS USED IN EYE SURGERY

Acetylcholine 1:10,000	Novocain-Suprarenin
Atropine	Pilocarpine
Cocaine	Ringer's solution
Cortisone	Saline solution
Dexametazone	Sodium Sulamyd 10% Ointment
Epinephrine	Suprarenin
Hyaluronidase	White's Ointment
Methylcellulose	Yellow Oxide of Mercury
Neosporin	Xylocaine

Simple Iridectomy

After satisfactory anesthesia, the eyeball was fixed with fixation forceps. The tip of the keratome was placed about 1 mm. above the limbus at the 12 o'clock position and gently directed forward until the point could be detected in the anterior chamber. The handle of the keratome was positioned downward somewhat until the blade was parallel to the plane of the iris and projected forward to a point approximating the center of the pupil. The handle of the keratome was lowered somewhat and the instrument gently withdrawn.

A closed iris forceps was inserted through the original incision to a point almost at the pupillary border where the forceps was opened to bite a small fold of iris. This tissue was brought out through the wound and removed with the aid of de Wecker scissors creating a small coloboma as the scissors were applied in the vertical meridian of the cornea.

The iris pillars were repositioned with the aid of a spatula. The anterior chamber was irrigated with saline.

Iridencleisis

Under local anesthesia and after a subconjunctival injection of 2% cocaine above the upper limbus, a conjunctival flap including the conjunctiva and episclera was made.

A limbal incision was made with a keratome through which an iris forceps was inserted. The iris was grasped near the edge of the pupil and drawn out until the pigment epithelium on the back of the iridial tent could be seen. The sphincter pupillae was cut on either side of the forceps. A piece of sclera adjacent to the limbal incision was snipped off with the use of a scleral punch. A continuous silk suture was placed through the conjunctival flap.

Peripheral Iridectomy

After routine preparation and draping of the lids, a 00000 black silk bridle suture was placed through the superior rectus muscle. A conjunctival flap was made approximately 5 mm. in depth and dissected down to the limbus. A keratome incision was made and enlarged slightly with scissors. The anterior capsule was grasped and pulled free. Lens material was expressed. A small basal iridectomy was performed. In attempting to remove more of the posterior capsule, a small amount of vitreous was lost.

The conjunctiva was closed with a running 00000 black silk suture. Sodium Sulamyd Ointment and atropine drops of 1% were instilled. An eye pad and shield were applied.

Extracapsular Cataract Extraction

After satisfactory anesthesia, preparation and draping of the operative area, a capsule forceps was introduced through the coloboma and the teeth of this forceps used to grasp the anterior capsule just below the pupillary center. A piece of capsule was removed from the lens in a gentle maneuver after the capsule was incised in two directions with a cystotome. A strabismus hook was used to express the lens, applying pressure from below. During this procedure the assistant pulled the corneal lip downward with gentle traction on the corneal suture and the surgeon held a spoon on the upper lip of the wound. The lens was delivered by elevating the lens from behind as it was withdrawn. The sutures were tied and the remnants of the lens washed out. The pillars of the iris were replaced with a spatula.

Atropine and White's Ointment were applied to the operated eye and both eyes were bandaged.

Intracapsular Cataract Extraction

After satisfactory akinesia of the lids and injection of Novocain-Suprarenin, the superior rectus was anesthetized by a cocaine soaked applicator.

A bridle suture was inserted beneath the superior rectus muscle. A Desmarres lid elevator was used to keep the eye open during the procedure.

A conjunctival flap was developed by dissecting the conjunctiva in the region of the upper limbus and undermining it. A needle of a double-armed suture was introduced through the episclera and superficial sclera horizontally at the 12 o'clock position about 3 mm. above the cornea. Another needle was then inserted through the superficial layers of the cornea in a vertical manner. Both needles were brought out through the conjunctival flap 8 mm. from its free border.

A Graefe knife was used for the corneal section being introduced into the cornea at the limbus. As the tip of the knife entered the anterior chamber, the handle was lowered somewhat and the blade advanced parallel to the plane of the iris to the opposite limbus. The knife was then advanced upward and section carried out in a back and forth fashion, bringing the cutting edge of the knife toward the surgeon. The lens was extracted with the use of Arruga's forceps in a tumbling fashion. The sutures were tied and the iris reposited.

Intracapsular Cataract Extraction With Iridectomy

The patient was admitted with a senile cataract of the right eye. She had a postsurgical aphakia of the left eye as well as a postoperative coloboma of the left iris.

After routine preparation and draping of the area, a 00000 black silk superior rectus bridle suture was placed. A Beaver blade was used to make a limbal groove superiorly from 3 to 9 o'clock. Three interrupted 0000000 black silk sutures were placed at 10, 12 and 2 o'clock.

A keratome incision was made and enlarged with scissors. A basal iridectomy was performed at 12 o'clock. The lens was delivered by a tumbling procedure with an erisophake. Sutures were tightened. Two additional sutures were placed to completely close the wound. An air bubble was instilled in the anterior chamber and the iris pillars replaced. An eye pad and shield were applied.

Recession of Ocular Muscles—correction for strabismus

Local anesthesia is obtained using cocaine instillation and 2% Novocain-Suprarenin injection into the muscle and its insertion.

A vertical incision is made through the conjunctiva 6 mm. from the limbus which is freed from the underlying Tenon's capsule. A strabismus hook is inserted under the muscle through a buttonhole made in Tenon's capsule, below the lower edge of the muscle. A similar opening is made where the point of the hook causes the capsule to bulge. The point of the hook is then introduced through this second opening following which another hook is also placed into this buttonhole. It is carried in the opposite direction, under the muscle, until its point comes up through the first hole. The muscle belly and tendon now rest on the hooks.

An incision is made on both edges of the tendon and the muscle tendon freed of its capsular sheath. The recession suture is placed at the proximal end of the tendon. The tendon is cut from its scleral insertion and the capsular adhesions under the muscle belly are lysed. The two ends of the sutures are passed through the superficial layers of the sclera and then through the tendon stump and tied.

The conjunctival wound is sutured and binocular dressing applied.

Kuhnt-Szymanowski Operation for Spastic Ectropion of the Lower Eyelid

After routine preparation and draping of the area and 2% Xylocaine local infiltration anesthesia, the lower lid was split between the skin surface and the conjunctivotarsal area in the lateral two-thirds of the lid. A skin triangle was then excised from the conjunctivotarsal surface of the lower lid and this surface was brought together with the other using 00000 black silk suture.

The skin was undermined so as to present a sliding flap which could be moved up into the triangular defect laterally and pulled up and closed with seven interrupted 00000 black silk sutures.

The previously split lid was then reapproximated by a through-and-through 00000 black silk suture onto a button.

Sodium Sulamyd 10% Ointment was instilled and pressure dressing was applied.

Flapping of Conjunctiva, Rt. Eye

After routine preparation and draping of the lids, the conjunctiva was excised at the limbus from 3 o'clock to 9 o'clock. It was then dissected free up into the superior cul-de-sac. Two 00000 black silk sutures were placed at 10 o'clock and 2 o'clock and hooked into the conjunctiva in the lower cul-de-sac so as to pull a flap of the conjunctiva over the corneal ulcer. The central suture was also incised so as to give complete corneal coverage. Sodium Sulamyd Ointment was instilled and an eye pad applied.

Excision of Chalazion

The area of the right eye was prepared and draped in the usual manner. Several drops of 4% cocaine were instilled. The portion of the eyelid containing the tumefaction was grasped in a chalazion forceps. The lid was everted and several drops of Novocain-Suprarenin were placed around the chalazion.

After a few minutes, a vertical incision was made on the conjunctival side, with care, to avoid injury to the lid margins. The contents of the chalazion were evacuated with a small curet. The cystic wall was gently removed with scissors. No excessive bleeding was encountered.

Transplant of Pterygium

Under general anesthesia, the head of the pterygium was grasped with a forceps and it was removed from the cornea on which it was encroaching with a fine knife. The portion of the cornea from which the pterygium had been removed was carefully curetted.

The pterygium was undermined along with the conjunctiva proximal to it. This extended toward the lower cul-de-sac. The head of the pterygium was then slightly elevated. A double-armed mattress suture was inserted through the head of the pterygium. Two needles were passed through the conjunctival pocket which had been formed beneath. The suture was tied and the pterygium buried.

Partial Penetrating Keratoplasty

With the trephine centered on the pupil and the host eye in myosis (or: miosis) the Paufique trephine was applied perpendicularly to the surface of the cornea and a graft removed with care to insure regular corneal margins. The graft measured 7 mm.

A vertical incision was made with the trephine and scissors in the host eye, without bevel. The graft was sutured in place using direct radial sutures, edge-to-edge, placed 1 mm. from the corneal margins and passing through the middle portion of the stroma.

A Grieshaber 83/4 needle with virgin silk and a Barraquer mosquito needle holder were used to seal the anterior chamber.

Three milligrams of Dexametazone were injected under the conjunctiva to reduce postoperative reactions.

Reattachment of Retina by Electric Cautery

A conjunctival incision was made inferiorly about 3 to 9 o'clock. The inferior rectus muscle was dissected free. The conjunctiva and Tenon's capsule were dissected back to the posterior globe area. Multiple ½ mm.

retinal cautery punctures were made with good fluid drainage in both inferior quadrants. The conjunctiva was closed with a running 00000 black silk suture. Sodium Sulamyd 10% Ointment was instilled in the conjunctival sac.

Discission of the Lens

A sickle-shaped Ziegler knife was introduced at the limbus subconjunctivally. Keeping its flat surface parallel to the plane of the iris, it was further introduced through the cornea until the tip of the instrument extended to the upper border of the pupil. The cutting edge was directed towards the lens making a deep vertical cut into the capsule and anterior lens. A horizontal incision was made and the instrument removed via the route of introduction.

Removal of Meshed Ball Implant; Insertion of Polyethylene Implant with mucous membrane graft to conjunctiva covering the implant

After routine preparation and draping of the lids, enucleation scissors were used to dissect free the meshed implant ball that showed about an 8 mm. exposure anteriorly. A 15 mm. polyethylene ball was inserted.

Tenon's capsule and the scleral area were dissected free from the conjunctiva. Interrupted 0000 chromic sutures were used to close this defect. A mucous membrane graft approximately 1 cm. wide by 3 cm. long was then removed from the inner side of the lower lip. It was attached to the existing conjunctiva so as to give a complete closure using interrupted 00000 black silk sutures. Gentle pressure bandages were applied.

Evisceration of the Right Eye; Insertion of Plastic Ball

The patient was given a local anesthetic and a topical anesthetic was introduced into the conjunctival sac. A Good retractor was introduced. It was noted that the eye was considerably engorged and the conjunctiva was quite reddened. The iris was cloudy and the eyeball was under considerable tension.

The conjunctiva was incised in an elliptical fashion near the limbus. Dissection was then continued to the region of the limbus where the anterior chamber was entered with a keratome. Fluid from the anterior chamber was released and the eyeball relaxed.

By means of forceps the retina was removed. The iris was scraped free. The incision was enlarged in a T-shaped fashion.

A Lucite plastic ball was introduced. The sclera was approximated with interrupted 00000 plain suture. The conjunctiva was sutured similarly and closed with 00000 silk suture.

Dacryocystorhinostomy (Toti Operation)

Anesthesia was obtained by blocking the infratrochlear nerve with 2 cc. of a 2% solution of Novocain Hydrochloride with epinephrine hydrochloride. In addition to this, a cocaine-Suprarenin pledget was inserted on the inside of the nasal mucosa against the middle turbinate. This was followed by packing of this side of the nose.

An incision was made in the skin beginning from 3 to 5 mm. above the internal canthal ligament, curving outward as it was carried downward along the anterior lacrimal crest to a point immediately below the nasal duct.

A Mueller speculum was then introduced into the wound. The canthal ligament was then identified, beneath which, we were able to identify the lacrimal sac. The ligament was then incised vertically. The sac was gently teased away from the ligament. A longitudinal incision was then made the entire length of the sac on its nasal side. The periosteum beyond the lacrimal crests was then elevated and the anterior crest chiseled away. The mucous membrane of the nose was exposed and care was taken to avoid injury to this tissue. A 2 cm. piece of bone was removed from the ascending process of the maxilla and lacrimal bone with the use of a chisel and mallet.

A longitudinal incision was then made in the nasal mucosa opposite the one made in the lacrimal sac. The anterior and posterior lips of the nasal mucosa were then sutured with the matching sides of the sac in apposition.

The outer wound was closed by a few deep catgut sutures. Interrupted silk was used for the outer wound edges.

McLaughlin Canthoplasty, Lateral, Left

Following suitable premedication, the patient was taken to surgery and the face prepared with pHisoHex and draped. 1% Xylocaine containing ½ cc. of adrenalin to the ounce was used for local anesthesia.

A wedge-shaped area of tissue on the lateral canthus of the left eye, to include some of the lash margin, was excised in both the upper and lower lid areas. These areas were based with the narrow portion of the triangle medially. They were trimmed so that they would overlap accurately and give a new canthus. This would permit tears to flow out over the cheek from the lateral angle of the eye.

A 00000 dermalon suture was used to close the canthoplasty. It was sutured through-and-through the lid and tied over a small piece of polyethylene tubing used as a bolster. The remainder of the incision was closed into a crow's foot using 00000 dermalon cuticular suture and twists to follow, as necessary.

An ellipse of tissue in the left nasolabial fold measuring 2 cm. in width and 4 cm. in length was excised with skin, subcutaneous fat and scar. This was suitably defatted and undermined. Closure was accomplished with interrupted subcutaneous nylon sutures followed by 00000 dermalon cuticular sutures and twists, as necessary.

Fine moistened mesh gauze was placed over the wound. Some Terramycin Ointment was placed in the eye and an eye pad applied. A light pressure dressing was placed over the wound and the mouth was immobilized on the left side.

EPONYMIC TITLES OF EYE OPERATIONS

Agnew canthoplasty
Ammon canthoplasty
Arlt epicanthus repair
Arruga cataract extraction
Arruga dacryostomy
Arruga keratoplasty
Arruga tenotomy
Bardelli lid ptosis operation
Barkan double cyclodialysis
Barkan goniotomy
Barrio iridencleisis
Basterra dacryostomy
Berens sclerectomy
Bielschowsky strabismus operation
Blasius lid operation
Blaskovics canthoplasty
Blaskovics dacryostomy
Blaskovics inversion of tarsus
Blaskovics lid operation
Blaskovics tarsectomy
Blatt pterygium operation
Bossalino blepharorrhaphy
Briggs strabismus operation
Büdinger blepharoplasty
Casanellas operation on lacrimal
  canaliculi
Castroviejo keratoplasty
Celsus lid operation
Celsus spasmodic entropion operation

Csapody orbital cavity repair
Czermak pterygium operation
Daviel cataract extraction
Dupuy-Dutemps dacryostomy
Dupuy-Dutemps lid operation
Dürr non-penetrating keratoplasty
Duverger and Velter dacryostomy
Elliott corneoscleral trephination
Elschnig blepharorrhaphy
Elschnig canthorrhaphy
Elschnig central iridectomy
Elschnig cicatricial entropian
  operation
Elschnig ptosis operation
Elschnig total keratoplasty
Filatov keratoplasty
Filatov-Marzinkowsky keratoplasty
Franceschetti keratoplasty
Franceschetti upward deviation of
  pupil
Fricke lid operation
Friede keratoplasty
Friedenwald ptosis operation
Fuchs canthorrhaphy
Fuchs transfixion of iris
Fukala lens extraction
Gayet operation for trichiasis
Georgariou cyclodialysis and
  sclerectomy

EPONYMIC TITLES OF EYE OPERATIONS (continued)

Gifford's delimiting keratotomy
Gomez-Marquez operation for
  obstructed lacrimal canaliculi
Gonin cautery of retinal detachment
Gradle keratoplasty
Gutzeit dacryostomy
Guyton ptosis operation
Hasner lid operation
Hess ptosis operation
Hippel (Von) keratoplasty
Hogan dacryostomy
Holth iridencleisis
Holth punch sclerectomy
Horay muscle and tendon
  advancement
Horvath muscle and tendon
  advancement
Hotz cicatricial entropion operation
Hughes lid operation
Imre blepharochalasis
Imre canthoplasty
Imre epicanthus operation
Imre keratoplasty
Imre lid plasty
Imre spasmodic entropion operation
Jaesche-Arlt trichiasis operation
Jameson tenotomy
Key iridodialysis
Kirby cataract extraction
Knapp lid operation
Knapp pterygium operation
Knapp-Imre lid operation
Kofler endonasal dacryostomy
Kraupa keratoplasty
Kreiker blepharochalasis
Kreiker blepharorrhaphy
Kriebig lid operation
Krönlein orbit operation
Kuhnt dacryostomy
Kuhnt lid operation
Kuhnt ectropion operation
Kuhnt epicanthus operation
Kuhnt tarsectomy
Lacarrere strabismus operation
Lagleyze cicatricial entropion
  operation

Lagrange sclerectomy
Lagrange modification of Arruga
Lagrange modification of Berens
Lagrange strabismus operation
Langenbeck plastic lid operation
Lindner corneoscleroconjunctival
  suture
Lindner posterior sclerotomy
Lindner shortening of eyeball
Löhlein keratoplasty
Londermann trephination of cornea
Lopez Enriquez trephine of the sclera
Löwenstein dacryostomy
Machek trichiasis operation
Magitot keratoplasty
Majewsky keratoplasty
Mauksch cyclodialysis
McGuire advancement in strabismus
McReynolds pterygium operation
Meller operation for coloboma of the
  lids
Morax keratoplasty
Mosher-Toti dacryostomy
Motais ptosis lid operation
Nida ptosis operation
Nizetic inversion of tarsus
Nizetic keratoplasty
O'Connor strabismus operation
O'Connor-Peter muscle operation
Paufique detachment of retina
Paufique lamellar keratoplasty
Paufique shortening of the eyeball
Peter tenotomy
Polyak endonasal dacryostomy
Poulard operation for spasmodic
  entropion
Raverdino dacryostomy
Richet cicatricial ectropion operation
Rowinski dacryostomy
Rubbrecht extirpation of cornea
  segmentally
Silva-Costa lacrimal operation
Smith extraction of cataract
Snellen entropion operation
Soria dacryostomy
Sourdille ptosis operation

EPONYMIC TITLES OF EYE OPERATIONS (continued)

Sourdille total lamellar keratoplasty
Spaeth pterygium operation
Speas strabismus operation
Spencer-Watson trichiasis operation
Stock dacryostomy
Suarez Villafranca plastic lid
  operation
Szymanowski spastic ectropion lid
  operation
Szymanowski-Kuhnt lid operation
Terson pterygium operation
Thomas keratoplasty
Thomas strabismus operation
Toti operation dacryostomy
Toti-Mosher dacryostomy
Trantas tarsectomy
Verhoeff advancement operation
Verhoeff corneoscleral trephination

Verwey epicanthus operation
Waldhauer trichiasis operation
Wecker, de anterior sclerotomy
Wecker, de posterior sclerotomy
Weekers iridencleisis
West dacryostomy
Weve dacryostomy
Weve shortening of the eyeball
Wheeler advancement of the inferior
  oblique
Wheeler advancement of the superior
  oblique
Wheeler operation for coloboma
Wheeler iridectomy
Wiener keratoplasty
Wilmer central iridectomy
Wolfe sclerectomy and cyclodialysis
Worth strabismus operation

10 ⎰ *Neurosurgery*

Neurosurgery, the specialty dealing with surgical lesions of the nervous system, might well be considered one of the most modern surgical specialties. Although archaeologic evidence has been uncovered to indicate the earliest efforts of man to operate on the brain, it was not until the beginning of this century that modern neurosurgery had its inception. In the half century which has followed, the scope of this specialty has been magnified many times and its store of knowledge enlarged to an extent which could not have been anticipated by its most enthusiastic forefathers.

Neurosurgery is no longer limited to the removal of brain tumors, treatment of brain and spinal cord injuries and alleviation of pain. Procedures are being performed today which thirty years ago would have been regarded as daringly experimental. Modern anesthesia, new drugs and modern supportive treatment based on advances in our knowledge of morphology, physiology, ultrabiophysics and biochemistry have made possible these more radical operations. Radioactive isotopes, electroencephalography, electrocorticography, depth recordings, bioelectric potentials and new radiographic methods have facilitated earlier detection and localization of neurosurgical lesions.

The fund of scientific knowledge relating to this specialty is being swelled by contributions from bioscientists and neurosurgeons all over the world, each lending his genius to unraveling the mysteries of this all important organ, the brain.

The complexity of the brain and its associated structures can be better appreciated if we consider the brain proper and the spinal cord separately. No attempt will be made to elaborate further on the nerves which have been discussed in Chapter 6.

238

THE SPINAL CORD (Myelon)

The spinal cord is the elongated portion of the central nervous system extending from the foramen magnum, at the level of the upper part of the atlas, down to the upper border of the second lumbar vertebra. At this level it gives off a terminal strand of nonnervous tissue called the filum terminale which projects extradurally down to the first coccygeal vertebra. At its upper (intradural) portion, the filum terminale is surrounded by the lumbar, sacral and coccygeal spinal nerve roots which are referred to collectively as the cauda equina (horse's tail).

The average length of the spinal cord is about 18 inches, extending from the base of the brain down to the upper border of the second lumbar vertebra. The cord is situated within the spinal canal of the vertebral column where it is invested by three layers of membranes (meninges) continuous with those covering the brain. The outermost layer is called the *dura mater* or dura; the middle layer is the *arachnoid mater,* and the innermost layer is the *pia mater*. The pia mater extends beyond the spinal cord and is joined with dura mater at the level of the third sacral segment.

Spinal fluid circulates between the meninges particularly in the subarachnoid space situated between the pia and the arachnoid membranes.

An epidural cavity separates the dura mater from the vertebral canal wall and an intervening space called the *subdural cavity* separates the dura from the underlying arachnoid. The arachnoid, in turn, is separated from the underlying pia mater by a wide space known as the *subarachnoid cavity* which is filled with spinal fluid.

The *ligamentum denticulatum* (dentate ligament) extends as a narrow band on either side of the spinal cord for its entire length. Its medial border is continuous with the pia mater and its lateral border with the dura mater, at intervals. It separates the anterior and posterior nerve roots.

The spinal nerves, consisting of thirty-one pairs, project from the spinal cord. Each of these nerves has a ventral (anterior) root and a dorsal (posterior) root. The dorsal roots contain a spinal ganglion. The spinal nerves are paired into 8 cervical, 12 thoracic, 5 lumbar, 5 sacral and 1 coccygeal.

A longitudinal median groove incompletely divides the spinal cord into halves. This groove is called the anterior median fissure and the posterior median sulcus.

The anatomic terms for structures associated with the spinal cord and for the cord proper have been listed below to provide a ready reference.

FEATURES OF THE SPINAL CORD AND ASSOCIATED STRUCTURES:

Anterior column
Anterior cornu
Anterior funiculus
Anterior gray commissure
Anterior median fissure
Anterior nerve roots
Anterior white commissure
Anterolateral region
Arachnoid
Cauda equina
Central canal
Cisterna magna
Conus medullaris
Dentate ligament
Dorsal nerve root
Dura mater (dura)
Epidural cavity
Fasciculus cuneatus
Fasciculus gracilis
Filum terminale
Filum terminale externum
Filum terminale internum
Formatio reticularis
Glial sheath
Lateral column
Lateral funiculus
Ligamentum denticulatum
Ligamenta flava (plural)

Ligamentum flavum
Medulla oblongata
Medulla spinalis
Meninges
Nerve rootlet
Pia-glial membrane
Pia mater
Posterior column
Posterior funiculus
Posterior gray commissure
Posterior median sulcus
Posterior nerve roots
Postero-intermediate sulcus
Posterolateral sulcus
Spinal ganglion
Subarachnoid cavity
Subarachnoid cisterna
Subarachnoid septum
Subarachnoid space
Subdural space
Substantia gelatinosa centralis
Substantia gelatinosa of Rolando
Terminal ventricle
Tract of Burdach
Tract of Goll
Tract of Lissauer
Transverse commissure
Vertebral canal

Lumbar Hemilaminectomy for Ruptured Disc (Herniated Nucleus Pulposus)

The patient was surgically prepared and draped in a prone, semiflexed position on the operating table.

A midline incision was made in the lower back over the spinous processes of the 3rd, 4th, and 5th lumbar and 1st sacral vertebrae. The spinous processes of L-4, L-5 and S-1 were exposed. An incision was made in the thoracolumbar fascia just lateral to the spinous processes on the side where the hemilaminectomy was planned. Bleeding was controlled by coagulation.

A periosteal elevator was used to separate the Erector spinae and Multifidus muscles from the spinous processes and laminae. The laminae and the articular processes of the vertebrae were exposed. A coagulating current was used to control bleeding. All bleeding from the cut ends of the bone was controlled with Horsley's bone wax. The interspaces were visualized after the muscle had been removed. The ligamenta flava were seen between the vertebrae.

The proposed hemilaminectomy was outlined on the 4th and 5th lumbar laminae on the left. A gooseneck rongeur was used to remove this portion of the lamina. After the hemilaminectomy had been performed at the 5th and 4th lumbar areas, the ligamentum flavum was grasped with a hook at the 4th interspace. Cottonoid was introduced under this area to protect the dura. The ligamentum flavum was excised by incision of its attachments. It was completely removed in its lateral attachment.

The nerve root was identified and retracted following which the ruptured disc was identified at the level of L-5. It was noted to be compressing the outgoing nerve. Using a Love retractor the 1st sacral nerve was retracted. The disc was removed piecemeal from the epidural space using pituitary forceps. Bleeding was controlled by electrocautery on vessels and Gelfoam at the sites of oozing.

The 4th interspace was then explored and no pathology was found. The dura was tightly closed with a running suture of fine silk with stitches 4 mm. apart. The Erector spinae muscles were closed with interrupted chromic catgut sutures. The fascia was treated in a similar manner. The subcutaneous tissues and skin were closed with interrupted silk sutures.

Hemilaminectomy for Cervical Disc

The patient was prepared and draped in a sitting position. An incision was made over the spinous processes of the 4th, 5th, 6th, and 7th cervical vertebrae to the 1st dorsal vertebra. Following the incision of the midline of the posterior neck and thorax, the ligamentum nuchae and the spinous processes of the lower cervical and 1st dorsal vertebrae were exposed. The incision was made on the side of the lesion. The spinous processes of the 7th cervical and the 1st dorsal were exposed. Bleeders were coagulated with electrocautery. Further dissection with scissors was carried out to expose the spinous processes of C-5 and C-6. The bifid portions of the spinous processes of C-5 and C-6 were separated from their muscle attachments on the side of the ruptured disc. A periosteal elevator was used to further dissect the muscles away from the spinous processes and the laminae. A Scoville self-retaining retractor was used to retract the muscles. The laminae were removed. A dental drill was used to bite off the shelf of bone on the lateral aspect of the opening.

By gentle palpation, the ruptured disc was located under the outgoing nerve; however, to avoid trauma to the outgoing nerve, a transdural approach was elected. The dura was transfixed with a pair of silk sutures at the ends of the proposed incision, following which, the dura was elevated and incised. Following retraction of the dura, the denticulate ligament was identified. This was cut with scissors exposing the ruptured disc. The outgoing nerve was gently retracted downward and the disc removed with pituitary forceps.

The anterior dural opening was closed with a single interrupted silk suture. The muscles and fascia were closed with a chromic catgut. The subcutaneous tissues and skin were closed with interrupted silk sutures.

ANATOMY OF THE BRAIN

The brain can be divided grossly into three parts: the forebrain, the midbrain and the hindbrain. Each of these sections is subdivided into major subdivisions as must be the case with an organ as complex morphologically and physiologically as the brain. No attempt can be made to review the anatomy of this system other than superficially in the confines of this chapter; however, salient features of the brain and its major divisions are listed to provide the secretary with an anatomic reference.

The forebrain comprises the largest portion of the brain. It consists of the diencephalon and the cerebrum. A longitudinal fissure divides the cerebrum into halves called *cerebral hemispheres.* Each of these hemispheres are further divided into lobes: *the insula* (island of Reil), *limbic, occipital, temporal, parietal,* and *frontal.* The outer surface (cortex) of the cerebrum consists of numerous convolutions or folds (gyri) separated by fissures or sulci.

The midbrain is a short section which connects the forebrain with the pons and cerebellum. It is situated just below the inferior aspect of the cerebrum.

The hindbrain consists of the pons, cerebellum and the medulla oblongata. The cerebellum is the second largest section of the brain. It is located just beneath the posterior aspect of the occipital lobe of the cerebrum, in the back of the skull. The medulla oblongata is a 3 cm. segment of brain connecting with the spinal cord below and with the pons above. The pons situated just above the medulla serves as a connection for the neural pathways between the cerebellum and the cerebral cortex.

The anatomy of the brain is more complex than that of any organ in the body. No attempt will be made to list all of its features; however, the structures which might be identified in a surgeon's report have been included in the following list.

SALIENT FEATURES OF THE BRAIN AND ITS INVESTING TISSUES

Accessory cuneate nucleus
Accessory nerves
Ala cinerea
Anterior central gyrus
Anterior cerebrospinal fasciculus
Anterior external arcuate fibers
Anterior median fissure
Anterior medullary velum
Anterolateral sulcus
Aqueduct of Sylvius
Arachnoid mater
Arachnoid space
Arbor vitae
Area acoustica
Area postrema
Calcarine fissure
Cerebellum
Cerebral aqueduct
Cerebral hemisphere
Cerebral peduncle
Cerebrum
Choroid plexus
Cingulate sulcus
Clava
Colliculus facialis
Corpora quadrigemina
Corpus callosum
Corpus cerebelli
Cortex
Corticopontile fibers
Corticospinal tract
Crura
Crusta
Cuneate tubercle
Deep transverse fibers
Dentate fascia
Diencephalon
Dorsal fasciculus of Schütz
Dorsospinocerebellar fasciculus
Dura mater
Epithalamus
Falx cerebri
Fasciculus cuneatus
Fasciculus gracilis
Fibrae propriae
Fissure prima

Fissure of Sylvius
Flocculonodular lobe
Foramen cecum
Formatio reticularis
Fornix
Fourth ventricle
Frenulum veli
Frontal lobe
Frontopontile fibers
Funiculus separans
Furrow
Fusiform gyrus
Geniculate body
Genu
Glia
Gyrus (gyri)
Gyrus of Broca
Hippocampal gyrus
Hook bundle of Risien Russell
Hypoglossal nucleus
Hypothalamic area
Hypothalamus
Incisura temporalis
Inferior cerebellar peduncle
Inferior fovea
Inferior frontal gyrus
Insula lobe (island of Reil)
Interpeduncular fossa
Interpeduncular ganglion
Interventricular foramen
Intraparietal sulcus of Turner
Lateral aperture
Lateral cerebral fissure
Lateral ventricle
Lateral cerebrospinal fasciculus
Lateral hemispheres
Lateral sulcus
Limbic lobe
Lingula
Lobus simplex
Locus caeruleus
Longitudinal cerebral fissure
Mammillary bodies
Marginal gyrus
Medial aperture
Medial eminence

SALIENT FEATURES OF THE BRAIN AND
ITS INVESTING TISSUES (Continued)

Medial frontal sulcus of
  Eberstaller
Medial lemniscus
Medial lobule
Medial longitudinal fasciculus
Median sulcus
Medulla oblongata
Medulla spinalis
Metathalamus
Middle cerebral peduncle
Middle frontal gyrus
Nucleus ambiguus
Nucleus arcuatus
Nucleus cuneatus
Nucleus gracilis
Nucleus lacrimalis
Nucleus of Schwalbe
Nucleus salivatorius
Occipital lobe
Oculomotor sulcus
Olive
Opercula of the insula
Orbital operculum
Paramedial sulcus
Parietal lobe
Parieto-occipital fissure
Pars optica
Pia mater
Pineal body
Pons
Posterior commissure
Posterior median fissure
Posteromedian lobule
Primary fissure
Pyramid
Pyramidal decussation
Raphe
Recess
Recessus infundibuli

Recessus suprapinealis
Restiform bodies
Rhomboid fossa
Rubrospinal tract
Septum pellucidum
Splenium
Striae medullaris
Subdural space
Substantia ferruginea
Substantia nigra
Subthalamus
Sulcus basilaris
Sulcus circularis
Sulcus limitans
Sulcus lunatus
Superficial transverse fibers
Superior fovea
Superior frontal gyrus
Taenia pontis
Tectospinal tract
Tegmental part of pons
Tegmentum
Tela choroidea
Telencephalon
Temporal lobe
Thalamus
Transverse occipital sulcus
Trigonum hypoglossi
Tuber cinereum
Tubercle of Rolando
Tuberculum acusticum
Uncinate fasciculus
Ventral spinocerebellar tract
Ventral spinothalamic fasciculus
Ventricle
Ventriculus quartus
Vermis
Zona compacta
Zona reticulata

ARTERIES OF THE BRAIN

Anterior cerebral
Anterior choroidal
Anterior communicating
Arterial circle of Willis

Basilar
Lateral striate arteries
Middle cerebral
Posterior cerebral
Posterior communicating

CRANIOTOMY

Unlike most surgeons, the neurosurgeon operating on the brain cannot reach his operative site by simply deepening his skin incision. He has the bony protective incasement of the brain confronting him before he can gain access to the cranial cavity and the brain. Limited access to his objective makes it necessary that he accurately localize the lesion through preliminary diagnostic examinations. Sometimes it is possible for him to operate through one or more bur holes; however, when a more extensive lesion is involved, it may be necessary to turn down a skull flap.

The operation in which a hole is cut in the skull is called a *trephination* or *craniotomy*. It is performed with an instrument resembling a corkscrew (trephine) which has a short nail-like tip above which is situated a threaded cutting disk. In this procedure an opening is made through which the surgeon may operate. These openings range in size from about 5/8ths of an inch to 1 1/2 inches in diameter and are enlarged, as necessary, with a rongeur. Such openings are adequate for the introduction of needles, exploring cannulas and the removal of subdural hematomas.

When a portion of the skull must be removed and cannot be replaced, the operation is called a *craniectomy*. When such a procedure is extensive as in certain skull fractures, the defect in the cranium is corrected by insertion of a vitallium skull plate such as the Hoen skull plate. Plastic materials, usually acrylics, are also used to cover cranial defects.

CRANIOTOMY INSTRUMENTS (for additional listings see Chapter 5)

Adson brain forceps
Adson brain suction tip
Adson dura hook
Adson hemostatic forceps
Adson saw guides
Allis forceps
Bayonet thumb forceps
Blair saw guides
Cone wire twister
Crile hemostatic forceps
Cushing brain retractor
Cushing brain spatula
Cushing flat drill
Cushing vein retractor
Dandy scalp hemostats
D'Errico bur
DeVilbiss cranial rongeur
DeVilbiss cranial trephine
Ferguson bone grasping forceps
Frazier dura elevator

Frazier dura hook
Galt trephine
Gigli saw
Hajek-Ballenger elevator
Horsley dura separator
Horsley bone wax
Hudson cranial drill
Kanavel exploring cannula
Kirmisson periosteal raspatory
Klemme retractor
Kolodny scalp hemostats
Langenbeck periosteal elevator
Love-Gruenwald rongeur
Lucae bone mallet
McKenzie clip applying forceps
Oldberg retractor
Raney cranial drill
Sachs exploring cannula
Seletz ventricular cannula
Senn small rake retractor

CRANIOTOMY INSTRUMENTS (Continued)

Smithwick clip applying forceps
Smithwick nerve hook
Spurling rongeur
Stille-Gigli wire saw
Stille-Liston bone cutting forceps
Stille-Luer cutting forceps
Stille-Luer rongeur

Stille osteotome
Strully scissors
Sweet clip applying forceps
Taylor scissors
Verbrugghen retractor
Volkman curet
Weitlaner retractor

HEMOSTATIC AGENTS AND METHODS IN NEUROSURGERY

Bone wax
Bovie electrocautery
    coagulating current
    cutting current
Cellulose gauze
Clips
    Adson
    Cushing
    Köln
    Mayfield
    McKenzie
    Michel
    Olivecrona
    Raney
    Silver

Tantalum
Tonnis
Crushed muscle
Fibrin film
Fibrin foam
Gelfoam
Gelita B
Horsley's bone wax
Ligatures
Muscle graft
Muscle stamp
Oxycel
Spongostan
Suction

Trigeminal Rhizotomy, Right

With the patient in a sitting position under general anesthesia, a vertical incision was made over the right temporal region about 2 cm. anterior to the external auditory canal on the right side. Retraction was obtained.

The squamous portion of the temporal bone was identified. A trephine opening was made. This opening in the temporal bone was enlarged with rongeurs until it was about 1½ inches in diameter. The dura was separated from the base of the middle fossa until the middle meningeal artery was identified. The middle meningeal artery was cauterized at its point of emergence from the foramen spinosum and the foramen spinosum was packed with cotton. The middle meningeal artery was then cut across.

The dura was reflected from the base of the middle fossa medial to the foramen spinosum until the foramen ovale was identified. The external dura was then stripped away from its trigeminal ganglion until the whole of the trigeminal ganglion was identified. The maxillary and mandibular roots of the trigeminal ganglion were then cut leaving the ophthalmic root intact.

Bleeding was controlled by packing.

Temporal Craniotomy with Exploratory Trephine

Under general anesthesia, the patient was placed in the supine position, prepared and draped in the usual manner.

A left frontal temporal craniotomy incision was marked out. After instillation of $\frac{1}{2}\%$ Xylocaine with ephedrine, local, a skin incision was made over the coronal suture approximately 3 cm. in length and held open with self-retaining retractors. No. 1, 2 and 3 burs were used and a trephine was done. The dura was not noted to be under tension. It was incised in a cruciate manner. Bleeding was controlled by the use of bone wax and electrocautery.

The surface of the brain was noted to be bulging somewhat. An exploratory needle was passed inferiorly, superiorly, anteriorly and posteriorly. The anterior horn of the lateral ventricle was entered and 10 cc. of air instilled. As the needle was passed inferiorly toward the middle fossa, increased resistance was encountered which possibly represented a tumor. It was felt that any such lesion in this area would be inoperable.

The wound was closed in two layers with 000 black silk interrupted sutures.

The biopsy specimen was sent to the pathologist for histologic examination. It was reported back as an Astrocytoma, Grade 1.

Left Temporal Craniotomy with Removal of Subdural Hematoma

Under general anesthesia, a horseshoe-shaped flap was turned down on the left temporal region. The flap was approximately $2\frac{1}{2}$ inches in diameter.

The dura was found to be under increased tension. The dura was opened and underneath it, a subdural hematoma was found. The membrane was ruptured. There was a gush of liquid, consisting of old changed dark blood, from the opening. The hematoma extended from the tip of the frontal lobe to the tip of the occipital lobe, over the whole surface of the hemisphere. The maximum depth of the subdural hematoma was approximately $1\frac{1}{4}$ inches.

The hematoma cavity was completely washed out. All bleeding points were controlled. There was no large single bleeding point.

A silver clip was placed on the surface of the left hemisphere for x-ray control in the future. The dura was closed with interrupted silk. The bone flap was replaced and the scalp closed in two layers with silk.

Exploration for Extracerebral Hematoma

The scalp was shaved and then surgically prepared and draped. Under local anesthesia using Avertin as a basal anesthetic, a vertical incision was made above and 2 cm. in front of the ear. The first bur hole was made just below the superior insertion of the temporal muscle. No hematoma was found. A similar bur hole was then made in the same position, on the opposite side. A clot was found. The bur hole was enlarged with rongeurs. The clot was removed in its entirety using suction.

Bleeding was traced and the incision extended down to the floor of the temporal fossa. Bleeding was noted to be originating from the foramen spinosum. The incision was extended, the bone rongeured away and the bleeding point exposed. Bleeding was controlled with electrocoagulation. All of the clot was evacuated by suction and irrigation. Bleeding was controlled from the emissary veins between the dura and the bone. Hemostasis was obtained.

The temporal muscle and scalp were closed in layers with interrupted silk. No drainage was necessary.

Craniectomy

The scalp was shaved, prepared and draped and the patient was positioned in the face down position. The head was supported on an Adson outrigger type headrest.

After local infiltration of the operative site with Novocain, a curved incision was made in the scalp, starting just opposite the middle of one mastoid process, curving upward and around to the middle of the other mastoid process. The incision paralleled the superior nuchal line. An incision was then made in the occipital muscle and fascia parallel to the scalp incision, 5 mm. below its insertion on the occipital bone. The musculocutaneous flap thus formed was reflected downward until the rim of the foramen magnum was exposed. The occipital muscles were divided in the midline down to the arch of the atlas.

A bur hole was made in the occipital bone, rongeuring away bone up to the insertion of the occipital fascia above, downwards to the foramen magnum and laterally to the mastoid processes. An accidental incision into the mastoid cells was immediately sealed with bone wax.

The dorsal rim of the foramen magnum was removed along with the arch of the atlas. Next, the bone in the middle was removed. This was followed by profuse bleeding which was controlled by generous application of bone wax.

The dura was noted to be under increased tension. The lateral ventricle was tapped.

A 4 cm. vertical incision was made in the scalp about 7 cm. above the external occipital protuberance and 4 cm. toward the midline followed by a bur hole with incision of the dura. A cannula was inserted into the posterior horn of the lateral ventricle. A flanged cannula was left in situ during the operation for continuous drainage.

The dura was opened down to the foramen magnum with ligation of the occipital sinus. Hemostasis was obtained. After exploration of the posterior fossa had been carried out, the dural flaps were replaced without sutures. The deep occipital muscles were sutured in the midline with interrupted sutures of silk being sutured back to the fascial margin along the superior nuchal line. The fascia was then sutured in a similar manner. The galea and skin were closed using interrupted sutures of silk. No drainage was used.

Chordotomy (Sectioning of the lateral spinothalamic tract)

After satisfactory preparation, draping and anesthesia, a median incision was made in the back and a laminectomy performed involving the 3rd and 4th thoracic vertebrae. Using a Kerrison rongeur the lateral portion of the canal was removed. Full exposure was accomplished on both sides. The dura was then opened and retracted with sutures. The outgoing anterior and posterior nerve roots as well as the ligamentum denticulatum were visualized. The attachment of the denticulate ligament was severed bilaterally and grasped with a hemostat on the side of the section. The spinal cord was carefully rotated by means of the denticulate ligament. In an avascular area, at a depth of 4 mm., the anterolateral portion of the cord was sectioned with a # 11 Bard-Parker blade. The arachnoid in the area for section was removed. The section was carried anteriorly at a point just medial to the outgoing anterior nerve roots.

The dura was closed with interrupted 0000 silk ties. The muscles were reapproximated with interrupted 00 chromic. The subcutaneous tissue was closed with interrupted chromic and the skin edges were brought together with interrupted silk. A dressing was applied.

Elevation of Depressed Skull Fracture

The scalp was shaved and the head surgically prepared and draped. A bur hole was made to one side of the depressed bone. All depressed fragments of the inner table were removed with rongeur forceps. It was noted that the fracture was situated above the superior longitudinal dural sinus. Hemorrhage followed removal of the bone fragments. This was controlled by application of a muscle stamp, held in place with a suction tip against wet cottonoid which adhered to the dura.

The bone fragments were fitted into place, the larger fragments being anchored by silk sutures passed through gimlet holes in the bone edges.

The scalp wound was closed with a layer of interrupted silk sutures in the galea and another row in the skin.

Subtemporal Decompression

After the scalp had been surgically prepared and the area draped, a hockeystick incision was made in front of the ear. The resulting scalp flap was reflected anteriorly. Using a vertical incision, the temporal fascia was incised by beginning at the zygoma. A 3 mm. horizontal incision at the zygoma from the vertical incision permitted better retraction of the temporal fascia. The upper end of the vertical incision was then converted into a Y-shape and the resulting flap retracted superiorly. The temporal muscle was incised in the direction of its fibers and the edges were retracted. A bur hole was then made in the exposed temporal bone, rongeuring away the bone in all directions. The underlying dura was opened by a cruciate incision.

Hemostasis was obtained. The exposed cortex was covered with fibrin film to prevent adhesions between the cortex and overlying structures.

The galea and then the skin were closed with interrupted silk sutures.

Clipping of Middle Cerebral Artery

Under general anesthesia, with the patient on his right side, a horse-shoe-shaped flap was turned down over the left temporal region. The incision was carried down to the zygoma. The bone flap, involving the squamous portion of the temporal bone, was reflected and the bone was further rongeured away down to the base of the middle fossa.

When adequate exposure of the dura over the temporal lobe had been obtained, a curved incision was made through the dura centering over the Sylvian fissure. The dura was reflected downward and the Sylvian fissure was identified. The arachnoid over the Sylvian fissure (sulcus lateralis cerebri) was then split so that the frontal lobe could be separated from the temporal lobe by splitting the tissues through the Sylvian fissure.

Small bleeding points were coagulated as the fissure was opened. The branches of the middle cerebral artery were identified. These were followed medially until the aneurysm was encountered. The aneurysm was carefully dissected away from its bed. It was found to be about 5 or 6 mm. in diameter. When the actual aneurysm had been identified along with its feeding branches, a clip was placed across the base of the artery. There was a hematoma in the tip of the temporal lobe. This was punctured and evacuated with suction. Bleeding points were coagulated and clipped.

The dura was closed with interrupted black silk. The bone flap was replaced and the scalp closed with silk throughout.

Cervical Sympathectomy

An incision was made in the skin parallel to the posterior border of the sternocleidomastoid muscle, extending from the tip of the mastoid process toward the lower border of the clavicle. The spinal accessory nerve was identified and retracted. The external jugular vein was divided and hemostasis secured. The muscle incision was made longitudinally. The carotid-vagus-jugular bundle was freed without entering its sheath and retracted medially along with the sternocleidomastoid muscle.

The cervical sympathetic chain was identified and followed up to the fusiform superior cervical ganglion. The superior cervical ganglion was freed and dissection carried downward. The superior ganglion was avulsed from its cranial attachments. The cervical chain was seen to course around the inferior thyroid artery and was found in proximity to the vertebral artery. The vertebral artery was freed and retracted. The thyroid axis, vertebral and subclavian vessels, scalenus anticus muscle along with the sternocleidomastoid muscle, pleura, carotid sheath and contents were likewise retracted. The lateral branches of the ganglion were divided and the sympathetic trunk followed upward to the first thoracic ganglion.

Following hemostasis, the wound was closed using fine silk.

Lumbar Sympathectomy

A midline incision was made through the skin and fat extending from the symphysis pubis to one inch below the umbilicus. The incision was extended into the shape of a Y with its upper limbs on either side of the umbilicus. The superficial fascia was then separated from the inner halves of the rectus sheaths on each side, in the lower incision, to a level in the same plane as the upper extensions of the incision. A longitudinal incision in each rectus sheath was then made in such a fashion that a third of the muscle was medial and two-thirds of the muscle was lateral to each incision.

The rectus muscle was incised in the same plane extending to the posterior sheath of the rectus in the upper three-fourths, and the peritoneum in the lower one-fourth of the incision. Using a finger, the posterior sheath was gently separated from the peritoneum. This was continued inward, toward the midline. The posterior sheath was incised just lateral to the deep epigastric artery, leaving the artery medial to the incision.

The patient was repositioned in a low Trendelenburg position. The peritoneum was then separated laterally from the abdominal fascia. The abdominal contents were retracted to facilitate exposure of the aorta and iliac vessels on the left and the vena cava and iliac vessels on the right.

The incision was closed in layers using a single continuous chromic catgut suture in the posterior sheath and muscle. Single chromic inter-rupted catgut sutures were used in the anterior sheath reinforced with figure-of-eight silkworm gut sutures. The Y extensions of the incision were closed with figure-of-eight sutures, the lower loops of these sutures alternating on opposite sides with one suture passing through the skin and fat and looping through the right rectus to exit through the skin and fat on the opposite side. The same procedure was carried out, in an al-ternating fashion, on the opposite side. After emerging from the skin, one end of each loop was passed through the margins of the skin incision and tied to one side of the skin incision. Dead space within the incision was obliterated by rubber tubing passed under the silkworm loops above the skin. The sutures were tied over the rubber tubes. The skin was closed with clips.

Thoracolumbar Sympathectomy (Smithwick's Technic for Essential Hypertension)

The patient was prepared and draped after being placed on his abdo-men with pressure relieved from the abdomen and lower chest by use of rolls.

Endotracheal anesthesia was used with careful watch of blood pressure readings.

A skin incision was made extending from the 10th spinous process level to a point just below the level of the 12th rib. It was carried parallel to the rib as far as the posterior axillary line.

The renal fascia was opened and the kidney packed away. The pleural fold was identified and traced. The diaphragm was incised in a trans-verse manner up to the level at which the splanchnic nerve emerged. The celiac ganglion was identified. Hemostasis was accomplished with silver clips.

Using blunt dissertion, the parietal and mediastinal pleura were stripped from the paravertebral gutter. The posterior mediastinum was ex-posed. Identification of the sympathetic chain was made and it was traced with further identification of the enlarged 11th ganglion. A fine nerve hook was used to raise the ganglion and the branches of the nerve to the ganglion were transected. The course of the sympathetic nerve was fol-lowed upward. Further retraction of the wound was accomplished with a

Deaver retractor. As the transection proceeded upward, care was exercised to avoid injury to the intercostal vessels. At the end of the transection, the chain was secured with a silver clip and transection below this point. The splanchnic nerve and its plexus were separated from the sympathetic chain and cut. Its lower portion was transected at its entrance into the celiac ganglion. The resection proceeded downward with excision of D-12 L-1. The Iliopsoas muscle was identified and retracted.

The adrenals were identified and explored for possible tumor. None was found. A pinch biopsy was taken from the renal cortex as well as from the intercostal musculature. The wound was closed in layers.

NEUROSURGICAL EXAMINATIONS

The following examinations are some of the procedures commonly employed by the neurosurgeon to localize and confirm the presence of space-occupying lesions as well as diseases of the brain.

Ventriculogram — **Posterior**

The posterior portion of the head was shaved, prepared and draped with the patient in the supine position. An Adson ventriculogram headrest was used to immobilize the head after it had been elevated to a 40 degree position.

Starting 7 cm. above the external occipital protuberance and 4 cm. from the midline, a 4 cm. incision was made on each side, parallel to the midline. A small Jansen retaining retractor was used to obtain retraction.

Bur holes were made on each side of the skull and through these holes cruciate incisions were made in the dura with the aid of a dural hook and small scalpel. Next, the arachnoid was nicked over the convexity of a convolution. A brain cannula was then introduced parallel to the plane of the tentorium cerebelli and the plane of the falx cerebri. It entered the posterior horn at a depth of 5 cm. Fluid was obtained on the initial attempt. The stylet was replaced and the other ventricle tapped. Fluid was collected from both ventricles simultaneously. The cannulas were then removed and hemostasis secured.

The scalp incision was closed in separate layers with interrupted silk sutures to include the galea and skin in layers with one layer of galea buried.

Cistern Puncture

With the patient on his side at the edge of the bed and the suboccipital area properly prepared, the spine of the second cervical vertebra was identified by palpation. A 2% Novocain solution was injected intradermally 1 cm. above this. An 18 gauge spinal puncture needle was inserted in the midline as well as in the plane of the outer canthus of the eye and external auditory meatus. The needle was advanced very carefully to a depth of 5 cm. until it was felt to penetrate the fused atlanto-occipital membrane and dura. The stylet was removed and fluid permitted to escape. The manometric pressure was measured and fluid was withdrawn for further studies.

11 } *Gynecology*

Gynecology is that branch of general surgery which concerns itself with diseases of the external and internal female genitalia. The gynecologist is also trained in the practice of obstetrics, gynecologic pathology and female endocrinology.

Some of the procedures performed in this specialty along with their eponymic titles are reviewed in this section to assist the secretary with her vocabulary.

EXTERNAL FEMALE GENITAL ANATOMY

Bartholin's glands
Bulbus vestibuli
Canal of Nuck
Clitoris
Crura of clitoris
Fourchette
Frenulum
Hymen

Labia majora
Labia minora
Mons pubis
Navicular fossa
Perineum
Vaginal orifice
Vestibule of vagina
Vulva

INTERNAL FEMALE GENITAL ANATOMY

Anterior ligament
Areolar tissue
Broad ligaments
Cardinal ligaments (Mackenrodt)
Cervical canal
Cervix
Cervix uteri
Corpus albicans
Corpus hemorrhagicum
Corpus luteum
Corpus of the uterus
Cul-de-sac of Douglas

Endometrium
Epoophoron
External os
Fallopian tubes
Fimbriae
Fimbriated ends
Follicular cysts
Fornix (pl. fornices)
Fundus of uterus
Graafian follicle
Hydatids of Morgagni
Infundibulopelvic ligament

INTERNAL FEMALE GENITAL ANATOMY (Continued)

Internal os
Interstitial tissues
Lateral ligament
Levator ani
Ligamentum ovarii proprium
Mackenrodt's ligament
Mesosalpinx
Mesovarium
Mucous membrane
Myometrium
Ovarian artery
Ovarian vein
Ovary (pl. ovaries)
Oviduct
Pampiniform plexus
Parametrium
Paroophoron

Pelvic floor
Portio supravaginalis
Portio vaginalis
Posterior ligament
Pouch of Douglas
Rectouterine ligaments
Round ligament of uterus
Sacrogenital ligaments
Sacrouterine ligaments
Suspensory ligament of ovary
Tunica albuginea
Uterine artery
Uterine nerves
Uterosacral ligaments
Uterus
Vagina
Vesicouterine ligaments

HYSTERECTOMY

Removal of the uterus is called a hysterectomy. This operation may be performed by an abdominal or vaginal route. It may be total or subtotal depending upon whether it includes the cervix. The high incidence of carcinoma in cervical stumps has prompted surgeons to include the cervix with the corpus uteri when removal of the uterus has been indicated. The supracervical hysterectomy is therefore performed rarely today.

The vaginal route for hysterectomy is performed in severe uterine prolapse particularly where childbearing functions are no longer a consideration. All vaginal hysterectomies are total except for the Spalding-Richardson vaginal hysterectomy.

An example of a vaginal hysterectomy and abdominal hysterectomy is presented here to illustrate the terminology and structures involved.

TYPES OF HYSTERECTOMY

Abdominal hysterectomy
Doyen's vaginal hysterectomy
Latzko radical abdominal
    hysterectomy
Panhysterectomy (total)
Radical hysterectomy

Ries-Wertheim operation
Spalding-Richardson
Supracervical hysterectomy
Vaginal hysterectomy
Wertheim radical

Vaginal Hysterectomy

The patient was placed in the lithotomy position with legs and hips elevated. The cervical canal was asepticized and the bladder catheterized.

The external uterine opening was closed with silkworm gut sutures which were tied and left long for tractors. Circumcision was carried out on the vaginal mucosa at its junction with the cervix uteri. The anterior vaginal cuff was separated from the bladder by sharp and blunt gauze dissection. This was carried out until the broad ligaments were exposed on both sides. The vesicouterine reflection was identified after the bladder was reflected upward and out of the way.

The peritoneal fold was identified and opened. Both indices were introduced and spread laterally. A warm lap sponge was introduced through the opening and the bowels packed away. The ureters were identified and displaced upwards and out of the way.

The cervix was pulled upwards. The anterior vaginal cuff was dissected away from the uterus up to the peritoneal pouch. The posterior cuff was treated similarly. The broad ligaments were isolated. The uterus was held suspended in the pelvis by the broad, uterosacral, infundibulo-pelvic and round ligaments.

A curved Mayo needle with a # 2 chromic catgut engaged the lower end of the broad ligament which was ligated, tied and left long to be used temporarily as a traction suture. This portion of the broad ligament was divided close to the uterus. Another segment of tissue above the first ligature was treated similarly. The needle was introduced under the guidance of the finger to suture a large segment of the broad ligament. The broad ligament on the other side was treated in a similar manner. A finger was hooked over the top of the broad ligament on the right. After placing safety sutures, the ligament was severed from the uterus. The same procedure was repeated on the opposite side.

A frequent check was made for thorough hemostasis. Inspection of the pedicles of the ligamentous structures held by the traction sutures disclosed no bleeding. The gauze pack was removed from the anterior cul-de-sac. The divided edge of the bladder peritoneum was isolated.

The sutures of the round ligament on each side were tied to each other. The same was done with the broad ligaments. The vaginal vault was closed with interrupted sutures. The vagina was lightly packed.

Total Abdominal Hysterectomy; Bilateral Oophorectomy; Left Salpingectomy

A right paramedian scar was present and excised. The right tube and the appendix had been removed previously. The anterior fascial sheath was incised in a vertical fashion. The recti muscles were separated. The posterior fascial sheath and peritoneum were picked up and incised vertically.

The pelvic and abdominal viscera were examined. Multiple uterine fibroids were noted. There was also a fibroid of the cervix, lying at the base of the broad ligament, measuring approximately 6 x 10 cm. in diameter. The uterus, the left tube and both ovaries were severely bound down with adhesions. The gallbladder was normal as were the kidneys and bowel. The pelvic adhesions were lysed.

The bowel was pushed back and the pelvic organs were exposed. The round ligaments were picked up with Kocher clamps, incised and ligated with chromic 00 catgut. The bladder reflection was peeled away from the lower uterine segment. The right ovary was picked up and the infundibulopelvic ligament clamped with Buies and the right ovary was removed. The infundibulopelvic ligament was sutured with a chromic 0 catgut suture. The left tube and ovary were then removed by clamping the infundibulopelvic ligament and tying same with chromic 0 catgut sutures. The uterosacral ligaments were then clamped, cut and tied with chromic 0 catgut sutures.

The uterine arteries were doubly clamped and cut using chromic # 1 catgut sutures. A double ligature was placed on each uterine artery. The pericervical vaginal fascia was then circumcised in a circular fashion and the uterus removed in toto. The vaginal mucosa was then sutured together utilizing chromic 0 catgut in a continuous suture.

The perivesical vaginal fascia was sutured together utilizing chromic 00 catgut suture in a continuous manner. The base of the left broad ligament and the left uterosacral ligament as well as the right uterosacral ligament and the base of the right broad ligament were sutured into the angles of the dome of the vagina. Reperitonealization of the pelvis was carried out with 0 intestinal suture. After a correct sponge count, the abdominal peritoneum was closed with a 00 chromic intestinal catgut everting type suture. The posterior fascial layer was then sutured with a continuous chromic 00 intestinal catgut suture. The recti muscles were then approximated with chromic 2 intestinal catgut suture. The anterior fascial layer was sutured together with figure-of-eight chromic 0 catgut sutures. The skin was approximated with 000 silk sutures.

DILATATION AND CURETTAGE (D & C)

The D & C consists of a scraping of the inside of the uterus for the purpose of removing endometrial tissue for histologic examination. It is also performed following incomplete abortion for removal of the remaining products of conception.

INSTRUMENTS USED FOR D & C:

Allis tissue forceps	Jacobs vulsellum forceps
Auvard weighted speculum	Kelly placenta forceps
Backhaus towel clamp	Ovum forceps
Bond placenta forceps	Schroeder uterine tenaculum
Bozeman uterine dressing forceps	Sims vaginal speculum
Braun uterine tenaculum	Sims uterine curet
Curet (curette)	Sims uterine probe
Deaver retractor	Sims uterine sound
Eastman vaginal retractor	Skene uterine spoon curet
Goodell dilator	Sponge forceps
Graves vaginal speculum	Starlinger dilator
Hegar dilator	Thomas uterine curet
Henrotin vulsellum forceps	Uterine sound
Hurtig dilator	Vulsellum forceps

Operative Technic (Diagnostic D & C)

The patient was placed in the lithotomy position. The lower abdomen, inner thighs, perineum and vaginal vault were prepared and draped in a sterile manner.

Bimanual examination revealed a parous outlet. The cervix was clear. The uterus was slightly enlarged, anterior, smooth and firm. The adnexa were negative.

The anterior lip of the cervix was grasped with a single tooth tenaculum and drawn downward. The uterine cavity was sounded to a depth of 4 inches. The cervical canal was dilated with Starlinger and Goodell dilators. The uterine cavity was then well curetted with large and small curets. A moderate amount of endometrial tissue was obtained and sent to the pathologist for histologic examination.

PROLAPSE OF THE UTERUS
(procidentia or descensus uteri)

When the anatomic structures supporting the uterus fail to maintain it in proper position, prolapse occurs with the uterus descending through the vagina and everting the vagina in the process.

A number of operations have been proposed for correcting this condition, the titles of which appear below. Vaginal hysterectomy is performed more universally for this condition than are some of the other procedures, but regardless of the technique chosen, the vaginal route of repair is the one generally agreed upon.

UTERINE PROLAPSE OPERATIONS

Donald operation
Fothergill
Gilliam suspension
Goodall-Power modification of LeFort
Heaney vaginal hysterectomy

LeFort operation
Manchester
Spalding-Richardson composite
  operation
Watkins transposition

Modified Gilliam Suspension of the Uterus

The patient is prepared and draped in the supine position. The abdomen is entered with a midline incision. The incision is carried through the anatomic layers of the abdominal wall. The peritoneum is picked up and incised. The peritoneal cavity is entered. Allis clamps are applied to the edges of the rectus fascia and the peritoneum at approximately the level of the anterior superior spine of the ilium. The uterus is raised and its round ligaments identified. A # 1 chromic gut ligature is placed around one of the round ligaments but not tied. This is elevated with a hemostat. The same procedure is carried out on the opposite round ligament and traction applied bringing the uterus up to the abdominal wall. Following this, the rectus muscle on the left is retracted toward the midline and the subcutaneous tissue retracted away from this. A curved Kelly clamp is introduced through the internal inguinal ring to the peritoneum. The clamp is open and the peritoneum extending over the clamp is opened. The clamp is introduced further through this rent in the peritoneum and picks up the traction ligature on the left. The ligature is pulled up through the opening and through the internal inguinal canal bringing the round ligament to the outside of the anterior rectus fascia. This brings the uterus up firmly to the abdominal wall. The round ligament brought up through the opening is sutured to the anterior rectus fascia with three interrupted cotton sutures. The ligature is then removed without damage to the round ligament. The same procedure is carried out on the right side.

The peritoneum is closed with 00 chromic catgut suture, continuous; the fascia with a continuous 0 chromic catgut, and the skin with vertical mattress 000 silk sutures.

OPERATIONS FOR SUSPENSION OF THE UTERUS

Abell modification of Gilliam
Alexander-Adams
Baldy-Webster (posterior
  implantation of round ligaments)
Coffey suspension
Gilliam suspension
Interposition operation

Leopold modification
Manchester operation
McCall-Schumann modification
Olshausen operation
Subperitoneal Baldy-Webster
Ventrofixation of uterus
Watkins interposition

Hysteropexy — Abell modification of Gilliam

The patient was prepared and draped in the Trendelenburg position. A four inch midline suprapubic incision was made.

Guy sutures of catgut were placed through each round ligament, midway between their origin and exit through the internal abdominal rings. Each suture was held by an artery forceps and not tied.

After the rectus sheath was opened on each side of the midline incision, the Rectus abdominis was separated from the under surface of the anterior rectus sheath. A curved artery forceps with blunt ends was passed under the fascia, above the rectus muscle, through the posterior end of the sheath of the rectus to the outer aspect of the internal ring. After the abdominal wall on the same side was elevated, the inner aspect of the internal ring was elevated by traction on the guy sutures in the round ligament. The artery forceps was introduced through the internal ring, under the peritoneum and on the upper surface of the round ligament, penetrating the peritoneum when well within the limits of the parietal peritoneum. After separation of the blades of the artery forceps, the guy suture in the round ligament was grasped and drawn through the internal ring, into the midline incision. By exerting further traction, the elongated round ligament was doubled on itself, through the internal ring, over the upper surface of the rectus and along the under surface of the fascia to the midline incision.

The round ligament was stretched out in the form of a triangle. It was tacked to the undersurface of the fascia with three catgut sutures with the apex at the cut edge of the fascia, in the midline incision, and the base looking outward toward the outside of the rectus. The procedure was repeated with the round ligament on the opposite side.

The midline incision was closed in tiers. The apex of each round ligament was sewn together with closure of the fascia. No. 1 chromic catgut was used to suture the round ligament. No. 2 chromic catgut was used for the peritoneum and fascia and stay sutures of silkworm gut were used to close the skin.

Shirodkar Operation for Incompetent Cervix

An injection of adrenalin and saline was performed under the bladder, at the sides of the cervix and posteriorly, where the incision was made. The incision was made in front of the cervix. The area above the external os was exposed by dissecting the anterior vaginal wall and bladder away from the cervix. A fold of posterior vaginal wall was raised with an Allis forceps and a vertical incision made in the fold. Curved artery forceps were used to stretch the incision.

A right Shirodkar isthmorrhaphy needle was directed in and under the right pillar of the bladder adhering to the cervix. It was introduced under the mucosa and backward toward the posterior incision. Linen thread holding one end of a Mersilene tape was placed on a Mayo needle and was threaded through the eye of the Shirodkar needle on a handle. The right limb of the Mersilene tape was then drawn forward.

A left Shirodkar needle was used to take up the other end of the Mersilene tape. The two ends of the tape were then tied into a reef knot and the knot transfixed with a fine linen suture. The redundant ends on either side were sutured to the circular part of the tape to prevent slipping. The vaginal mucosa was then closed with interrupted 00 chromic. Blood loss was minimal.

Electrocoagulation of the Cervix

With the patient in lithotomy position, the perineum was prepared and draped. I.V. Sodium Pentothal was used for anesthesia.

With the tip of the coning instrument placed against the cervical external os, the combined cutting and coagulating current was used. As the wire cut into the cervix the instrument was twisted to enucleate a cone of tissue. Crucial incisions were made with coagulation at the 12, 9, 6 and 3 o'clock points.

Lash Operation for Incompetent Cervix

The patient was prepared and draped in the lithotomy position. A semicircular incision of 3 cm. was made above the external os. A vaginal mucosal flap was elevated and the urinary bladder retracted from the cervix. A stay suture was introduced above the upper border of the defect, the defect excised and the cervical canal opened.

A Hegar dilator was introduced through the cervical canal to the uterine cavity. Four interrupted # 1 surgical gut sutures were taken through the inner half of the cervical wall, avoiding the endocervix. Interrupted sutures were then placed in the outer half of the cervical wall. The anterior portions of the cardinal ligaments were then approximated and sutured in the midline to the cervical wall. The vaginal flap was closed. No blood replacement was necessary.

Insertion of Radium into the Cervix Uteri

The anterior lip of the cervix is grasped with a tenaculum and drawn downward. The cervical canal is dilated with Hegar dilators up to # 10. Using an Ernst applicator, a tandem containing radium is inserted into the uterine cavity and cervical canal. The cervical canal is firmly packed with ½ inch gauze and the vagina packed with a 1 inch gauze. The cord extending from the tandem is attached to the inner thigh with adhesive. Paracervical irradiation is obtained by means of a colpostat comprised of three corks containing radium tubes. One cork is placed in the right vaginal vault and another in the left vaginal vault. The third cork is placed midway between the other two. The two lateral corks are connected by a rubber covered spring.

A 2 inch gauze packing is placed between the rectum and the colpostat, into the vaginal fornices and between the bladder and the anterior lip of the cervix.

A total of 4,000 roentgen gammas is delivered by intracervical tandem and 4,000 more by colpostat.

Sturmdorf Amputation of the Cervix

Following a routine D & C, the cervix is grasped with a tenaculum and drawn downward with the uterus. A circular incision is made around the vaginal mucosa just above the external os. The vaginal mucosa is separated from the cervix. A cone of cervix is removed near the internal os.

A tenaculum is used to grasp the anterior lip of the cervix and a Hegar dilator is used to dilate the cervical canal. Bleeding is controlled by ligation of the cervical branches of the uterine arteries.

Coverage of the raw surface with vaginal mucosa is accomplished by use of the Sturmdorf stitch. Using a large cutting needle and # 1 chromic surgical gut, a bite is taken in the posterior vaginal mucosa at its edge. The needle is inserted inside the cervical canal and a suture passed from the inside of the cervix, through the cervical tissue, and through the posterior vaginal mucosa about 2 cm. from the edge. Another cutting needle is used and the remainder of the suture threaded on this needle about 0.5 cm. from the other suture in the cervical canal. This suture is brought out in the same manner as the previous one, at the same distance from the edge of the posterior vaginal mucosa, 1 cm. from the first suture. The two sutures are pulled down securely and tied bringing the posterior vaginal mucosa into, the cervical canal. A second Sturmdorf is placed on the anterior aspect of the new cervix. The two Sturmdorf sutures are pulled together almost covering the entire cervix with mucosa. A few interrupted 0 chromic surgical gut sutures are used to further approximate the anterior and posterior vaginal mucosa. Included in these stitches is the vaginal mucosa with its underlying cervical tissue.

A gauze pack is placed in the cervical canal to be removed in 24 hours.

COLPORRHAPHY

Common surgical problems of the vaginal wall include the cystocele and rectocele; less often they also include the enterocele and urethrocele. Repair of the vaginal wall (colporrhaphy) is designated as anterior or posterior.

In a cystocele there is a protrusion of the urinary bladder through the anterior vaginal wall. In the rectocele there is a protrusion of the rectum through the posterior vaginal wall. These defects usually occur together and are repaired surgically in a procedure called an anterior and posterior colporrhaphy (A & P colporrhaphy).

Anterior and Posterior Colporrhaphy

Under spinal anesthesia the patient was placed in lithotomy position and sterilely prepared and draped.

Bimanual pelvic examination was performed. The uterus was found to be normal in size. No descensus uteri was found by traction with a tenaculum. A large cystocele, urethrocele and rectocele were noted. The uterus was otherwise normal in size, shape and form. No adnexal masses were palpable.

The vaginal mucosa surrounding the external cervix was incised transversely. The mucosa was incised at the midportion creating an inverted T up to the urethral meatus. The vaginal mucosa was sharply dissected from the fascia. The bleeders were clamped and tied with 000 chromic suture. The pubocervical fascia was reapproximated in the midline using 00 interrupted chromic sutures. The urethra was plicated with 000 chromic intestinal suture. A Kelly type suture was placed at the angle of the neck of the bladder using 00 chromic intestinal suture. The bladder was well elevated with good angulation and absence of the urethrocele. The excess vaginal mucosa was excised in a triangular fashion bilaterally. The vaginal mucosa was then reapproximated in the midline with interrupted 000 chromic sutures. The mucosa was resutured to the cervix at the inverted T with interrupted 00 chromic suture.

Posterior repair was performed with an incision at the mucocutaneous portion of the posterior fourchette. The vaginal mucosa was freed from the perirectal fascia in a tunneling fashion thus creating two pillars laterally which were clamped with Kochers. The vaginal mucosa was incised. The pillars were approximated in the midline with figure-of-eight chromic sutures. The excess vaginal mucosa posteriorly was then excised in an angular manner. The vaginal mucosa was approximated with a continuous locked 00 chromic suture. The Levator ani were reapproximated in the midline with interrupted 00 chromic. The perineal bodies were approximated with the same material and the skin was closed with interrupted figure-of-eight 00 chromic suture.

A vaginal pack was introduced into the vagina. A Foley catheter was left in the bladder. The urine was clear and no bleeding was encountered following this procedure.

Excision of the Left Fallopian Tube (for ruptured ectopic tubal pregnancy)

Under general anesthesia and after blood was started on the patient, a midline suprapubic incision was made approximately 4½ inches in length. The external fascial layer was incised vertically. The recti muscles were separated. The posterior fascia and peritoneum were picked up and incised in vertical fashion following which the abdominal cavity was entered.

Approximately 1,500 cc. of whole blood and clotted blood was evident in the abdominal cavity. The pelvis was examined and the left fallopian tube was found to be ruptured in the distal one-third.

The left tube was picked up and the base of the tube clamped with hemostats. The distal end was clamped with a hemostat. A small fetus and sac were found in the cul-de-sac. This was sent to the laboratory.

The uterus could not be delivered upward properly due to dense adhesions on the posterior aspect of the uterus between the uterus and the sigmoid portion of the rectum. This was believed to account for the severe third degree fixed retroversion of the uterus.

After the tube was clamped at its base, it was excised from its cornual portion. A figure-of-eight suture was placed in the cornual portion of the uterus for closure and hemostasis. The portions of the broad ligaments were clamped and tied with 000 chromic catgut suture. Blood was aspirated from the abdomen and pelvis and the clots were extracted.

The sponge count was correct. The abdomen was closed in layers. The peritoneum and posterior fascial layer were closed with a continuous everting type mattress 00 intestinal catgut suture. The recti muscles were approximated with 00 intestinal chromic catgut suture. The anterior fascial layer was sutured together with figure-of-eight chromic 0 Gyn. sutures. The skin was closed with vertical mattress 000 silk sutures.

A total of 1,500 cc. of whole blood was given during the operation.

Hirst Operation for Dyspareunia

Under general Surital anesthesia, the patient was prepared and draped in the usual manner in a lithotomy position. The bladder was catheterized.

Preliminary examination under anesthesia revealed a uterus located in the midline, anteflexed, normal in size and consistency. The adnexal areas were negative. The marital introitus only admitted two fingers with difficulty.

The posterior lateral aspect of the introitus was grasped with Allis forceps and a skin incision made in the midline in the posterior vaginal wall and perineal body. The mucosa was reflected away from the underlying tissue until the levator muscle on each side was identified. These were cut bilaterally. Following this, the apex of the posterior vaginal wall was approximated to the midline of the posterior fourchette and the corresponding edges were approximated with interrupted 0 Gyn. sutures without difficulty.

There was a moderate blood loss. A vaginal pack was placed in the vagina for purposes of hemostasis. Furacin Cream was applied to the vaginal pack.

CESAREAN SECTION

Cesarean section consists of the delivery of the newborn infant through the abdominal rather than the vaginal route. Numerous indications for this operation include: CPD (cephalopelvic disproportion), previous cesarean section, previous incisions in the uterus which might have left a weakening scar, previous cervical repairs, placenta previa and other conditions which might prevent delivery of a living child from the normal vaginal route.

TYPES OF CESAREAN SECTION

Cervical cesarean section   Low cervical cesarean section
Classical cesarean section   Poro cesarean section
Extraperitoneal   Transverse cervical section
Latzko operation   Waters' operation (extraperitoneal)

DRUGS USED IN CESAREAN SECTIONS:

Ergonovine   Pituitrin
Ergot   Silver nitrate 1% (baby eyes)
Pituitary extract

Cervical Cesarean Section Technic

The patient is placed in the Trendelenburg position and catheterized. A midline incision is made extending from a point immediately below the umbilicus to the symphysis pubis. The wound edges are retracted to expose the lower uterine segment along with the bladder and its uterine reflection. The vesicouterine peritoneum is incised transversely just below the firm attachment of the peritoneum to the upper uterine segment. Using finger dissection, the inferior flap is gently dissected toward the pelvis along with the bladder. A rounded retractor is used to hold the bladder out of the operative field.

The lower uterine segment is incised at the upper pole of the intended incision. Care is taken to avoid opening the amniotic sac. Bandage scissors are used to extend the incision to the lower pole. Bleeding is controlled with ring forceps.

A finger is introduced into the baby's mouth and the infant's face is brought into the incision. The chin is delivered first, over the upper angle of the incision, and then the rest of the head by flexion.

Bleeding is controlled with hemostatic clamps. Pituitrin is injected into the uterus. The placenta is removed manually after delivery of the infant. The uterus is packed with gauze with an end allowed to project out through the vagina.

Interrupted sutures of # 1 20-day catgut are placed down to the mucosa. A second row of sutures is placed external to the first which also include the fascia. The fascia is closed with interrupted sutures with one side slightly overlapping the other. Insert mattress sutures are used as required to control bleeding. The reflected vesicouterine peritoneum is closed by fastening the superior flap over the upper pole of the uterine incision with a few stitches and then bringing the inferior flap over the entire incision, closing it with continuous suture of # 1 chromic catgut. The knot is buried under the peritoneum.

EPONYMIC TITLES OF GYNECOLOGIC OPERATIONS

Abell modification of the Gilliam uterine suspension
Aldridge temporary sterilization
Alexander-Adams uterine suspension
Baldy-Webster uterine suspension
Ball technic for omentectomy
Basset radical vulvectomy
Coffey uterine suspension
Donald operation for uterine prolapse
Donald-Fothergill operation for uterine prolapse

EPONYMIC TITLES OF GYNECOLOGIC
OPERATIONS (Continued)

Doyen vaginal hysterectomy
Falk technic for vesicovaginal fistula
Fleming instrument conization of cervix
Fothergill operation for uterine prolapse
Frangenheim-Goebell-Stoeckel operation for urinary incontinence
Freund operation for uterine prolapse; cystocele
Fritsch modification of Freund operation
Gilliam uterine suspension
Giordano operation for urinary incontinence
Goodall-Power modification of LeFort operation
Grant-Ward operation for vaginal prolapse
Green-Armytage pursestring cervical closure
Heaney technic for vaginal hysterectomy
Hirst operation for dyspareunia
Irving sterilization
Kelly operation for urinary stress incontinence
Kennedy operation for urinary stress incontinence
Lash operation for incompetent cervix
Latzko repair of the bladder
LeFort colpocleisis
Leopold uterine suspension
Madlener technic for sterilization
Manchester operation for uterine prolapse
Marshall-Marchetti-Krantz operation for urinary stress incontinence
McIndoe reconstruction of the vagina
Moschowitz enterocele repair
Munnell bilateral oophorectomy
Olshausen uterine suspension
Peterson insufflation of tubes
Pomeroy sterilization operation
Poro cesarean section
Radium application technics, intrauterine and intravaginal
   Ernst applicator method
   Manchester ovoid method
   Stockholm box method
Ries-Wertheim hysterectomy
Rizzoli operation for congenital rectovaginal fistula
Rubin tubal insufflation
Schauffler removal of bartholin cyst
Schauta radical vaginal hysterectomy
Schuchardt incision in carcinoma of the cervix
Shirodkar operation for incompetent cervix
Spalding-Richardson composite operation
Spinelli operation for inversion of the uterus

EPONYMIC TITLES OF GYNECOLOGIC
OPERATIONS (Continued)

Stockholm radium application
Strassman-Jones operation for double uterus
Sturmdorf amputation of the cervix
Sturmdorf trachelorrhaphy
Taussig-Morton node dissection
TeLinde operation for vaginal prolapse
Twombly operation for vulvar carcinoma
Twombly-Ulfelder operation for carcinoma of the cervix
Waters cesarean section
Watkins interposition uterine suspension
Watkins-Wertheim operation for uterine prolapse
Wertheim radical hysterectomy and node dissection
Wharton technic for construction of an artificial vagina
Whitacre sterilization operation
Williams vaginal occlusion
Williams-Richardson operation for vaginal prolapse

12 { *Orthopedic Surgery*

Orthopedics is that branch of surgery which is concerned with preservation and restoration of the function of the skeletal system, its articulations and associated structures.

Tables of the bones, joints, ligaments and muscles are presented in Chapter 6.

In this chapter we will include a consideration of fractures, dislocations, bony deformities, amputations, arthroplastic procedures and surgery of the muscles, ligaments and tendons. This material is designed primarily to assist the secretary with technical terms encountered in dictations of these various procedures, including eponymic titles of the operations.

APPROACHES TO ORTHOPEDIC OPERATIONS

Abbott
Abbott and Lucas
Avila
Badgley
Banks and Laufman
Bosworth
Boyd
Callahan
Cave
Coonse and Adams
Cubbins
Darrach and McLaughlin
Fahey
Fisher "U"
Gatellier
Gibson
Guleke–Stookey
Harmon
Henderson
Henry
Heuter
Jones and Brackett
Kocher

Koenig
Luck
Ludloff
MacAusland
McFarland and Osborne
McWhorter
Milch
Ollier
Osborne
Osgood
Phemister
Putti
Radley, Liebig and Brown
Ralston
Roberts
Rowe
Saber-cut
Smith-Petersen
Thompson
Van Gorder
Wagoner
Watson-Jones
Yee

AMPUTATIONS

In the broadest consideration of amputations of the extremities, they may be divided into two main types: *open* and *closed*. The open amputation is a temporary procedure where the surface of the wound is not covered over with skin. The wound is left open to promote drainage. The closed type of amputation is a final operation where the resulting stump may be fitted with a prosthesis.

A further refinement of the closed amputation is a *cineplastic amputation* in which the stump is formed to permit the patient to activate the prosthesis directly by a muscle "motor" placed within the muscle belly. The "motor" consists of an inverted tube skin flap, lined on the inside by skin, which is pulled up transversely through a muscle canal, at right angles to the line of muscular pull, and attached to the opposite end. A peg is fixed in the tube, with cables attached to either end, for the purpose of transmitting muscle action to the prosthesis. The amputee thus obtains active control of the artificial limb or hook. This is specialized orthoplastic surgery usually confined to orthopedic centers equipped for proper limb fitting and rehabilitation.

An amputation may be performed through the body of a bone or through a joint. When the latter method is used, the operation is termed a *disarticulation*.

The "phantom" limb phenomenon, where pain and sensation is experienced in the limb which has been removed, is one of the undesirable effects following some amputations. The development of a painful terminal neuroma is another such occurrence. Revision of the amputation stump is often necessary when these conditions exist.

AMPUTATION TECHNIQUES

Aperiosteal supracondylar
  tendoplastic
Batch, Spittler, McFadden
Boyd
Callander
Carnes
Chopart's
Gordon-Taylor
Holscher and Warner
King and Steelquist
Kirk
Kutler
LeMesurier

Lisfranc's
Littlewood
Pedersen and Day
Pirogoff
Rogers
Silbert and Haimovici
Slocum
Sorondo and Ferre
Spittler
Stokes-Gritti
Syme
Vasconcelos
Woughter

Amputation Through the Surgical Neck of the Humerus

The patient was placed in the dorsal decubitus position with the back supported by a sandbag. The arm and adjacent areas were sterilely prepared and draped.

The skin incision was started at the level of the coracoid process and extended along the anterior border of the deltoid muscle down to its point of insertion. An incision was then carried along the posterior aspect of the deltoid muscle to the axillary fold. A separate incision was carried through the axilla to join the previous incisions.

The Pectoralis major muscle was identified and traced to its insertion where it was sectioned and reflected medially. The neurovascular bundle between the Pectoralis minor and the Coracobrachialis muscles was exposed. The axillary artery and vein were sectioned just below the Pectoralis minor muscle. Next, the radial, ulnar, median and musculocutaneous nerves were isolated, gently drawn down and sectioned in such a way that they were able to fall above the Pectoralis minor muscle. The deltoid muscle was then sectioned at its insertion and reflected upward together with its attached lateral skin flap. Further sectioning was carried out of the Latissimus dorsi and Teres major at the bicipital groove near their insertions. At a point about 2 cm. distal to the saw line, the Coracobrachialis, biceps tendon and triceps were severed. A Gigli saw was used to cut through the humeral neck. After the bone was severed, the Coracobrachialis and long head of the biceps were sutured over the end of the remaining humerus. The Pectoralis major was carried laterally and sutured to the inferior pole of the bone. This was covered by the deltoid muscle and a skin flap carefully outlined to provide a well aligned closure. Interrupted skin sutures were used to approximate the wound edges.

Above Knee (A-K) Amputation

The patient was placed on the operating table in the supine position after infiltration of spinal anesthesia. The entire leg, groin and abdomen were prepared with alcohol and Zephiran and draped. A site for A-K amputation was chosen. Anterior and posterior skin flaps were fashioned.

The incision was carried down through the fascia and muscle layers to the femur. It was noted that the blood supply was quite adequate. The superficial femoral artery was divided and had an excellent pulsatile flow. This artery was doubly ligated, both with a free ligature and suture ligature. The sciatic nerve was identified and placed under traction. A 00 chromic ligature was placed high around the nerve and the nerve was then transected and allowed to retract high up into the thigh.

The femur was transected with a hand saw and the edges filed. The marrow cavity was packed with bee's wax. All bleeding was controlled by clamping and fine chromic ligatures. After good hemostasis was achieved, the deep fascia of the thigh was approximated with interrupted 00 chromic sutures and the skin reapproximated with interrupted 00000 Tevdek sutures.

A through-and-through thyroid drain was passed through the thigh to the fascial layer. A pressure and occlusive dressing was applied.

Revision and Closure of Partial Amputation, Right Index Finger

After the usual sterile preparation and draping and with a pneumatic tourniquet on the arm elevated to 300 mm. of mercury, the wound was thoroughly lavaged with copious amounts of saline. Meticulous debridement was carried out.

The amputation had occurred at the distal joint causing a disarticulation of the joint and a comminuted fracture of the distal end of the middle phalanx.

The skin of the dorsal aspect of the finger was amputated at the level of the joint while the volar aspect of the remaining flap extended about 1 cm. beyond the amputation level. It was shredded and severely lacerated. A midline incision was made on the radial and ulnar aspect of the finger, approximately 1 cm. from the distal end of the middle phalanx. Dorsal and volar skin flaps were retracted. The middle phalanx was amputated at the level of the flare of the condyles, at its distal end. The amputation site was smoothed off and the edges rounded.

The extensor tendon and the Flexor digitorum profundus were both pulled down and severed allowing them to retract proximally. The neurovascular bundle on each side was identified. The artery and vein were ligated. The nerve was dissected free and amputated proximal to the level of the amputated phalanx.

The skin flaps were revised in such a manner that the volar flap was brought back over the dorsal end of the stump and sutured to the end of the dorsal flap. This produced a tactile pad without a scar over the volar surface of the distal end of the stump.

A pressure dressing and dorsal plaster of Paris splint were applied.

ARTHRODESIS

Arthrodesis (fusion) is an operation performed to induce immobilization (bony ankylosis) in a joint where motion is not desired. These fusions may be intra-articular, intra- and extra-articular, or extra-articular in type. An extra-articular arthrodesis is performed when union is desired between normal bony surfaces outside of the joint capsule. A spinal fusion is the best example of this type of arthrodesis.

Intra-articular arthrodesis is performed when fusion of cancellous bony surfaces is the surgeon's goal. The articulating surfaces are devested of diseased tissue to facilitate union of cancellous bony surfaces. Autogenous cancellous bone grafts are sometimes used to promote fusion.

In the intra- and extra-articular arthodeses bone grafts are used across the joint after the articular surfaces are stripped of their investments.

SEE: Listing of orthopedic operations at the end of this chapter for assistance with the titles of specific operations.

Charnley Arthrodesis of the Ankle

An incision extending from 1 cm. proximal to the tip of one malleolus to the same point on the other is made across the anterior aspect of the ankle joint. The incision curves out distally in a semicircular fashion at its midpoint. A thick flap is formed by dissection of the skin and subcutaneous tissues proximally. The extensor tendons are thus exposed. The Extensor digitorum communis, the Extensor hallucis longus and the Tibialis anterior tendons are divided. Care is exercised to avoid the distal portion of the Peroneus tertius tendon.

The anterior tibial vessels are cut and tied, the nerve is sectioned and the joint capsule is incised transversely. Subperiosteal exposure of the posterior surfaces of the malleoli and lower portion of the tibia is carried out. Traction is obtained by introducing a periosteal elevator behind each malleolus.

The fibular and tibial collateral ligaments are divided and the foot is plantarflexed. Using a saw, the lower ends of the tibia and fibula are cut horizontally. An osteotome is used to complete the bone division. The foot is then placed in the position of choice. A one-fourth of an inch thick piece of bone is removed from the talus. A Steinman pin is then introduced through the talus and open wound, well anterior to the axis of the bone. It is positioned in such a way that it will counterbalance the pull of the tendo calcaneus posteriorly. Care is taken to avoid puncturing the subtalar joint. An upper pin is inserted through the shaft of the tibia using the compression clamps on the lower pin as a guide. The clamps are tightened to assure proper position. The sutures in the tendons are tied and the skin incision closed. A thickly padded plaster cast is applied from below the knee to the toes.

Ischiofemoral Arthrodesis of the Left Hip (Brittain Technique)

The patient was anesthetized with Pentothal Sodium and placed on the fracture table. The left leg was prepared from the hip to the ankle with G-11 and the operative area draped free in the usual fashion.

First, an incision was made parallel to an old incision of the hip. It was carried directly to the tensor fascia lata. This structure was then sectioned with a clean scalpel. The Vastus lateralis was then incised and separated from the shaft of the femur by a sharp periosteal elevator. A single guide wire was drilled through the area of the femur, just above the lesser trochanter, and an x-ray was made. The wire was found to lie in a satisfactory plane in relation to the ischium.

Next, an incision was made over the tibial crest, beginning one inch above the ankle joint, and carried proximally to the tibial tubercle. The margins were reflected. The periosteum was incised and separated from the entire tibial shaft by a sharp periosteal elevator. With a Stryker bone saw, a large arrow-shaped graft was cut from the entire width of the surface of the tibia, measuring $6\frac{1}{2}$ inches in length. The wound was closed by approximating the periosteum with interrupted 00 chromic catgut. The subcutaneous tissue was closed with interrupted 000 plain catgut and the skin with interlocking black silk suture. Dry sterile dressings were applied to this wound.

The femur was osteotomized along the wire osteotomy plane that had been established. The femur was then driven into the ischium and this bone was also osteotomized. The previously cut graft was then inserted into the osteotomy area and driven well into the ischium. The femoral shaft was displaced medially.

The wound was closed by approximating the Vastus lateralis with interrupted 0 chromic catgut, the tensor fascia lata with interrupted 00 chromicized catgut, the subcutaneous tissue with 000 plain catgut and the skin with interlocking black silk suture.

Dry sterile dressings were applied. A left hip spica was applied from the costal margin to the toes on the left leg with the leg in abduction and the knee in slight flexion. The ankle was kept in a neutral position.

Shoulder Arthrodesis

With the patient in Fowler's position with the knees flexed and the feet braced against a padded foot rest, the area of the shoulder was prepared and draped.

An incision was made over the glenohumeral joint and carried through the anatomic layers to the joint. The joint was entered anteriorly and superiorly. It was stripped of cartilage. The acromion was prepared and fitted into a depression formed in the greater tuberosity of the humerus. Satisfactory positioning was obtained. A shoulder spica was applied. The upper arm was placed in a position of 70 degrees abduction from the scapula with 30 degrees forward flexion and 30 degrees internal rotation.

Arthrodesis L-4 — Sacrum With Autogenous Right Iliac Graft (Modified Hibbs Technique with H-grafts)

After administration of satisfactory general anesthesia, the patient was placed in the prone position on the operating table and positioned for spinal fusion. The back area, including the posterior aspect of the right ilium, was prepared and draped in the usual fashion.

The lumbosacral spine was approached through a midline vertical skin incision which was carried down to the investing lumbar fascia. This was divided vertically in the midline. The spinous processes and lamina of the 3rd, 4th and 5th lumbar vertebrae and the upper sacral segments were exposed by subperiosteal dissection of the paravertebral muscles.

A Downing muscle retractor was positioned so as to afford proper exposure of the area. Investigation of the stability of this portion of the spine revealed that the L-4-5 segment was the most significant area of instability, although the L-5 and S-1 area did show mild instability. An arthrodesis from the 4th lumbar segment to the upper sacrum was elected and performed by the modified Hibbs technique with superimposition of two H-grafts. The spinous process of L-5 was carefully cut and prepared to act as an intermediary between the two H-grafts. The 4th lumbar spinous process was also prepared as was the upper sacral process. The laminae were carefully dissected with sharp osteotome to expose raw cancellous bone. Small shingles of cortical bone were turned over to permit this. All extraneous soft tissue was carefully removed by rongeur dissection. The facet joints were exposed and destroyed by dissection with an osteotome and prepared for packing with cancellous bone graft. The entire area of fusion was prepared for reception of the bone graft. When this preparation was completed and the area lavaged, the site was packed with sponges.

Attention was directed to the posterior crest of the right ilium. A curved skin incision was made directly over the crest. Subperiosteal dissection of the muscles on the outer aspect of the crest was utilized to expose a sufficient area from which a bone graft could be taken. Only outer table grafts were taken. Two relatively large pieces were cut in the usual fashion to be used as H-grafts. Multiple strips of cortical cancellous and cancellous bone were removed with a gouge and curet for additional bone graft material. When sufficient bone grafts had been obtained, the area was lavaged with sterile saline.

Bleeding from the bone was controlled by Gelfoam packing and a closure accomplished with 00 chromic to reapproximate the musculature, 0000 chromic for the subcutaneous tissue and interrupted 000 silk for the skin.

Attention was then directed to the arthrodesis site where cancellous bone graft was packed into the facet joint spaces. Previously prepared strips of cancellous and cortical cancellous bone were laid down in the usual barrel stave manner to afford a satisfactory fusion bed. The H-grafts were carefully cut to the proper size. The patient's spine was then hyper-flexed. The two H-grafts were fitted into place, one between L-4 and 5 and one between L-5 and S-1. The patient's spine was extended. The H-grafts were locked into place satisfactorily. Remaining bone graft was packed in and about the area. Another sterile lavage with saline was per-formed.

Anatomical closure was accomplished using 00 chromic for the muscle and lumbar fascia, 000 chromic interrupted for the subcutaneous tissue and 000 silk interrupted for the skin. A sterile compression dressing was applied over the entire area. The patient was then turned on his back on the Stryker circOlectric bed and extubated.

The patient was transfused during and after the surgical procedure with 1000 cc. of whole blood.

Harrington Spinal Instrumentation With Multilevel Spinal Fusion

The patient, a 15 year old white female with known idiopathic scoliosis, was placed on the operating table in the prone position. General anes-thesia was administered and both of the patient's legs were wrapped with 6 inch Ace bandages. The chest was protected with chest pads to allow free breathing of the abdominal wall. The entire width of the back and its entire length from the neck to below the buttocks were prepared with Septisol and draped free.

A long skin incision, extending from the level of T-6 to L-4, was carried through the skin, subcutaneous tissues and overlying fascia. Just before the skin incision was made, 120 cc. of $1/4\%$ Xylocaine and epinephrine were injected into the area to decrease the amount of bleeding. The in-cision was carried down through the underlying fascia to the spinous processes of the vertebrae. The fascia and periosteum over the vertebrae were incised with each tip. Using two periosteal elevators, one team work-ing each side of the table, the spine was simultaneously stripped of its muscle attachments by subperiosteal dissection extending from the ver-tebral spines back to the transverse processes and facet areas. This was accomplished from the level of T-7 down to the level of L-4. All soft tissues were removed from this area.

A partial laminectomy, removing approximately 2 or 3 mm. of the superior surface of the left lamina L-3, was carried out which allowed the lower distraction hook to seat easily, gripping sufficient bone for strength. Attention was then directed to the upper portion of the wound at the level of T-7 where another distraction hook was placed between the facet area of T-7 and T-8. Attention was then turned to the right side of the body where compression hooks were placed at T-8, 9 and 10, and at the bottom of the wound in T-12 and L-1 and 2.

The operation was then directed to the right iliac crest. A long incision, approximately 5 inches in length, was carried through the skin, subcutaneous tissues and overlying fascia. All bleeders were clamped and cauterized. Dissection was carried down to the fascia which was incised and to the periosteum of the iliac crest which was also incised. This was stripped with a periosteal elevator revealing the external surface of the iliac bone. Using a curved and straight osteotome, a large graft measuring approximately 4-5 inches square was removed, taking only the outer table of the iliac crest and all cancellous bone to be used later in the graft area. Bleeding was minimal. The periosteal and fascial layers were closed with 00 chromic interrupted sutures. The subcutaneous tissue was closed with 000 plain interrupted sutures.

The operation was again focused on the original wound. The facets between the two distracting hooks were removed, from the facet at T-8-T-9, all the way down the left side of the spine to L-2. The facets between these areas were removed and cancellous bone packed into the area. The facets were also removed on the right side of the body between T-11 and 12 and this was also packed with cancellous bone. Now a 7 inch distraction rod was placed between the distraction hooks and directed partially into position. A completed compression rod assembly, utilizing 6 hooks and a small threaded rod, was taken to the right side of the body and the individual hooks which had been placed previously were removed. This new compression assembly was placed in the same areas. Tightening was then accomplished. First, the distraction hook was jacked out one or two notches until tightness was felt. Compression hooks were then directed in until tightness was felt. This was carried out until stability was achieved. The curve appeared straight, perhaps a little overcorrected. A point was reached where it was unwise to apply any more pressure to these hooks. The ends of the threaded rod were removed and the wire crimped so that the nuts would not back off.

The graft, originally taken from the right iliac crest, was cut up into many small segments. Using sharp gouges and osteotomes, the lamina and posterior elements of all the processes involved in the fusion were scarified and elevated into a modified Hibbs type fusion. At the same time, the spines of the vertebrae were split vertically and bent laterally and portions of the graft were inserted between the split and turned over spines and along the gutters of the vertebral bodies.

The wound was inspected for bleeding. The sponge count was correct. The deep fascia was closed with 00 chromic interrupted sutures, the subcutaneous tissue with 000 plain interrupted sutures and the skin closed with 0000 dermalon interrupted sutures as was the skin over the graft site.

The patient tolerated the procedure well. She received 5 bottles of blood for a total of 2500 cc. of whole blood. A large compression dressing was placed on her back. She was placed in a circOlectric bed and taken to the recovery room in good condition.

ARTHROPLASTY

Arthroplasty is a plastic or reconstructive operation on the joints for the purpose of restoring motion to the joint and function to the component parts of the articulation. Such operations are performed on joints where abnormal immobility (ankylosis) has occurred as a result of trauma or pyogenic infection. Ankylosis is seen most often in the joints of the hip, knee, elbow and jaw and it is in these joints that the operation can be performed most effectively. Arthroplastic procedures include plastic revisions of the soft parts and the introduction of autogenous tissues between the articular surfaces of the joint in addition to reconstruction of the osseous parts.

Reconstructive Arthroplasty of the Left Knee (including primary reconstruction of the anterior cruciate ligament, the deep medial collateral and superficial medial collateral ligaments and excision of the dislocated medial meniscus)

After administration of a satisfactory general anesthetic, the left lower extremity was prepared and draped in the usual fashion. A pneumatic tourniquet was inflated about the left thigh. A modified median parapatellar skin incision was utilized of sufficient length to permit ready inspection of the entire medial compartment and a good share of the lateral compartment. After dissection of the subcutaneous tissue and investing deep fascia, the ruptured medial collateral ligament (superficial portion) was seen. Continuing the dissection and carefully identifying both ends of the ligamentous rupture, the deep injured portions were visualized. The medial meniscus was dislocated into the adjacent soft tissue. The capsule of the joint was then very carefully opened in a median para-patellar fashion and the remaining portion of the joint inspected. The anterior cruciate ligament was obviously also involved.

The knee was flexed to 90 degrees and the patient was properly positioned for continuation of the procedure and repair. The inner surface of the patella was not significantly injured. The patella was dislocated laterally to permit better exposure. There were areas of the articular cartilage of the femur which had been acutely injured with the ligament. The medial meniscus was sharply dissected and removed, care being taken at the margins to insure removal of the total dislocated meniscus. The anterior cruciate ligament had ruptured just at its origin from the lateral femoral condyle, but there were sufficient portions of the fibers present to permit reconstruction of the ligament and end-to-end anastomosis with the proximal and distal fragments. This was accomplished with interrupted 00 cotton suture material. A satisfactory reconstruction of the ligament was obtained. The deep medial collateral ligament was repaired with interrupted 00 cotton suture and reinforcement of the superficial ligament was also performed. The wound was then lavaged with sterile saline and the knee brought into a neutral position and redraped.

A standard closure of the knee incision was performed with interrupted 00 chromic for the capsule and investing fascia and a continuous 00 nylon subcuticular suture for the skin. A Sommers compression dressing with anterior and posterior plaster molds was applied. The tourniquet was deflated.

Austin-Moore Endoprosthetic Arthoplasty

The patient was placed in the right lateral position and the left hip prepared and draped from the iliac crest to below the knee.

Under general anesthesia, a long Gibson approach was carried out with a skin incision approximately 12 inches long. The incision started posteriorly and traveled anteriorly into the previous incisional area in the old hip nailing site of two years ago. The incision was carried down through the skin, subcutaneous tissues and overlying fascia. All bleeders were cauterized.

The fascia lata was opened and the nail palpated underneath. The fascia lata was further opened in the line of the incision and the nail was visible. All five screws were removed from the Jewett nail. There was no sign of corrosion. As soon as the five screws were removed the nail could be easily extracted. This hip nailing was performed two years ago for an intertrochanteric fracture.

The reason for this operation was the pathologic fracture of the femoral neck which would not allow the Jewett nail to protrude into the superior part of the acetabulum, causing the patient a great deal of pain.

With the nail removed, attention was directed to the area of the femoral head. One half of the abductors of the Gluteus maximus and medius were released from the trochanteric region. The leg was rotated and flexed. Blunt and sharp dissection was carried over the anterior portion of the hip capsule.

It was believed that the pathologic fracture of the left femoral neck was 2½ weeks old. With some difficulty, the capsule was located and incised onto the femoral neck and head area. The femoral head was very soft. In some areas it was of egg shell thickness and had to be removed in pieces. The femoral neck was now high riding. There was no question about tumor in the femoral neck. Posteriorly, there was very little bone left.

Using what remained of the femoral neck, it was cut down and notched to admit the Austin-Moore prosthesis. A 1⅞ prosthesis was inserted and fixation accomplished with a #18 wire through the bone and prosthesis.

There was considerable bleeding from the tumor area with a drop in blood pressure which was rectified by the administration of additional blood.

Closure was carried out with 00 chromic for the capsule and 00 chromic for the overlying muscle and fascial layers. The incision of the fascia lata and Vastus lateralis where the Jewett nail had been removed was closed in a similar manner. The subcutaneous tissue was closed with 00 chromic interrupted sutures and the skin closed with sutures of 0000 dermalon. A large compression dressing was placed on the wound. The heels were wrapped with ABD and Ace bandages and the lower extremities immobilized with three pillows between the legs. The legs were held in a position of function.

Magnuson Modified Arthroplasty, Rt. Knee

The right lower extremity was prepared and draped following which a pneumatic tourniquet was applied and inflated to 500 mm. of mercury. It was sustained at that pressure.

The right knee was approached through a median peripatellar skin incision carried through the subcutaneous tissue down to the investing deep fascia of the thigh. This was also incised in the course of the skin incision.

The insertion of the Vastus medialis muscle into the rectus and the medial patella was sharply incised and allowed to retract medially. The incision was continued along the medial border margin of the patella down to the joint line and this curved distally following the patellar tendon insertion. The capsular joint was thereby opened as was the synovium up to and including the suprapatellar pouch. Very thick redundant synovium filled the suprapatellar pouch and was therefore resected as completely as possible.

Inspection of the medial and lateral compartments was accomplished with the patella dislocated laterally, revealing detachment of the anterior third of the medial meniscus, with evidence of a chronic process. The undersurface of the patella was inspected and found to have undergone both subacute and chronic chondromalacial change. Very careful recontouring of the undersurface of the patella was accomplished, including osteotome dissection of the margins and sharp knife condyleplasty of the articular surface of the patella. The femoral condyles were treated in like fashion producing smooth, gliding articular surfaces. The medial meniscus was then removed almost totally under direct vision with the knee flexed at 90 degrees. Inspection of the anterior and posterior cruciate ligaments revealed no pathology. The two-thirds of the lateral meniscus, which could be visualized, appeared normal.

A very copious lavage of the joint was performed and all small bits of cartilage and synovium were removed. The knee was extended and the patella replaced in its normal position.

An anatomical closure was performed. The Vastus medialis muscle was reattached to the Rectus femoris tendon and the medial aspect of the newly contoured patella under a normal amount of tension. The capsule of the joint was closed with interrupted 00 chromic suture material. The subcutaneous tissue and deep fascia were approximated with interrupted 00 chromic and the skin was closed with 0000 nylon interrupted and vertical mattress sutures. A bulky Sommers compression dressing was applied with a posterior plaster splint. The tourniquet was deflated.

BONE GRAFTS

The use of autogenous and homogenous bone grafts as a means of providing fixation with osteogenesis is becoming more widely accepted. The availability of material from bone banks has further promoted the use of this technique in preference to other methods of fixation where union is apt to progress more slowly.

Bone grafts are used in a variety of situations: to promote union, to fill defects in delayed union, in cases of nonunion, to provide fixation, to bridge joints and provide arthrodesis, to fill defects following excision of lesions, to provide bone blocks which limit joint motion, and in numerous other circumstances.

Grafts are divided into three categories based on their source of origin, as follows:

Autogenous   Bone removed from one site and implanted in another site in the same individual.

Homogenous   Bone obtained from a human other than the patient. Bone bank specimens belong in this group.

Heterogenous   Use of material such as boiled ox bone upon which the host deposits his own tissues.

TYPES OF BONE GRAFTS

Diamond inlay graft
Dual onlay
Hemicylindrical
Inlay
Intramedullary and spongiosa
Massive sliding
Medullary

Onlay
Osteoperiosteal
Peg
Single onlay cortical
Sliding inlay
Whole bone transplant

BONE GRAFT TECHNIQUES

Albee sliding inlay
Banks
Boyd dual inlay
Flanagan & Burem massive apposing
Gallie diamond inlay
Haldeman

Henderson
Hey-Groves and Kirk self-sustaining
Hoglund medullary bone
Phemister onlay
Ryerson medullary bone
Soto-Hall

Bone Graft to the Femur

The area of the right femur was prepared and draped. The tissues covering the site of the fracture were dissected bluntly and the tissue between the fragments carefully removed. Eburnized bone ends were trimmed until cancellous bone was reached. The fragments were pared with a motor saw, reaming out the medulla.

The site of the donor area was selected on the tibia and the periosteum stripped to each side of the proposed graft site for about an inch. A large graft was removed. The cortex and spongiosa were separated. A strip of the spongiosa along with its endosteum was inserted in the medulla, bridging the fragments. The graft was fitted into place on the cortex.

Drill holes were made in the graft and receiving sites. Autogenous bone nails which had been developed from the cortical graft were then driven through the holes into the cortex.

The wound was closed in layers and dressed. A hip spica was applied.

Autogenous Bone Graft to Right Tibia   **Donor site: Left Anterior Ilium**

After administration of a satisfactory general anesthetic, a pneumatic tourniquet was inflated to 500 mm. of mercury and sustained about the right leg. The right lower extremity and the anterior crest of the ilium were prepared and draped in the usual manner.

The area of delayed union in the proximal third of the right tibia was exposed by a curvilinear incision following one of the previous skin incisions. The incision was carried directly to the bone. The periosteum was divided in the course of the skin incision. Very careful soft tissue dissection was utilized to bring the delayed union site into view. The subperiosteal dissection was carried around to the lateral aspect of the tibia. The delayed union site was then prepared in fenestra fashion by roughening and shingling the cortex by sharp osteotome dissection. Multiple drill holes were made in different directions to stimulate and provide access for new blood vessel growth. This area was then lavaged and packed and the tourniquet deflated.

Attention was then directed to the left anterior iliac crest which was exposed through a skin incision directly over the crest. Strips of autogenous cancellous and cancellous-cortical bone graft were obtained in the usual fashion and placed in a sterile saline basin. The donor site wound was then packed with Gelfoam over the bone and closed with interrupted 00 chromic to approximate the musculature over the crest. Interrupted 00000 nylon was used for the skin closure.

The bone grafts were carefully cut to proper proportion and packed in and about the area of nonunion, especially in the lateral and posterior aspects, with some anteromedially also. The periosteum was then loosely closed over the bone grafts and the skin was brought into its normal position and closed with interrupted 00000 nylon suture material.

After satisfactory lavage of the area, a sterile dressing was applied and a long leg anterior-posterior plaster mold with a Sommers compression dressing. The tourniquet was deflated. A dressing was also placed over the previously closed donor site.

Removal of Tibial Bone Grafts

With the patient in the supine position, the area of the lower right leg is prepared and draped in a sterile manner.

An incision is made along the flat portion of the tibia and carried through the skin and tissues. An osteoperiosteal graft is removed and an incision is then made through the periosteum following the shape of the proposed graft. The desired graft is further outlined with a Luck bone saw. A motor drill is then used to drill the ends. A sharp, thin osteotome is used to connect the drill holes and the tibial graft is removed. Some cancellous bone is curetted out of the medullary cavity.

The periosteum is closed with plain catgut and the wound closed in layers. Dressing and stockinette are applied.

DISLOCATIONS

The displacement of a bone from its normal anatomic position is termed a *dislocation*. Most acute or fresh dislocations are amenable to manual reduction through proper manipulation; however, dislocations which resist closed reduction or which have become habitual are treated by open reduction. Dislocations are often attended by fractures of varying degree which complicate conservative management and require surgery. The most frequently encountered injury of this type is dislocation of the shoulder with fracture of the surgical neck of the humerus. The shoulder is also the joint in which recurrent dislocations are most likely to occur. These dislocations usually occur anteriorly constituting a subcoracoid type displacement.

Numerous operative techniques have been adopted to correct dislocation, with or without fractures, by methods of open reduction. Some of the more popular methods are listed here.

OPERATIONS FOR DISLOCATION

Bankart (shoulder)
Blount osteotomy
Campbell (patella)
Campbell shelf operation
Cave (capitate bone)
Cave and Rowe (shoulder)
Conn operation
Cubbins (shoulder)
Dickson (shoulder)
Eden-Hybbinette (shoulder)
Evans (ankle)
Haas
Hauser (patella)
Kapel (elbow)
King and Richards (hip)
Levine (hip)
Lorenz bifurcation
MacAusland (lunate)

Magnuson-Stack (shoulder)
Mahorner and Mead (lunate)
McLaughlin (shoulder)
Milch (elbow)
Mumford and Gurd (clavicle)
Nicola (shoulder)
Palmer and Widen (shoulder)
Pheasant (elbow)
Putti-Platt (shoulder)
Reichenheim and King (elbow)
Reversed Eden-Hybbinette (shoulder)
Roux-Goldthwait (patella)
Schanz
Slocum (metacarpal joint-thumb)
Speed (elbow)
Watson-Jones (ankle)
Wilson-McKeever (shoulder)

Watson-Jones Operation for Dislocation of the Ankle

The operative area is sterilely prepared and draped. Under general anesthesia, a lateral incision is made over the posterior border of the lower third of the shaft of the fibula. It is carried around the tip of the lateral malleolus and brought out on the lateral aspect of the foot. Proximally, the Peroneus brevis tendon is freed from its muscular attachment. The muscle fibers are sutured to the Peroneus longus tendon. The Peroneus brevis tendon is released as far as the lateral malleolus distally, care being taken not to disturb the annular fibers.

Beginning about one inch above the tip of the malleolus, an antero-posterior tunnel is developed for the tendon through the fibula. A vertical drill hole is made through the outer margin of the neck of the talus, just in front of the articular surface. The drill emerges in the roof of the sinus tarsi. The drill is then introduced in the outermost tip of the lateral malleolus and directed from the anterior aspect, upward and backward. The tendon is then brought from a posterior position forward, is threaded through the first hole in the lateral malleolus, through the second hole in the talus, in a direction from above downward, and then back through the hole in the malleolus. The end of the tendon is sutured to the periosteum on the posterior aspect of the external malleolus.

A cast is applied from the toes to the tibial tubercle.

Bankart Operation for Chronic Dislocation of Shoulder

The patient was placed in Fowler's position with the knees flexed and the feet supported by a padded foot rest. Sterile preparation and draping was carried out.

A deltopectoral incision was made extending from the tip of the acromion to the middle and distal third of the clavicle. The incision was curved downward following the course of the cephalic vein. A groove was created between the pectoral and deltoid muscles. The cephalic vein was ligated and retracted mesially.

Using a No. 3/32 drill, the tip of the coracoid process was drilled and an osteotomy performed.

Medial retraction of the muscles of the coracoid process was carried out. Lateral retraction of the Deltoideus and Pectoralis major muscles was obtained. The Subscapularis muscle was reflected from its insertion. The capsule was opened along the glenoid labrum. The torn glenoid labrum was attached to the bone with wire sutures which were pulled through a drill hole in the neck of the scapula and tied over a button and felt pads posteriorly.

The Subscapularis muscle was reattached to its original insertion using a heavy chromic catgut. A suture placed through a previously made drill hole served to reattach the tip of the osteotomized coracoid process. The muscles were repaired and the wound closed in layers with plain catgut.

A Velpeau dressing was applied.

FRACTURES

A partial or complete interruption in the continuity of a bone is referred to as a *fracture*. Such a break may assume many and varied forms. Definitions of the more frequently used designations for fractures are listed below to familiarize the secretary with the precise connotation of these terms.

BENNETT	A fracture through the first metacarpal of the wrist involving the carpometacarpal joint and associated with subluxation.
CLOSED	A fracture which does not involve a break in the skin.
COLLES'	Fracture of the radius at the wrist with displacement of the lower fragment.
COMMINUTED	A crushing fracture in which the fragments are splintered to pieces.
COMPOUND	Fracture of a bone with an open wound of the skin.
COMPRESSION	Fracture caused by compression and usually seen involving the spine.
COTTON'S	Trimalleolar fracture of the ankle.
DEPRESSED	A type of skull fracture where fragments are pushed inward.
GREENSTICK	An incomplete fracture of a bone.
LEFORT	Fracture of the maxilla, bilaterally, in a horizontal plane.
LINEAR	A fracture running the length of a bone.
MONTEGGIA'S	Dislocation of the head of the radius associated with fracture of the ulnar shaft.
OPEN	Same as compound fracture where there is a wound through the skin.
PATHOLOGIC	Fractures caused by disease such as malignancy.
POTT'S	Bimalleolar fracture of the ankle.
TRIMALLEOLAR	Fracture of the ankle. Cotton's fracture.

Occasionally, fractures occur near a joint resulting in a dislocation of the joint. Such an entity is referred to as a *fracture-dislocation*.

Surgical Techniques in the Treatment of Fractures

Fractures are treated by closed or open reductions. A variety of screws, nails, plates and prostheses are used to perform internal fixations of fractures. Such equipment and instruments are listed in Chapter 5.

This section will be devoted primarily to a presentation of sample operative reports and listings of techniques employed in fracture management.

SOME REDUCTION TECHNIQUES

Crutchfield (cervical spine)
Essex-Lopresti (axial fixation of
 calcaneous)
Lottes (tibia)
Magnuson (patella)

Martin (patella)
Speed and Boyd (Monteggia fracture)
Thomson (patella)
Wagner (Bennett fracture)

Lottes Technique for Medullary Nailing of the Tibia

After sterile preparation and draping and after the administration of a general anesthetic, the leg is supported on a fracture table. The hip is flexed 130 degrees and the knee to 90 degrees. A traction apparatus is used.

The tibial crest is palpated. Proper alignment and apposition of the fracture is obtained by manual manipulation.

A small skin incision is made and extended proximally one finger-breadth medial to the tibial tubercle. The incision is carried through the subcutaneous tissues; however, the bone is exposed only in the distal 3 cms. of the incision. With a three-eighths inch drill, a perforation is made in the cortex opposite the mid-portion of the tibial tubercle. The drill is introduced at right angles to the bone. The handle of the drill is gently depressed after entry into the medullary canal. The drill is kept parallel with the shaft of the tibia. A small metal shield is placed in the incision proximally to prevent soft tissue damage. A carefully positioned slotted hole is then made. The driver is attached and the tip of the nail inserted into the slotted hole with its dorsal fin pointed forward. The tip of the anterior flange is aligned with the middle and lower thirds junction of the tibial shaft. The nail is tapped down into place until resistance is encountered. The tip of the nail is then brought forward by depressing the mid-portion of the nail with the palm of the hand. The nail is driven down the medullary canal and its progress checked by a nail of the same length. Rotation and reduction of the fracture are checked again and the nail driven through the fracture site.

Roentgenograms are made to determine the course of the nail. Satisfactory position having been obtained, the nail is driven in further until the driver strikes the cortex. A small threaded portion of the nail is allowed to protrude to facilitate future extraction.

A temporary plaster cast is applied extending from the toes to the midthigh.

Open Reduction of Left Humerus with Rush Rod Insertion

With the patient under general anesthesia, the left shoulder, chest, and arm were prepared and draped in a sterile manner. A pillow was inserted under the shoulder to elevate the operative area.

An incision was made anteriorly and longitudinally between the pectoral groove. The cephalic vein was not identified. The incision was carried down to the fracture site. A moderate amount of hematoma was evacuated.

The head of the humerus was dislocated posteriorly and the base of the fracture site pointed in a lateral direction. By means of manual manipulation the head of the humerus was placed back into the glenoid fossa and rotated. Traction was applied to the extremity and by means of bone hooks the fracture was reduced. The post-reduction position was satisfactory.

A stab wound was made just lateral to the acromion tip on the shoulder and carried down to the intercondylar groove. Two 8 inch Rush rods were driven down into the humeral shaft. This stabilized the fracture.

The operative area was thoroughly irrigated with saline and the wound closed in layers with interrupted 000 chromic.

Check films of the shoulder showed it to be in satisfactory position. The extremity was bandaged in a Velpeau sling.

Open Reduction—Smith-Petersen Nailing with a Lawson-Thornton Plate, Left Hip

With the patient under suitable anesthesia, the left hip was manipulated and satisfactory reduction óbtained. This was verified by x-ray examination.

A lateral incision, approximately 10 inches in length, was made starting at the level of the greater trochanter and extending distally. This was deepened through the fascia. The Vastus lateralis was reflected subperiosteally. There was marked subtrochanteric comminution.

With some difficulty, the spikes were manipulated into position and held in place with a Wilman clamp. The inferior trochanteric fossa was osteotomized and a guide wire passed. Due to the x-ray appearance of bending of the guide wire, it was removed and a 4 inch Smith-Petersen nail inserted into the neck and head of the femur. X-ray examination revealed adequate alignment of this nail. A Lawson-Thornton side plate was suitably fastened to the nail and attached to the femoral cortices with stainless steel screws. Stability was solid following this procedure.

The muscular and fascial layers were closed with interrupted 00 chromic catgut. The subcutaneous tissue was closed with 000 plain catgut and the skin with a running suture of black silk. A dressing was applied.

Austin-Moore Prosthesis, Right Hip

With the patient under spinal anesthesia in a left lateral position, the right extremity was prepared and draped in a sterile manner.

A hockey-stick incision was used to expose the capsule and head of the femur. The Gluteus maximus attachment was then separated. The capsule was entered. Using a periosteal elevator, the broken femoral head was removed. After chipping the bone over the greater trochanter, the reamer was driven into the shaft of the femur. The acetabulum was then tested for the size of the prosthesis to be used. This was inserted into the femur after packing it with cancellous bone. It was then fitted into the socket and a snug fit obtained.

The capsule was reapproximated with interrupted 00 chromic. The muscles were reattached with interrupted chromic. The skin was also closed with chromic.

OTHER ORTHOPEDIC PROCEDURES

In addition to the types of orthopedic procedures already presented, there exist a wide variety of other procedures which include osteotomy, ostectomy, osteoclasis and operations on the bursae, muscles, tendons, ligaments, and fasciae. Examples of some of these operations have also been included in this section to provide the secretary with additional exercise in orthopedic terminology.

Bunionectomy and Hammer Toe Correction

With the patient under general anesthesia, a bloodless field was created by using a blood pressure cuff on the right leg, inflated to 500 mm. of mercury, as a pneumatic tourniquet. The operative field was prepared and draped.

A semilunar incision was made just dorsal to the presenting bunion and skin flaps were raised. The subcutaneous presenting synovial cyst was removed and a triangular flap of synovium was raised exposing the joint cavity. By means of an osteotome and mallet, the exostosis was removed. An incision curving laterally and beginning at the webs of the first and second toes was made. By means of blunt dissection the sesamoid bone on the medial aspect of the first metatarsal head was removed.

A hemostat was passed beneath the first and second metatarsal heads and a 00 chromic suture was threaded completely around the first two metatarsals. It was tied snugly on the medial aspect of the first metatarsal. This helped in the correction of the metatarsus varus.

A wedge-shaped piece of skin over the interphalangeal area of the second and third toes was raised and removed. The extensor tendon was divided proximal to the joint and raised distally until the joint was exposed. By means of an electric saw the articular surface, both proximally and distally, was removed.

Hammer Toe Correction

The hammer toe defect was then corrected. A Kirschner wire of appropriate size was introduced into the joint from the tip of the distal phalanx. This held the joint in position. A Kirschner wire was also introduced into the metatarsophalangeal joint of the first toe from a distal and a medial direction. The wires were then cut leaving them exposed for a brief distance on the second and third toes and burying them subcutaneously on the first toe. The tendons of the toes were then repaired with interrupted 000000 cotton and the synovial flap was resutured in place with interrupted 000000 cotton.

A Jones procedure was performed on the second and third hammer toes. This consisted of tying the long and short extensors of the second and third toes together with a 000000 cotton, freeing the long extensor of the second and third toes approximately to this point, and abrading the surface of the tendon with a knife. The second and third metatarsals were exposed and the periosteum was raised on the lateral aspect of the metatarsal. The extensor tendons of the second and third toes were divided and threaded through a Keith needle with a 00 cotton. This was tunneled between the bone and periosteum ventrally. The sutures were then brought out through the skin in the plantar aspect of the foot.

The foot was padded with a sponge over the cotton sutures which were tied on a button. All skin incisions were closed with interrupted 00000 dermalon. A plaster boot was applied with the foot in a neutral position, maintaining compression on the metatarsal head. The blood pressure cuff was deflated.

Hauser Procedure — **Bilateral transfer of tibial tubercle medially**

After adequate anesthesia had been obtained, both lower extremities were prepared and draped in the usual fashion.

The right knee was corrected first. The tourniquet was inflated about the right thigh to 500 mm. of mercury and sustained.

A curvilinear skin incision crossing the knee joint in the flexion crease from the medial to the lateral aspect was utilized to expose the patella, patellar tendon and tibial tubercle. Sharp and blunt dissection were used to outline the area. A flap was cut in the periosteum about the tibial tubercle. Multiple drill holes were used to outline a small rectangular area including the tibial tubercle and the insertion of the patellar tendon. These drill holes were joined by sharp osteotome dissection and the patellar tendon insertion, including the tibial tubercle and the fragment of bone there, were lifted away from the tibia. The new insertion site for the tibial tubercle was prepared 1 cm. distally and 1 cm. medially from the previous insertion.

A sharp H incision was made and periosteal flaps raised. Multiple drill holes were used to outline the rectangular bone block. The drill holes were joined by sharp osteotome dissection and the bone block was gently elevated.

The bone block removed from the new insertion was then placed in the defect left by removing the tibial tubercle. The patellar tendon with its bone block was then inserted in this new site. It was internally fixed by means of one large bone screw. The periosteum was sewn carefully to the tibial tubercle periosteum and to the patellar tendon at its new insertion to provide additional security.

The area was lavaged with copious amounts of sterile saline. The lateral portion of the patellar retinaculum was carefully divided with a scissors up to the Vastus lateralis crossover. The medial portion of the retinaculum was then imbricated with interrupted 00 chromic. Subcutaneous tissues were closed with interrupted 000 plain suture and the skin with interrupted 00000 cotton. A compression dressing was applied. The tourniquet was deflated. Another tourniquet was inflated about the left thigh.

The same procedure was repeated on the left lower extremity with the exception that a stainless steel bone screw was not necessary to secure the tibial tubercle transplant. This was done by geometrically cutting the block and placing it in its new bed. It was fixed securely enough and therefore did not require a bone screw.

When both knees had been finished, dressings were applied. Long leg plaster splints were utilized to secure immobilization of the knees.

Medial Meniscectomy

Under general anesthesia, with tourniquet control, an arthrotomy of the left knee was performed through a medial peripatellar skin incision. The medial meniscus was found to be completely detached posteriorly with a large bucket-handle caught in the joint. A total meniscectomy was performed. The remainder of the knee appeared normal.

Following lavage with saline, an anatomical closure with 000 nylon subcuticular sutures for the skin was accomplished. The tourniquet was deflated and a Sommers compression dressing applied.

Primary Tenorrhaphy

Under general anesthesia the patient was placed in the supine position. Routine sterile preparation and draping was carried out.

Initially, the wound was irrigated with normal saline. Mild debridement of the necrotic and bruised tissue was done. The various tendons were then located and held in place with a Keith needle. Inspection of the wound made it apparent that the Flexor digitorum sublimis, the Flexor carpi radialis and ulnaris as well as the Palmaris longus tendon had been completely severed. After these tendons were found, a primary tenorrhaphy was carried out by approximating the respective tendons to their counterparts with interrupted 000000 cotton sutures.

After adequate hemostasis had been maintained, the wound was closed using interrupted 000000 cotton sutures for the subcutaneous tissue and continuous running 00000 dermalon suture for the skin. The hand was then dressed with a compression dressing and splinted in flexion and partial ulnar deviation.

500 cc. of 5% glucose in water was used during the operation.

Tendon Graft

The Flexor digitorum sublimis (superficialis) tendon was used for a graft to the Flexor digitorum profundus tendon.

Under general anesthesia, the entire right hand and forearm were thoroughly prepared with soap and water for 10 minutes. A pneumatic cuff was used as a pneumatic tourniquet to control bleeding.

A midline incision was made on the ulnar aspect of the right middle finger. It was found that the Flexor digitorum profundus and sublimis tendons had been cut into two parts. The ends were divided and separated. The proximal end of the profundus and sublimis tendons had retracted into the palm.

A longitudinal semicurved incision was made in the palm and the proximal ends of the tendon were identified here. A transverse incision was made in the wrist and the sublimis tendon removed at the wrist. Considerable scarring was present throughout the tendon, in the finger as well as in the palm.

The Flexor digitorum sublimis tendon was used as a graft. It was united to the insertion of the Flexor digitorum profundus in the distal phalanx of the right middle finger. The graft extended from the distal phalanx to the volar area of the palm. A pulley was reconstructed out of the remaining portion of the sublimis tendon over the middle finger.

The blood pressure cuff was removed at half hour intervals. The skin edges were carefully closed with interrupted fine 00000 nylon sutures. Several small rubber drains were inserted in each operative site. A large compression type dressing with a posterior metal splint was applied.

Split Thickness Skin Graft to Index Finger With Repair

With the patient under general anesthesia, in the supine position, the right hand and forearm were prepared and draped in the usual manner. A bloodless field was secured by means of a pneumatic tourniquet about the right arm. The tourniquet was elevated to 300 mm. of mercury.

There was an avulsion of skin and subcutaneous tissue on the tactile pad of the finger. A split thickness skin graft was taken with a razor blade from the volar aspect of the forearm, transferred to the index finger amputation stump and sutured in position with interrupted 000000 nylon.

In the case of the middle finger there was an amputation through the distal phalanx. There was adequate skin and subcutaneous tissue for direct primary closure which was performed after the digital sensory nerves had been resected back into healthy soft tissue.

In the ring finger, there was a laceration on the tactile pad. This laceration was repaired with interrupted 000000 nylon.

Section of Transverse Carpal Ligament, Right Wrist

The patient presented a carpal tunnel syndrome of the right wrist.

Under general anesthesia a tourniquet was applied to the right upper arm and the hand was surgically prepared and draped.

A curved incision was made across the flexor palmar crease extending into the palm of the hand. The dissection was carried down to the palmar fascia. The Palmaris longus was identified and retracted. An incision was made through the fascia and the transverse carpal ligament identified. With a hemostat under the transverse carpal ligament to protect the median nerve, it was sectioned. It was found to be hard and gritty. There was evidence to indicate compression of the median nerve.

A small portion of the transverse carpal ligament was removed to insure adequate passage of the Flexor sublimis and Flexor profundus tendons as well as the median nerve. The median nerve was not disturbed in any way. Except for the swelling and thickening noted proximal to the transverse carpal ligament, no abnormalities were encountered.

The wound was closed with three sutures of plain catgut for the subcutaneous fascia. The skin was closed with a subcuticular suture of 000 nylon. This was followed by the application of Telfa, dry sterile gauze and a heavy compression bandage, after the tourniquet had been removed.

OTHER ORTHOPEDIC OPERATIONS

Eponymic titles often pose a problem for the medical secretary and for this reason we have included the following list of orthopedic procedures. The surgeons whose names appear in these titles often have numerous operative techniques to their credit, many of which have not been indicated here. This list is intended primarily as an index to some of the more important contributions to operative orthopedics. It will also serve to familiarize the secretary with the names of the men after whom operations in this field have been named.

Abbott arthrodesis
Albee fusion of the spine
Albee reconstruction operation
Albee shelf operation
Badgley arthrodesis of the hip
Bateman denervation of the knee
Bateman tendon transference of the shoulder
Bickel and Moe translocation of Peroneus longus
Blocker operation for elephantiasis
Blount rotation osteotomy
Blount technique for ununited fractures
Blundell Jones varus osteotomy
Boyd dual onlay bone graft
Boyd patellectomy
Brackett osteosynthesis of the femur
Brett technique for genu recurvatum
Brisement Force manipulation
Brittain extra-articular arthrodesis
Brittain fusion of the knee
Brockman operation for equinovarus
Bunnell repair of ligaments
Bunnell repair of tendons
Bunnell technique for malunited Bennett's fracture
Burman tendon transfer
Campbell bone block for paralytic equinus

ORTHOPEDIC OPERATIONS (Continued)

Campbell shelf operation
Carrell replacement of distal end of fibula
Cartilaginous cup arthroplasty
Chandler fusion of hip
Charnley compression arthrodesis
Clothespin "H" or Prop graft in spinal fusion
Cole operation for cavus deformity of the foot
Colonna arthrodesis of the wrist
Colonna arthroplasty for congenital dislocation of the hip
Colonna reconstruction operation
Colop ostectomy
Compere operation for lengthening the femur
Credo operation for congenital dislocation of the hip
Darrach resection of the distal end of the ulna
Denuse operation for congenital dislocation of the hip
Dickson shelf operation
Dickson-Diveley operation for clawtoe deformity
Dunn-Brittain arthrodesis of the ankle
Durman osteotomy and bone graft
Eden-Hybbinette bone graft
Eggers neurectomy
Eggers transplantation of hamstring tendons
Ellis Jones operation for displacement of peroneal tendons
Elmslie-Cholmeley double tarsal wedge osteotomy
Eyler flexorplasty
Fowler capsulotomy of metacarpophalangeal joints
Fritz Lange operation for congenital dislocation of the hip
Gaenslen split heel incision
Garceau anterior tibial tendon transfer in clubfoot
Ghormley arthrodesis of the hip
Ghormley osteotomy and bone graft
Ghormley shelf operation
Gibson arthroplasty
Gill arthrodesis of the shoulder
Gill operation for paralytic foot drop
Girdlestone laminectomy
Girdlestone-Taylor tendon transfer for clawtoe
Grice-Green extra-articular arthrodesis of subtalar joint
Hammond operation for hallux equinus
Hark operation for flatfoot
Harmon osteotomy
Harris-Beath operation for flatfoot
Hauser lengthening of tendo-calcaneus
Heifitz operation for ingrown toenail
Henderson arthrodesis of the hip

ORTHOPEDIC OPERATIONS (Continued)

Hendry posterior bone block of elbow
Henry and Geist spinal fusion
Heyman operation for genu recurvatum
Hibbs arthrodesis of the hip
Hibbs spinal fusion
His-Hass operation for brachial plexus injury
Hohmann operation for tennis elbow
Hoke pes planus operation
Horwitz and Adams transfibular arthrodesis
Howorth open reduction for congenital dislocation of the hip
Hueter-Mayo toe operation
Inclan bone block
Inclan osteotomy and bone graft
Joplin bunion operation
Judet prosthetic replacement arthroplasty
Judet technique for stem prosthesis
Kelikian arthroplasty of temporomandibular joint
Keller bunion operation
Kellogg-Speed operation for spondylolisthesis (anterior fusion)
Kidner pes planus operation
Kirkaldy-Willis ischiofemoral arthrodesis
Koenig-Wittek operation for congenital elevation of the scapula
Kutler plastic closure in transverse fingertip amputations
Lambrinudi drop-foot operation
Lapidus bunion operation
Lapidus operation for hallux equinus (dorsal bunion)
Legge spherical prosthesis technique
L'Episcopo osteotomy
Liebolt operation for radioulnar joint stability
Linton and Talbott operation for removal of gouty tophus
Littlewood's forequarter amputation
Lorenz bifurcation osteotomy
Lorenz operation for congenital dislocation of the hip
Lucas and Cottrell notched rotation osteotomy of the tibia
Ludloff incision for psoas abscess
MacAusland arthroplasty of the elbow
Macey technique for elephantiasis
Magnuson arthroplasty of the knee
Mayo bunion operation
Mazur patellectomy
McBride bunion operation
McCarroll rotation osteotomy
McElvenny neuroma operation
McElvenny operation for hallux varus
McLaughlin repair of musculotendinous cuff

ORTHOPEDIC OPERATIONS (Continued)

Milch cuff resection of ulna
Moyer transplantation of Trapezius
Mozicki spinal fusion
Mustard transference of Iliopsoas tendon
Naughton-Dunn arthrodesis of the ankle
Ober forward transference of Tibialis posterior tendon
Ober operation for congenital elevation of the scapula
Osgood osteotomy of the femur
Parkes tendon transplantation of Volkmann's contracture
Pauwels adduction osteotomy
Pauwels Y-osteotomy
Platou rotation osteotomy
Putti arthrodesis of knee with tibial bone graft
Putti arthrodesis of shoulder
Ridlon operation for congenital dislocation of the hip
Riordan tendon transfer of the thumb
Ruiz-Mora operation for overlapping 5th toe
Schanz osteotomy in congenital hip dislocation
Schede rotation osteotomy
Seddon arthrodesis of the wrist
Shrock operation for congenital elevation of the scapula (Sprengel's deformity)
Smith-Petersen acromioplasty
Sofield operation for congenital pseudarthrosis of the tibia
Soutter transference of crest of ilium
J.S. Speed osteotomy and bone graft
Stamm arthrodesis of the hip
Staples arthrodesis of the elbow
Steele-Stewart operation for equinovarus
Steindler flexorplasty
Steindler operation for pes cavus
Steindler operation of the shoulder joint
Trethowan operation for tennis elbow
Trumble arthrodesis
Vulpius-Compere lengthening of tendo-calcaneus
Whitman reconstruction operation
Whitman talectomy
Wickstrom arthrodesis of the wrist
Wilson trochanteric arthroplasty
Wilson-Jones arthrodesis of the shoulder
Wilson-Straub spinal fusion
Woughter sliding flap graft in transverse fingertip amputations
Yount posterior capsulotomy
Zodik operation for ingrown toenails
Zahradnicek biplane cuneiform osteotomy

13 { *Plastic Surgery*

Plastic surgery is a surgical specialty concerned with repair and reconstruction of congenital, developmental and traumatic deformities of the external body for the purpose of restoring function and providing the individual with a more acceptable physical image of himself. Numerous techniques are employed to achieve this end including tissue grafts, foreign implants, tattoo, dermabrasion, repair and reconstruction.

Some of the most interesting and impressive advances in surgery have been made in the use of tissue transplants. Genetic compatibility between the host and the transplant has been established as one of the most important factors in success with certain tissues, notably the skin. Whenever possible, the patient acts as his own donor; however, avascular tissues such as the cornea, cartilage and epidermis may be transplanted from one human to another.

Tissue transplants are classified into three main types based on the donor source.

AUTOGRAPHS — (autogenous transplants) In these grafts, tissue is transplanted from one site to another on the same individual. The tissues used most successfully include split skin, cornea, bone and cartilage.

HOMOGRAFTS — (isografts, homogenous transplants) These grafts consist of tissues transplanted from one human to another and include those composed of avascular tissue such as cornea, cartilage and epidermis. Tissues are exchanged between single ovum twins, but grafts utilizing tissues other than the avascular types mentioned have not been used successfully. Skin homografts, at the present time, are used primarily as biologic dressings over severe burn areas to prevent loss of body fluids. They are also utilized as temporary coverings in reconstructive surgery where defects have been created in donor sites. Such skin grafts are usually rejected by the host between the ninth and fifteenth day after transplantation although the survival time of the graft can be prolonged by using a closely related individual as the donor. *ZOOGRAFTS* — (animal tissues) Transplant of tissues from animals to man was regarded as an experimental curiosity a few years ago. Today, successful use is made of bovine fascia, ox bone as well as calf bone and cartilage.

SKIN GRAFTS

In the light of our present knowledge, it is the patient who serves as his own donor for skin grafts when a lasting result is desired. Such grafts assume the form of free grafts or pedicle grafts.

The *free graft* is removed entirely from one area and implanted into another area. The *pedicle graft,* as distinguished from the free graft, is raised from its bed except for one or more points at which it remains attached. These points of attachment are called pedicles and serve to provide the flap with an adequate blood supply until a circulation can develop at the recipient site. This graft remains attached to both the donor and recipient sites. It is severed at a later date when viability and a satisfactory vascular supply have been assured at the site of implantation.

A particular type of pedicle graft frequently used is the *tube pedicle.* In this method of skin transfer, the skin is formed into a tube and advanced by descriptive techniques known as caterpillaring, waltzing or conveyance. One of the extremities is used as the carrier in the latter method.

When skin grafts are referred to by the physician they are usually designated as being of full thickness or split thickness. These terms are defined below with two less often used grafts.

FULL THICKNESS (Wolfe graft)   Whole thicknesses of skin ranging in thickness from .030 to .050 inches are used for replacing large areas of tissue loss. This type of graft is frequently used for the face.

SPLIT THICKNESS   These grafts range in thickness from 0.010 to 0.020 inches and are used for repair of skin defects on the face. They also serve the purpose of epithelial inlays.

CHESSBOARD (Gabarro)   Small split thickness grafts cut into 5 to 10 mm. squares from a large sheet of skin are placed on a wound 1 cm. apart.

PINCH GRAFT (Reverdin)   Rounded bits of skin are used to cover the granulating surface of a wound such as that which follows a burn. This technique is seldom used today. These grafts often resulted in cobblestone-like scarring.

Skin Graft Techniques — **By Eponymic Title**

BLAIR-BROWN ....Split thickness graft of medium thickness.

BRAUN ....Thick skin graft.

BRAUN-WANGENSTEEN .Smaller implanted skin grafts obtained from a larger graft.

DOUGLAS ....A mesh-like graft.

DRAGSTEDT ....A corrugated type graft.

ESSER (Stent) ....A full thickness graft applied over a resin plastic (stent material) with which the graft is fitted into the recipient site.

GILLIES ....A rope-like graft.

KONIG ....A composite graft from the ear (skin and cartilage).

KRAUSE-WOLFE ....A full thickness graft.

OLLIER-THIERSCH ......A thin epidermal graft with some dermis present.

REVERDIN ....A pinch graft.

THIERSCH ....A very thin epidermal graft.

VAN MILLINGEN ....A lip graft.

WOLFE ....Full thickness graft.

SKIN FLAPS

Skin flap techniques are used when a thick graft with subcutaneous fat is desired. This method of tissue transfer has already been discussed in the opening of this chapter and therefore we will confine ourselves here to distinguishing between the various procedures through which this method is applied.

Types of Flaps

Bilobed ....A two lobed flap on a single pedicle.

Compound ....Addition of bone or cartilage to the flap before transfer.

Compound lined ....A flap with a lining and covering of epithelium between which bone or cartilage are inserted.

Delayed ....A flap raised from its bed except for a pedicle attachment. It is replaced to promote dependence on its pedicle and is transferred at a later operation.

304

Double pedicle ......A flap with two vascular attachments.

French (sliding) .....A flap with one pedicle which is advanced by sliding it over from an adjacent area.

Indian (rotation) ...A flap taken from a site near enough to the recipient site to permit transfer by simple turning or rotation.

Italian (distant) .....A distant donor site made possible by bringing the donor and recipient sites together. An arm may be brought to the forehead, etc.

Jump ....A chest or abdominal flap lined with a hinge flap turned down from the forearm.

Marsupial ....An abdominal flap is folded on itself to provide a lining and in stages is attached to the forearm and then the forearm freed from the abdomen.

Tumbler ....A hinge or folding flap.

In addition to skin, other tissues are used successfully in grafting including avascular animal tissues. Some of these tissues include the following:

Bone

The most common site from which bone grafts are taken is the ilium of the hip. This bone has a large surface area which consists of compact as well as cancellous elements. The ribs afford another source of bone graft material. Bone is preferred to cartilage by many surgeons because of its ability to replace lost bone in function as well as in structure.

Cartilage

Cartilage grafts are usually obtained from the septum, auricle of the ear and costal cartilages. Such grafts are used to fill in contour defects resulting from loss of bone. Some of the sites in which cartilage is used include the malar bone (cheek), nose and chin. It is interesting to note that autogenous cartilage need not be placed in contact with host cartilage in order to survive. In this respect cartilage differs from bone which becomes one with its host.

Cornea

Corneal grafts are classified as either penetrating (deep) or lamellar (superficial). The penetrating graft requires a fresh and transparent cornea which should have been enucleated not more than 5 hours after death and transplanted not more than 12 hours after enucleation. Eye donors are preferred in the age range between 12 and 45 years; however, occasionally an older donor with good eyes will be accepted. Preserved specimens can be used for lamellar grafts.

Fascia

Autogenous fascia lata and bovine fascia are being successfully used.

Hair Bearing

Grafts must be taken from hair bearing areas such as the scalp or eyebrows to replace tissue in hair bearing areas. New hope is being offered to men who regard their baldness as a cosmetic detriment.

Mucous Membrane

Mucous membrane may be taken from the lower lip, inner cheek, upper eyelid or vaginal mucosa to replace conjunctiva of the eye or vermilion border of the lip.

Nerve

Autogenous nerve grafts are the only ones which survive.

Tendon

Autogenous free tendon grafts are used successfully and grow with the recipient site.

TISSUE BANKS

The INTERNATIONAL EYE BANK (MEDICO, a service of CARE), a non-governmental, non-sectarian, non-profit organization, financed by contributions of citizens, has its headquarters and laboratory at the Washington Hospital Center in Washington, D.C. This agency receives eye donations from eye banks all over the U.S.A. and ships them, free of charge, to foreign countries all over the world, where eye banks do not exist.

A great need for eye donors exists. All persons associated with the field of medicine should be made aware of this need to recruit prospective donors. Eye donors are preferred in the age range between 12 and 45 years but an older donor may be considered. Where demise is anticipated within this age span, arrangements should be made through the nearest large city hospital eye department or the International Eye Bank for donation of the eyes. Preliminary registration of the donor is necessary in order that the next of kin be properly instructed in the procedure to be followed in assuring satisfactory specimens.

A TISSUE BANK is located in the U.S. Naval Hospital at Bethesda, Maryland, just outside Washington, D.C., from which tissues may be obtained free of charges other than those necessary for shipping. Tissues stored in the bank are obtained by sterile autopsy from donors who arranged for the removal of salvageable tissues prior to death.

The following surgical reports have been included in this chapter to further familiarize the secretary with the terminology of plastic surgery.

Split Thickness Skin Graft To Right Posterior Auricular Surface and Sulcus

With the patient in the supine position, under excellent general endotracheal anesthesia, the left leg and head were prepared and draped in the customary manner.

A split thickness skin graft of 10/1000 of an inch in thickness was taken from the left thigh with a Brown dermatome and preserved in saline moistened gauze.

The right auricle was then released from the scar tissue binding it down by sharp dissection. The dissection was continued along the posterior aspect of the auricle until the entire right ear lobe was freed to the sulcus. Hemostasis was well controlled with electrocautery.

An Esser inlay stent graft was then made by suturing the split thickness graft to the posterior aspect of the right auricle and to the posterior auricular skin. The graft was sutured in the sulcus with a continuous suture of 0000 chromic catgut. After a small saline moistened gauze stent was placed behind the ear, the auricle was sutured down to the skin with the skin graft using a continuous suture of 00000 monofilament nylon.

A moderate pressure dressing was applied. One piece of Adaptic was placed over the donor site and this was then covered with several saline moistened gauze flats. The wound was dressed with a 4 inch Kerlix bandage.

Excision of Scar and Old Graft
(Closure by means of interpolated nasolabial full flap)

The operative area was prepared with pHisoHex and water and draped in the usual manner. General anesthesia was used with oral endotracheal intubation.

Six months prior to admission, a full thickness postauricular graft was used to cover a defect on the left side of the nose. The resulting scar and deformity in the area caused some blockage of the airway. Patient re-admitted for a more definitive plastic repair.

The scar and old graft were removed from the left side of the nose leaving a defect approximately 1 inch in diameter. A flap was designed from the left nasolabial fold area superiorly in order to fit into the defect with better coverage and a more satisfactory cosmetic result. The flap was developed by means of sharp dissection. All bleeding points were clamped and tied with 00000 plain surgical catgut free ties. The skin edges of the nasolabial area were undermined and the subcuticular tissue approximated by means of interrupted 00000 white nylon sutures. Skin edges were approximated by interrupted 00000 blue nylon suture.

The flap was shaped to conform to the defect and was sutured in place by means of interrupted 00000 nylon sutures. Dry sterile dressing was applied.

Fascia Lata Graft (For residual Bell's Palsy of right face)

The upper left thigh was completely prepared with soap and water as was the entire face, following anesthesia. General anesthesia was supple-mented with 1% Xylocaine.

The first approach was to obtain fascia lata from the left thigh. This was done through a four inch incision over the greater trochanter. With our fascia stripper, we removed three long pieces of fascia about $\frac{1}{4}$ of an inch in width by about 8 inches in length. The wound on the hip was closed with 0000 plain and 00000 nylon. A drain was left in place. A pressure dressing was applied along the entire leg.

Attention was turned to the face. An attempt is being made here to support the entire right side of the face and the right lower eyelid. First, a piece of fascia lata was inserted which extended from the left side of the lower lid, beyond the midline to the angle of the mouth, and up to the Temporalis muscle. The second strip extended from the upper lid, beyond the midline, through the left side (the good side), up to the cor-ner of the mouth and to the temporalis region of the right side. The third strip of fascia extended from the left Frontalis muscle, which is good, down to the inner canthus along the lower eyelid margin and up to the Temporalis muscle. An incision made over the left Temporalis muscle was used to expose the fascia and the muscle. The three strips of fascia were then drawn up tightly to overcorrect the deformity. The fascia was sutured to the muscle with 0000 plain nylon.

The wound in the face was closed with 000000 nylon and in the scalp with 00000 nylon. All suturing of the fascia to the muscle on the face and Frontalis was done with 0000 nylon. A pressure dressing was applied to the face.

THE EXTERNAL EARS

The operation for plastic repair and reconstruction of the external ear is termed an otoplasty. A variety of techniques are used to correct deformities of the external ear which result from congenital errors in shape, size and position or traumatic deformities with loss of substance. Corrective surgery may range from alteration of the shape of the ear to complete reconstruction. By reconstruction of the external ear, it must not be construed that the surgeon can perfectly duplicate the intricate design of the external ear when total reconstruction is necessary.

Anatomic terms encountered in otoplasty reports, a listing of some of the more popular techniques and representative operative dictations follow to assist the secretary with this phase of terminology peculiar to plastic surgery.

ANATOMIC STRUCTURES OF THE EXTERNAL EAR

Antihelix
Antitragus
Auricle
Auricular tubercle of Darwin
Cauda helicis
Cavum conchae
Cephalo-auricular angle
Concha (pl. conchae)
Conchal fossa
Conchal mastoid angle
Crus of the helix
Cymba conchae
Eminentia conchae
Eminentia triangularis
External acoustic meatus
Fissure antitragohelicina

Fossa of the antihelix
Fossa triangularis
Helix
Incisura intertragica
Inferior crus of the antihelix
Intertragic notch
Lobule
Ponticulus
Retro-auricular sulcus
Scapha
Scaphoconchal angle
Scaphoid fossa
Sulcus antihelicis transversus
Superior crus
Tragus
Tympanic sulcus

SOME TECHNIQUES FOR OTOPLASTY

Adams
Alexander
Barsky
Becker
Binnie
Converse
Davis and Kitlowski
Demel and Ruttin
Dieffenbach
Eckstein-Kleinschmidt
Eitner

Erich
Fomon
Gavello
Gersuny
Holmes
Joseph
Kitlowski
Kolle-Lexer
Lexer
Luckett
Monks

SOME TECHNIQUES FOR OTOPLASTY (Continued)

Morestin
Nelaton
Ombredanne
Parkhill
Straith

Swenson
Szymanowski
Vogel
Young

Otoplasty, Bilateral

The patient presented bilateral protrusion of the ears with absence of the posterior crus of the antihelix and a poorly formed antihelix on each side.

Under adequate preoperative sedation, the operative area was prepared with pHisoHex and draped. The ear was blocked by means of 1% Xylocaine which was infiltrated anteriorly and posteriorly to the ear.

An elliptical piece of skin was excised from the posterior aspect of the ear following the curve of the antihelix. This ellipse extended the full length of the ear and was approximately 6 mm. in width. By means of Keith needles, which were inserted from the anterior to the posterior aspect of the ear, the new posterior crus of the antihelix and the new antihelix itself were marked.

An incision was made through the cartilage to form the new posterior crus and antihelix. The excess cartilage was trimmed, as needed, in order to restore the ear to its correct position. The cartilage was approximated by means of a continuous suture of 00000 multiple filament white nylon. The skin was then closed by means of a subcuticular suture of 0000 monofilament nylon with interrupted sutures of this material where necessary.

The same procedure was carried out on the other side. A modified compression dressing consisting of a moist 4 x 4 Kerlix and 2 inch roller bandage was applied.

THE EYELIDS

Plastic repair of defects of the eyelid is termed a *blepharoplasty*. There are many variations of the blepharoplasty, performed for a wide variety of anomalies, ranging from congenital defects to traumatic deformities. Ptosis of the eyelid (blepharoptosis) is one of the most prevalent defects. The popular techniques for correcting this condition have been listed separately in this section.

ANATOMIC FEATURES OF THE EYELID

Aponeurosis
Canthus
Caruncula
Ciliary margins
Conjunctiva
Fibers of Orbicularis oculi
Fornix
Inferior tarsus
Lacrimal ducts
Lacrimal sac
Lacus lacrimalis
Lamina
Lateral canthus
Levator palpebrae superioris
Medial palpebral ligament
Meibomian glands
Mueller's muscle
Nasojugal

Nasolacrimal duct
Orbital margins
Orbital septum
Palpebral fissure
Palpebral furrow
Palpebral raphe
Palpebrarum
Plica semilunaris
Posterior lamina
Riolan's muscle
Superior fornix
Superior tarsus
Tarsal glands
Tarsal muscles
Tarsal plate
Tarsus (pl. tarsi)
Tarsus orbital septum
Tunica conjunctiva

TECHNIQUES FOR EYELID REPAIR

Alsus-Knapp
Arlt
Beard-Cutler
Blair
Blaskovics
Burow
Cutler
Derby
Duke-Elder
Dupuy-Dutemps
Essers
Everbusch
Fox
Fricke's
Gaillard
Gifford
Hess
Hotz
Hughes
Jaesche
Jones
Krönlein
Kuhnt-Szymanowski
Lagleyze
Langenbeck

Lexer
Malbec
Minsky
Motais
Mueller
Panas
Reese
Sayoc's
Smith
Snellen
Spaeth
Stallard
Straith
Szymanowski
Tripier
Truc
Van Millingen
Verhoeff
Verweys
von Blaskovics-Doyen
Wheeler
Wicherkiewicz
Wiener
Wies lid fracturing

PTOSIS CORRECTION TECHNIQUES

Allport
Alvis
Angelucci
Berke
Berke-Motais
Blair
Blaskovics
Crawford
Elschnig
Fergus
Friedenwald-Guyton
Gayet
Gifford
Grimsdale
Guyton
Harman
Iliff
Johnson
Lancaster
Leahey
Lexer

Machek
Magnus
Malbran
Motais
Mules
Pagenstecher
Panus
Reese
Rosenburg
Savin
Schimek
Snellen
Sourdille
Spaeth
Tansley
Trainor-Nida
Wiener
Wolff
Worth
Wright
Young

ANESTHETICS USED IN LID SURGERY

Carbocaine
Cocaine hydrochloride
Hyaluronidase (adjunct drug)
Lidocaine
Mepivacaine 2%

O'Brien Akinesia
Pontocaine
Procaine with epinephrine
Tetracaine
Van Lint Akinesia

DRESSINGS

Cikloid
Collodion
Fluffed gauze
Pressure

Telfa
Telfa plastic film
Tie-over
Wet

Blepharoplasty, Upper and Lower

The excess skin of the upper eyelid was picked up at the inner and outer portion of the lid by means of thumb forceps. This produced a bridge of tissue which was clamped with a Hunt clamp. A few drops of 1% Xylocaine with ½ cc. of adrenalin to the ounce was infiltrated into the lid for anesthesia.

By means of a #11 Bard-Parker blade the upper lid tissue, which was held in a Hunt clamp, was incised. The clamp was then removed and at the inner and outer angle of the lid the skin was further trimmed so that the whole excision was moderately fusiform in shape. After it had been determined that sufficient excess skin had been excised, the skin of the lid was reapproximated by means of a subcuticular suture of 00000 dermalon.

Bleeding throughout the procedure was controlled by means of cautery. The same procedure was repeated on the opposite eye.

Terramycin Ophthalmic Ointment was placed in the eye and a modified pressure dressing applied.

The skin of the lower lid was then infiltrated with 1% Xylocaine containing adrenalin as was the lateral canthal region. A curvilinear line was carefully made along the lower lid approximately 3 cm. inferior to the tarsal plate edge. Undercutting was then carried out of the entire lower flap of skin from this incision. The lateral end of this incision was then extended in an oblique angle parallel to a line of crowfeeting. This skin was completely raised from the underlying muscle. The fat pads were then easily isolated through the Orbicularis oculi muscle fibers. The assistant applied moderate pressure to the eyeball so that this fat would herniate. The excess was carefully estimated and removed. Several 00000 white nylon stitches were used to reapproximate the muscle fibers.

A lower skin flap was then carefully smoothed in position so that no wrinkles remained in the lower lid. An excess could then be determined where it overlapped the upper skin edge. This was carefully removed.

Closure was accomplished by one subcuticular stitch of white nylon through both edges of the incision at the outer canthus of the eye angle. A 00000 dermalon subcuticular stitch completed both closures. A similar procedure was performed on the opposite eye.

A moderate pressure bandage was then built up over both eyes.

THE LIPS

An operation designed to correct a deformity of the lip (s) is called a *cheiloplasty*. A number of various type operations are performed to correct defects and deformities of the lip.

Some of the more frequently seen lip deformities are listed here with a listing of the more commonly used methods of cheiloplasty. Anatomic structures involved in cheiloplasty procedures are also given to assist the secretary with transcriptions.

Deformities of the Lip

CLEFT LIP   — A congenital fissure of the lip; also called a harelip.
DOUBLE LIP   — Hypertrophy (enlargement), usually of the upper lip with a longitudinal groove running parallel with the lip giving the appearance of a double lip.
ECTROPION   — Turning out of the lip.
ENTROPION   — Inward curling of the lip.
FLAT LIP   — Flatness of the upper lip.
MACROCHEILIA — Abnormal enlargement of the lip.
MACROSTOMIA — An abnormally large mouth.
MICROSTOMIA — Abnormally short lips and small mouth.

ANATOMIC STRUCTURES OF THE LIP

Areolar tissue
Buccal mucosa
Frenulum
Frenum labiorum
Gingivolabial sulci
Labial

Mucocutaneous border
Orbicularis oris muscle
Philtrum
Sphincter oris
Vermilion border

ARTERIES SUPPLYING THE LIP

Lower lip:
  inferior labial
  mental
  submental

Upper lip:
  infra-orbital
  superior labial (coronary)

CHEILOPLASTY TECHNIQUES

Abbe I & II stage
Bell
Brauer
Brown-Blair
Cronin
Esmarch
Gillies
Giralde
Hagedorn
Hagedorn-LeMesurier
Hagerty
Joseph
Kowalzig
LeMesurier
Lexer
Marcks
McCash-Randall

McDowell
Millard
Mirault
Mirault-Brown-Blair
Owens
Pierce-O'Connor
Randall
Rose
Simon
Teale
Tennison
Thompson
Veau
von Langenbeck
Webster
Wolfe

Tennison Harelip Repair

1% Xylocaine with adrenalin was infiltrated about the mouth, in the upper lip and base of the nose region.

The edges of the cleft were freshened by removing the mucous membrane and excess skin at the lower end of the incision on the medial cleft. A ⅛ inch incision was made into the lip from the mucous membrane border. This allowed the cupid's bow to rotate downward leaving a triangular defect with the apex in the center of the lip. The opposite mucous membrane was pared and trimmed. A small flap with its base laterally and inferiorly was rotated into the triangular defect.

Three sutures were inserted using a 0000 nylon figure-of-eight and were tied in the mucous membrane. The excess mucous membrane was then excised and approximated with 000000 silk. A subcuticular 00000 nylon suture was used to approximate the skin edges. Interrupted nylon sutures were used to close the floor of the nostril and reshape the nostril and ala.

A Logan Bow was applied. A wet Streptomycin dressing was placed over the skin edge.

THE NOSE AND PARANASAL SINUSES

Some of the more commonly used anatomic terms encountered in operative dictations describing procedures performed on the nose and accessory sinuses are listed here to assist the secretary with her transcription.

ANATOMIC STRUCTURES
Nose and Paranasal Sinuses

Ala (pl. alae)
Alanasi
Alar cartilages
Aponeurosis
Atrium
Bridge
Bulla ethmoidalis
Cartilaginous septum
Cartilaginous vault
Choana (pl. choanae)
Clinoid process
Columella
Columna

Concha (pl. conchae)-(turbinates)
Cribriform plate of ethmoid
Crista galli
Crura
Crus laterale
Crus mediale
Dorsum nasi
Ethmoidal air cells
Frontal processes of maxillae
Greater alar cartilage
Hamular process
Hiatus semilunaris
Hypophyseal fossa

ANATOMIC STRUCTURES—Nose and Paranasal Sinuses (Cont.)

Inferior meatus
Infundibulum
Kiesselbach's plexus
Lateral crus
Lateral wall
Lesser alar cartilage
Medial crus
Middle meatus
Mucoperichondrium
Mucous membrane
Nares
Nasal bones
Nasal conchae
Nasal crest
Nasal spine
Nasion
Nasolabial junction
Nasopalatine recess
Nostrils

Ostium maxillare
Palatine bone
Perpendicular plate of ethmoid
Piriform opening
Plica nasi
Rostrum of sphenoid
Septum
Septum mobile nasi
Sesamoid cartilages
Sinus groove
Sphenoethmoidal recess
Sphenoidal process
Superior meatus
Turbinates
Uncinate process
Vestibule
Vomer
Vomeronasal cartilage
Vomeronasal organ of Jacobson

PARANASAL SINUSES

Ethmoidal
Frontal

Maxillary
Sphenoidal

ARTERIES OF THE NOSE

Alar branches of ext. maxillary
Alveolar br. of int. maxillary
Anterior ethmoidal br. of ophthalmic
Dorsal nasal br. of ophthalmic
Infraorbital br. of int. maxillary

Pharyngeal br. of int. maxillary
Posterior ethmoidal br. of ophthalmic
Septal br. of ext. maxillary
Septal br. of superior labial
Sphenopalatine br. of int. maxillary

NERVES OF THE NOSE

Ant. alveolar br. of maxillary
Anterior ethmoidal
Anterior palatine
External nasal
Facial
Infraorbital of maxillary
Infratrochlear branch of ophthalmic

Nasal branches of sphenopalatine
    ganglion
Nasociliary branches of ophthalmic
Nasopalatine
Nerve of pterygoid canal
Olfactory

Rhinoplasty and Submucous Resection

Under adequate preoperative sedation, the face was prepared and draped in the usual manner. Under local infiltration and bilateral infraorbital block anesthesia, the usual intercartilaginous incision was made bilaterally and the skin of the nose was elevated by sharp dissection. After the intended nasal bridge had been measured with a profilometer, the saw was inserted through the incision and the nasal bone sawed through according to the measurements. This was repeated on the opposite side. The knife was inserted through the saw cut and the septum was cut through and separated from above, downward at the same level as the bone cut. The bony hump was removed. Irregularities were removed with a rasp.

The upper lateral cartilages on both sides were then cut free from the septum from below, upward and were lowered. The upper lateral cartilages were then shortened bilaterally.

By use of the scalpel, the septum was shortened by excising a wedge of septum and mucous membrane from the lower end of the septum, the base of the wedge being upward.

The lower lateral cartilages were then trimmed and a small amount of cartilage removed from the superior edge of each. A 1/32 of an inch saw was inserted into the intercartilaginous incision and a vertical saw cut was made on each side of the septum.

Bilateral osteotomies of the nasal processes over the maxillary bones were done extending from the lower limits of the maxillary bone to the region of the medial canthus of the eye. The bones were infractured.

The mucous membrane of the nose was anesthetized as required. A curved vertical incision was made through the mucous membrane and 1 cm. from the anterior end of the septum the cartilage was cut through to the opposite side. The mucoperichondrium on each side was elevated by means of a sharp and blunt dissector. The cartilage of the septum was then cut through with scissors leaving a 1 cm. dorsal strut to support the nasal bridge. Intervening cartilage was removed with a rongeur. The mucoperichondrial flap was then approximated with interrupted sutures of 0000 chromic.

* * * * * *

The following procedure is sometimes performed in conjunction with a rhinoplasty.

Bilateral Weir

The ala on each side was cut free from its attachment to the face. A piece of wedge-shaped tissue approximately 3/16th of an inch in width was excised. The base of the ala of the nose on each side was resutured by means of two figure-of-eight sutures using 00000 dermalon. The dog-ears of the upper extremity of the incisions were excised. The skin was approximated with a subcuticular suture using 00000 dermalon. Occasional twists were put in for more accurate approximation of the edges.

THE PALATE

The roof of the mouth consists of a structure called the palate. The anterior portion of this covering is designated as the *hard palate* in contradistinction to the posterior portion which is called the *soft palate*. Both the hard and soft palates sometimes exhibit a congenital defect referred to as a *cleft palate,* where proper fusion of the palate has failed to occur. This deformity is sometimes associated with a cleft lip or a cleft velum. Investigators believe that heredity is an important factor concluding that cleft palate alone may be attributed to a simple dominant gene with sex limitation to the female.

Repair of defects of the palate is termed a *palatoplasty* and may include pharyngeal flaps and pharyngoplasty. The techniques for repair which have received popular acceptance are listed here with anatomic terms used in reporting surgery of the palate and pharynx.

ANATOMIC FEATURES OF THE PALATE AND PHARNYX

Alveolar arches
Alveolar ridge
Alveolus
Aponeurosis of the velum
Foramina of Scarpa
Fossa(e) of Rosenmüller
Greater palatine foramen
Gums
Hamulus
Hard palate
Incisive canal
Incisive foramen
Incisive papilla
Isthmus faucium
Lesser palatine foramina
Linear raphe
Major palatine artery
Maxilla (pl. maxillae)
Maxillary tubercles
Medial pterygoid plate
Median raphe
Mucoperiosteum
Muscles of the palate
  Glossopalatinius
  Levator veli palatini
  Musculus uvulae
  Pharyngopalatinus
  Tensor veli palatini

Nasopharyngeal area
Neurovascular bundle
Oral mucosa
Palatal shelves
Palates, primary and secondary
Palatine aponeurosis
Palatine arches
Palatine bones
Palatine process
Palatine tonsil
Palatine uvula
Palatine velum
Palatum durum
Palatum mole
Passavant's cushion
Periosteum
Pharyngeal aperture
Pharyngeal bursa
Pharyngeal hemisphincter
Pharyngeal ostium
Pharyngeal recess
  (fossae of Rosenmüller)
Pharyngeal tonsil
Pillars of fauces
Posterior pharynx
Pterygoid plate
Pterygomandibular raphe
Pterygopalatine canal

ANATOMIC FEATURES OF THE PALATE AND PHARYNX (Cont.)

Salpingopalatine fold
Salpingopharyngeal fold
Salpingopharyngeus muscle
Soft palate (velum)
Sphenopalatine artery
Sphenopalatine nerve

Superior constrictor muscle
Torus (cushion)
Transverse mucosal rugae
Uvula
Velopharynx
Velum

CLEFT PALATE INSTRUMENTS

Also: See Chapter 5

Austin dental knife
Barsky double-end elevator
Brophy bistoury
Dott mouth gag
Freer elevator

Kilner suture carrier
Latrobe soft palate retractor
MacKenty cleft palate knife
McIndoe hawk's-beak elevator
Reverdin needles
Sluder palate retractor
Veau elevator

PALATE REPAIR TECHNIQUES

Barsky pharyngoplasty
Brown's push-back
Dieffenbach-Warren
Dorrance push-back
Gillies-Fry
Palatoplasty
Pharyngeal flap

Staphylorrhaphy
Uranoplasty
V-Y operation
Veau
von Langenbeck
W-Y retroposition
Wardill-Kilner four flap

Modified von Langenbeck Repair of Cleft Palate

The patient presented a Veau Type II cleft of the palate which included all of the soft palate and approximately ¾ths of the hard palate. The palate was separated approximately 1 cm. at its widest part.

Under nasal endotracheal anesthesia, the skin of the face was prepared and draped. A Dott mouth gag was inserted after the mouth and throat had been packed with gauze which contained 5% cocaine and adrenalin. This pack was allowed to remain in place for 15 minutes. 1% Xylocaine with ¼ cc. of adrenalin to the ounce was injected along the edges of the defect in the soft and hard palate and around the point of exit of the anterior palatine artery. By means of a Veau elevator, the mucoperiosteum was elevated from each side and the front of the underlying palatine bone. The palatine aponeurosis was cut by means of scissors and the soft palate elevated. The edges of the mucoperiosteum of the hard palate, soft palate and uvula were trimmed on each side by means of a #11 Bard-Parker blade.

An incision was made through the mucous membrane of the posterior tonsillar pillar approximately ⅛ of an inch from the anterior surface of the pillar. This mucous membrane was then split for a distance of approximately ¼ inch. At this time Brophy plates were inserted on each side of the soft palate just anterior to the uvula and were held in place by means of silver wires. The plates were not tied down tightly at this time.

The mucoperiosteum was approximated by means of interrupted vertical mattress sutures of 0000 black silk. The soft palate was approximated in the same manner. The anterior and posterior surfaces of the uvula were approximated by means of plain interrupted sutures of 0000 black silk. The posterior tonsillar pillars were approximated for a distance of about 2½ cm. by means of interrupted vertical mattress sutures of 0000 black silk. At this time the Brophy plates were set into position and held there by means of hemostats and the wires tightened. Care was taken not to wire the plates down too tightly. The excess wire was cut off and the ends bent in order that they not stick into the tongue.

Wardill Repair of Cleft Palate

Adequate anesthesia was obtained with oral endotracheal intubation. The patient was prepared with pHisoHex and water to the skin and Aqueous Zephiran intraorally. The patient was then surgically draped and a nasopharyngeal pack applied to catch any bloody drainage. Some local infiltration with 2% Xylocaine with epinephrine was performed along the course of incision of the palate.

The mucoperiosteal flap was raised on the right side after the method of Wardill. The dissection was carried down to the greater palatine neurovascular bundle. Care was taken not to disturb the neurovascular bundle in this area. The posterior lip of the pterygoid canal in this area was removed by means of an osteotome. The hamular process was fractured. This mobilized the right side of the flap sufficiently so it could be brought across the midline. The same procedure was carried out on the left side of the palate.

The edges of the cleft were freshened by means of a # 11 Bard-Parker blade, removing a portion of the edge down to normal tissue. After this had been performed, the nasal septum which was evident was split down its center. Repair of the nasal portion of the mucous membrane was carried out to the mucosa of the nasal septum by means of interrupted 0000 chromic catgut sutures. This also required repair of the soft palate by means of interrupted 0000 chromic catgut suture down to the uvula. The oral surface of the mucosa of the soft palate was repaired by means of interrupted 000 chromic catgut vertical mattress sutures.

A push-back procedure was performed by repairing the edge of the Y closure with interrupted 000 chromic catguts with the Y-suture being used to tack the upper portion of the flap down to the nasal septum in that area.

RESTORATION BY FOREIGN MATERIALS

Over the years a variety of synthetic materials have been tried in different body sites to fill defects and restore a more normal contour to the area. These have included the use of paraffin, rubber, plastics, polyvinyl sponges and others which, for numerous reasons, were eventually discarded. A new material called silastic is being used currently in the form of implants and liquid with satisfactory results. The following two operative reports illustrate two examples of popular application.

Silastic Injection into Area of Malar Bone Deficiency

The patient presented a Treacher-Collins Syndrome. Attention was focused this time on the deficiency of the malar bones.

An incision was made at the supra-auricular hairline and through this incision the dissection was deepened, separating the fibers of the temporal muscle. The temporal bone was then exposed.

Using periosteal elevators, the zygomatic arch was followed. The malar bone was freed from its underlying soft tissues which were elevated. Into this pocket a liquid silastic with a catalyst was injected. The material gradually filled up the deficiency of bone to the lower rim of the orbit and to the malar bone.

Closure of the wound was accomplished using a white nylon interrupted suture to reapproximate the temporal muscle fibers. Three interrupted white nylon sutures were placed subcuticularly. A running 00000 dermalon suture was placed intracuticularly. Interrupted sutures for the skin were placed as needed.

Eye patches and a moderately compressive pressure dressing were applied to the operative area.

Augmentation Mammoplasty, Bilateral

The patient presented small, shrunken, atrophic breasts, the left slightly larger than the right.

After adequate sedation with the patient under general endotracheal anesthesia, the anterior chest was prepared and draped in the usual manner. A very long strand of 000 Zytor suture was stitched to the skin at the midportion of the suprasternal notch. This was used for measuring the breast position of both nipples. A slightly curved incision was marked in the line of the submammary sulcus. An incision was made through the dermis and subcutaneous tissue and deepened to the fascia of the Serratus anterior. It was carried upwards until the border of the Pectoralis major was encountered. The deep muscle fascia was opened and lifted forward along with the breast and skin. Care was taken not to expose breast tissue. Final dissection was completed by inserting two index fingers and working them against one another in order to bluntly enlarge the pocket.

Careful hemostasis was obtained by packing the pocket with several 4 x 4 sponges and by use of electrocoagulation.

The larger size silastic implant was inserted into the pocket on the right with a twisting motion and carefully placed to lie against the Pectoralis major muscle. An antibiotic solution was applied over this implant.

The wound was closed in layers using 00000 white nylon stitches to approximate the implant to the fascial layers. The skin was approximated with interrupted 00000 white nylon subcutaneously and running 00000 Ethicons for subcuticulars. Antibiotic solution containing Bacitracin was injected into the pocket containing the implant. Careful pressure dressing was applied to the breast by using Kerlix and Ace bandages.

The operation was repeated on the opposite breast.

OPERATIONS ON THE FACIAL SKIN

In addition to reconstructive and repair operations performed on the face, a number of other procedures are employed for the purpose of improving the cosmetic image. Such operations include dermabrasion of acne scarred complexions, tattoo of discolored areas of the skin, rhytidectomy for the removal of wrinkles, revision of scars, etc.

Operative reports to illustrate several of these procedures appear below.

Total Facial Dermabrasion

The patient presented severe pitting and scarring of the cheeks and chin with a few superficial pits on the forehead. There was a very large amount of inspissated sebaceous material present throughout the entire face. Pressure was used to remove as much of this material as possible from the pores.

Under general nasal endotracheal anesthesia, the skin of the face was cleansed with pHisoHex and draped.

By means of an Iverson dermabrader, the entire face was sanded deeply. Bleeding was controlled by means of wet sponges containing saline and adrenalin. After completion of the sanding, the face was covered with fine mesh gauze soaked in saline and adrenalin. This was covered with moist 4 x 4's and a 2 inch roller bandage.

Face Lift

The skin of the face and scalp were prepared with pHisoHex and Aqueous Zephiran.

The frontal scalp, on the right, was locally infiltrated with $\frac{1}{2}\%$ Xylocaine containing 8 drops of adrenalin to the ounce. This subcutaneous infiltration was carried down in front of the ear and behind the ear, throughout the upper neck region, and across the entire anterior portion of the face and forehead. A one inch swath of hair had previously been shaved across the frontoparietal area extending from approximately one inch lateral to the midline down to the supra-auricular area.

An incision was carried along the posterior margin of this shaved area down to the supra-auricular area and then carried preauricularly down the cheek to the inferior pole of the attachment to the ear. The incision was then carried posteriorly just within this hairline to a position approximately $3\frac{1}{2}$ inches behind the ear. The forehead and the entire right cheek were elevated by means of sharp and blunt dissection, care being taken to remain in as superficial a plane as possible to guard against injury to the branches of the 7th nerve. Subcutaneous elevation was similarly carried out inferiorly throughout the upper two-thirds of the cervical region on the right side.

The skin of the forehead and face were then drawn up to a position of new snugness and contour, where it was secured by means of two 00 monofilament dermalon sutures placed in a pulley mattress fashion in a position just above the ear.

Closure was performed throughout the hair bearing areas with interrupted 0000 black silk braided sutures placed in central and vertical mattress fashion after removal of a small dog-ear triangle at the superiormost position of the scalp excision defect. In the preauricular region and in the retroauricular region the closure was carried out with buried white nylon and subcuticular 0000 dermalon with twists as needed.

The exact procedure was carried out on the left side. Following completion of the operation, a large pressure dressing was applied to the entire scalp, face and neck, leaving only the mouth exposed.

Hemostasis was obtained by means of clamping and white nylon ties. Blood loss was considered minimal for this type of operation.

REPAIR OF HYPOSPADIAS

A congenital abnormality sometimes occurs in the male in which the urethra opens on the underside of the penis or on the perineum. Such an anomalous opening is called a *hypospadias*. The counterpart of this condition in the female consists of an anomalous opening of the urethra into the vagina.

Hypospadias in the male is often associated with a condition known as *chordee* in which there is a downward bowing of the penis. A hooded prepuce often is seen with hypospadias

The techniques proposed for the repair of this condition are legion. Only some of the more frequently used methods are listed here.

REPAIR TECHNIQUES FOR HYPOSPADIAS

Blair-Byars
Broadbent
Cecil
Cloutier
Culp
Davis
Denis Browne
DesPrez
Devine
Dieffenbach-Duplay
Duplay I and II
Farmer
Havens

Heineke-Mikulicz
Humby
Marion-Perard
Marshall-Spellman
McCormack
McIndoe
Memmelaar
Nesbit
Nove-Josserand
Ombredanne
Thiersch-Byars
Wehrbein
Young-Benjamin

Second Stage Cecil Procedure for Hypospadias

The patient already has had an operation for correction of chordee and a first stage Cecil procedure for correction of the hypospadias.

Under general anesthesia the scrotum and lower abdomen as well as the upper thighs were cleansed with pHisoderm and then draped.

A traction suture of 5 monofilament nylon was placed through the glans penis. A # 12 French catheter was inserted into the bladder. By means of a # 15 Bard-Parker blade an incision was made releasing the penis from the scrotum. Care was taken to leave sufficient tissue so that the reconstructed urethra would not be entered. After the penis was released, there were two raw areas, one on the posterior aspect of the penis and another on the anterior surface of the scrotum. Bleeding was controlled by means of cautery.

The skin was reapproximated with a subcuticular suture of 0000 chromic catgut with twists of the same material where necessary.

A small incision was made into the glans penis. Bleeding was controlled by means of cautery. An attempt was made to transplant the meatus into the glans penis. The meatus was sutured into position in the glans with interrupted sutures of 0000 chromic catgut. The incisional line was covered with Achromycin gauze and a modified compression dressing consisting of fluffs and Elastoplast was applied. The French catheter was left in the bladder.

14 〉 *Thoracic Surgery*

CHEST

The specialty of thoracic surgery is concerned with diseases of the thorax involving the tracheobronchial tree, lungs, and mediastinum. Expert roentgenography, physical examination and bronchoscopy are the principal diagnostic procedures in this specialty.

Radiologic examinations of particular value in thoracic disease include fluoroscopy, roentgenography, bronchography, tomography, magnification, angiography, cineradiography, roentgenkymography, photofluorography and radioactive isotopes.

Laboratory examinations constitute an important adjunct to the diagnostic work-up when these findings are correlated with the clinical evaluation. Pulmonary secretions are obtained by sputum collection, tracheal, bronchoscopic and gastric lavage and by laryngeal swabs. These specimens are examined for acid-fast bacilli and malignant cells. Gram stains are performed on the sputum along with cultures, guinea pig inoculations and microscopic examinations. Serologic tests, important in confirming thoracic diseases, include the Youman's-Parlett serologic test for tuberculosis, tests for coccidioidomycosis, syphilis and viral diseases. The aspiration of secretions and lavage of the bronchi for the purpose of obtaining specimens is most effectively accomplished by bronchoscopy. Malignant cells can often be detected in specimens obtained bronchoscopically when such cells are not observed in expectorated sputum studies.

Scalene lymph node biopsy also represents another valuable diagnostic aid. Diseases of the mediastinum and lungs that can be transmitted by way of the lymph channels tend to involve the lymph nodes of the supraclavicular fossa from which the scalene node biopsy is taken. This procedure is of value in discovering sarcoidosis, diffuse pulmonary disease and undifferentiated types of bronchogenic carcinoma.

Bronchoscopy is one of the most important and frequently employed diagnostic procedures performed by the thoracic surgeon. Endoscopic examination of the bronchus may also be performed by trained internists and surgeons, but is usually referred to a thoracic surgeon because of his special understanding and experience with thoracic diseases.

Bronchoscopic examination enables the physician to examine the entire tracheobronchial tree, from the larynx to the orifices of the segmental bronchi. Most of the observed lesions are accessible for biopsy with the possible exception of those situated distal to the orifice of the upper lobe bronchi. Angled-vision lens systems are used to visualize these more remotely situated areas. The right-angle telescope is particularly useful in examining the upper lobe segmental orifices.

The secretary should be acquainted with the nomenclature for the tracheobronchial tree and the standard numbering system used to designate the segmental bronchi. There is a growing preference among radiologists and thoracic surgeons to refer to the segmental bronchi by number rather than by name.

RIGHT BRONCHIAL TREE	LEFT BRONCHIAL TREE
Right Upper Lobe Bronchus	**Left Upper Lobe Bronchus**
Apical	Apical posterior 1, 2
Posterior	Anterior 3
Anterior	Superior lingular 4
Middle Lobe Bronchus	Inferior lingular 5
Lateral	
Medial	(no middle lobe on the left)
Right Lower Lobe Bronchus	**Left Lower Lobe Bronchus**
Superior (apical)	Superior (apical) 6
Medial basal	Anteromedial basal 7, 8
Anterior basal	Lateral basal 9
Lateral basal	Posterior basal 10
Posterior basal	

The American terminology for the segmental bronchi is identical to that of the British except that they refer to the superior segments of the lower lobes as apical segments.

BRONCHOSCOPIC EXAMINATIONS

Bronchoscopy is an endoscopic examination in which a scope (bronchoscope) is introduced beyond the larynx and into the bronchus for the purpose of examination, biopsy and/or aspiration of secretions for cell study.

BRONCHOSCOPES

Broyles telescopes
Bruening
Chevalier Jackson
Davis
Double channel irrigating
Emerson
Foregger
Haslinger
Holinger
Holinger-Jackson
Hook-on
Jackson full lumen

Jackson standard
Jesberg
Kernan-Jackson coagulating
Michelson infant
Moersch
Negus
Pilling
Safar ventilation
Staple
Tucker
Yankauer

Bronchoscopy

The pharynx, larynx and trachea were anesthetized with 5% cocaine. The larynx was inspected first by means of a laryngeal mirror. The cords were found to move normally and the intrinsic larynx appeared entirely normal. Direct inspection of the larynx was also made with a laryngoscope. The arytenoids were normal except for moderate hyperemia. The ventricular bands were entirely normal in appearance. The cords were normal and appeared to approximate well on phonation. There was no evidence of disease in the intrinsic larynx. The laryngoscope was removed.

A 7 x 40 Chevalier Jackson bronchoscope was passed through a normal appearing larynx and trachea. The carina was sharp and freely movable in the midline. There was no evidence of subcarinal lymphadenopathy. There was normal flexibility of the bronchial tree. The mucosa of the trachea appeared essentially normal throughout, having been inspected from the carina to immediately under the glottis.

The bronchial trees were examined to their secondary divisions. The right upper lobe (RUL) bronchial orifice was normally patent as was the orifice of the middle lobe and of the right lower lobe on this side. There was no evidence of endobronchial tumor. The left stem bronchus was also examined. There was mild hyperemia. The upper lobe bronchial orifice and the orifices of the lower lobe and its divisions were visualized and found to be normal.

Secretions were collected for cell block and histologic examination. Cytologic studies were ordered.

Conclusion: This is an essentially normal tracheal tree and entirely normal intrinsic larynx. There is no evidence of endotracheal or endobronchial tumor. There is no evidence of laryngeal tumor. No evidence was found of any extrinsic pressure encroaching upon the trachea.

Left Thoracotomy — Mediastinal Tumor Excision

The patient was placed in the lateral position with the left side uppermost. A curved periscapular incision was made and deepened. The periosteum overlying the fifth rib was incised and stripped away and a long segment of the fifth rib was removed. The pleural cavity was then entered.

There were no adhesions except at the left upper lobe where it was adherent to the chest wall. As this was dissected free, a degenerated tissue gushed forth. Specimens of this tissue were sent to the laboratory for frozen section. It was the feeling that this might possibly represent a fibrin ball which had been encapsulated between the lung and the chest wall. After all of this tissue had been evacuated and a rather granulomatous lining had been dissected free from the posterior aspect of the left upper lobe and chest wall, there was no evidence of any residual tissue which appeared abnormal.

The pathologist reported that the lesion was quite cellular and could possibly be a lymphoma, but more likely, was a neurofibroma or neurolemoma. He felt that no further distinction could be made until the permanent sections were obtained.

If this were truly a malignant tumor, it would require a left upper lobectomy and excision of a portion of the chest wall. Since it was believed that this was actually a benign process, the operation was discontinued. Hemostasis was obtained.

An intercostal tube was placed posteriorly just above the diaphragm and connected to a water-seal drainage bottle.

The intercostal muscles, extracostal bundles, subcutaneous tissues and skin were closed with interrupted silk. Dry sterile dressings were applied.

Left Lower Lobectomy of the Lung

After satisfactory positioning of the patient in the right lateral position with the arm extended anteriorly and upward, the patient is sterilely prepared and draped. Artificial scoliosis is created by placing a sandbag under the right chest for support. Just prior to draping, the course of the 7th rib is marked.

A skin incision, extending from the spine to the cartilage, is made along the upper edge of the 7th rib. The incision is deepened through the musculature. The fascia of the sacrospinalis muscle is likewise incised. The 7th rib is removed from the cartilage to the costal angle. The pleura is opened and adhesions between the visceral pleura and the parietal pleura are separated by blunt and sharp dissection. A rib spreader is inserted and the thoracotomy wound is gently widened. Hemostasis is accomplished with the use of silver clips.

The interlobar fissures are opened in their entirety. The phrenic nerve is crushed. The hilar vessels are exposed as is the bronchus. The visceral pleura is then incised for about 5 cm. The three branches of the great artery supplying the basal segment are ligated with No. 1 silk after the placing of clamps. The inferior pulmonary vein is then ligated after having been identified by transillumination. The lower lobe is retracted anteriorly. A single ligature is placed around the main trunk of the vein and a second suture around each of the three branches. The vessel is cut between clamps. Shenstone's tourniquet is used to temporarily clamp off the bronchus and the bronchial artery. Two centimeters distal to this, heavy clamps are applied. A small piece of lung tissue is left with which to cover the bronchial suture. The lumen of the bronchial artery is clamped and cut. The bronchus is closed with 000 chromic catgut mattress sutures and the suture line covered with the pedicle of lung tissue. The 7th intercostal nerve is then resected.

100,000 units of penicillin in 20 cc. of saline is introduced into the pleural cavity. A drain is placed through a separate stab wound in the 9th intercostal space in the posterior axillary line. The lung is inflated and the thoracotomy wound closed with approximation of the ribs adjacent to the incision by pericostal sutures. The intercostal drain is clamped and the wound closed in anatomic layers. The tube is then connected to underwater drainage and the clamp released.

Pneumonectomy, Right

After the patient had been sterilely prepared and draped in the supine position, an incision was made anteriorly in the third interspace. A self-retaining retractor was introduced to spread the 3rd and 4th ribs apart. The mediastinal pleura was incised. The right pulmonary artery and the right superior pulmonary vein were exposed. The azygos vein was identified at the level of the bifurcation of the trachea. Just below the azygos vein, the right primary bronchus was noted.

The right azygos vein was doubly ligated and then sectioned. The mediastinal pleura was then incised at its transition into the visceral pleura and it was reflected medially. Retraction of the vena cava was then carried out. Careful dissection of the areolar tissues overlying the hilar structures was accomplished and using fine curved dissectors the artery was freed. Two silk threads were placed around the artery but not tied yet.

The superior pulmonary vein was isolated and cut between ligatures, utilizing two proximal ligatures and one at the distal end of each branch. The caudal branches of the artery were then identified and ligated. Better exposure was obtained of the pulmonary vein which was identified at the upper end of the divided pulmonary ligament. The pulmonary vein was ligated and transected. A transfixion ligature was placed over the central stumps of the doubly ligated artery and veins.

Attention was then turned to the bronchus where a pair of light Kocher forceps were applied below the clamps. Several interrupted fine silk sutures were inserted and the closure completed using a running suture of chromic catgut.

Sulfa was powdered over the raw area and the pleural edges approximated over the divided hilar structures with continuous catgut sutures. The stump of the bronchus was covered with a pad of viable tissue. A small opening was left at the upper and lower angles of the mediastinal suture to permit escape of air should the bronchial stump separate. The wound was carefully rechecked and hemostasis secured. The incision was closed anatomically.

Decortication of Right Lung

The patient was placed in the recumbent position before anesthesia was administered. With the electrocardiograph running, it was noted that the patient had a pulsus bigeminus. This was corrected. The patient was then anesthetized. An endotracheal tube was inserted and the patient was turned in the lateral position with the right side uppermost. The pulse continued at a normal rate and the blood pressure remained stabilized.

The thoracic area was sterilely prepared and draped. A curved periscapular incision was made and deepened. The periosteum overlying the sixth rib was incised and stripped away. A long segment of the sixth rib was removed. The pleural cavity was entered. There was a copious gush of purulent fluid encountered. This was aspirated. Cultures were taken and sent to the laboratory. Palpation then revealed that there were numerous pockets of pus and a thick visceral peel. Considerable difficulty was encountered in removing the peel. The process consumed about three hours. During this procedure, at least six large separate pockets of pus had been evacuated. The visceral peel overlying all of these areas had been removed. The lung was capable of full expansion.

No underlying disease was palpable in any segment of the lung or in the mediastinum. No bronchopleural fistula was found.

Copious flushing with saline and aspiration were then carried out. Bleeding points were coagulated. Oxycel gauze was used over areas which were bleeding diffusely. An intercostal tube was placed posterolaterally just above the diaphragm and an intercostal catheter was placed in the midaxillary line at the third interspace. Both were connected to water seal drainage bottles. Intercostal bundles were approximated with interrupted silk sutures. The extracostal muscles and subcutaneous tissues were approximated with interrupted cotton sutures. The skin was closed with interrupted silk sutures. Dry, sterile dressing was applied.

Thoracotomy and Cardiac Massage

The patient was given a spinal anesthetic and during the preparation the anesthesiologist announced that there was no blood pressure or pulse.

The surgeon struck a sharp blow to the precordial region with no effect. Two external cardiac compression maneuvers were performed with no reaction.

An incision was made in the left chest through the fourth interspace. The heart was found to be greatly dilated and in diastole. By means of massage the heart was reduced to normal size and effective carotid pulse was obtained by massage. A total of 10 cc. of calcium gluconate was then introduced into the right ventricle. A normal heart beat was then obtained. It was felt that an effective pulse rate was obtained in approximately three minutes from the time that arrest was noted. The chest was left open and the heart observed for approximately 15 minutes. It continued to beat normally. The thoracotomy wound was therefore closed using 00 silk.

The patient gradually began to regain consciousness to a semiconscious level. There was considerable difficulty with secretions at this point. The patient was quite excited. It was noted that there were choreic athetoid movements of the right arm.

A tracheostomy was performed following the usual skin preparation. It was felt that the patient was having convulsions and therefore I.V. Pentothal was given.

A midline skin incision was made over the base of the neck overlying the trachea. By means of sharp and blunt dissection the trachea was reached. A segment of the third ring was excised. A #6 tracheostomy tube was inserted and the patient thoroughly suctioned.

A left cephalic vein cutdown as well as a left greater saphenous vein cutdown were performed during the course of treatment.

The patient's level of consciousness never reached that of normal in the three hours of treatment and observation in the operating room. Following stabilization of the blood pressure and pulse the patient was sent to the recovery room.

Esophagectomy (Cor Carcinoma of the Esophagus)

The patient was prepared and draped in the right lateral position with the left arm pulled upward above the head.

A skin incision was made at the level of the third spinous process and extended down parallel to the spine to the seventh intercostal space. The incision was carried around the lower angle of the scapula to the midaxillary line. The chest muscles were opened and retracted and the thorax opened in the 6th intercostal space. Bites of the 5th, 6th and 7th ribs were taken close to the spine proper. Intercostal vessels were ligated and the 4th, 5th and 6th intercostal nerves cut. Rib spreaders were used to enlarge the wound. The pleura was opened. Upon separation of the leaves of the mediastinal pleura the esophagus was exposed.

The tumor in the esophagus was identified. A strip of rubber tubing was gently placed above and below the tumor. There were no structures outside the esophagus intimately adherent to the tumor mass. Arteries branching off the aorta were ligated between silver clips. The portion of the right pleura involved in the tumor was resected. The defect was closed by suturing the edges of the right lung over it with fine interrupted silk sutures.

The esophagus was cut between two heavy silk ligatures. The stump was carbolized. The cardiac stump was inverted into the stomach using a few silk sutures. The hiatus was likewise closed with the same type sutures. The remaining stump of the esophagus was covered by a firmly tied rubber finger.

Dissection of the esophagus was continued until the jugular notch could be felt. The wound in the chest was then closed and the patient repositioned on his back with the head and neck in an extended position.

After a complete change of drapes, gown and instruments, an incision was made along the anterior margin of the sternocleidomastoid muscle. The tumorous portion of the esophagus was gently brought into view. A tunnel was created subcutaneously extending from the lower cervical incision down to the second rib. A transverse incision about 3 cm. in length was made at the end of the tunnel. A forceps was passed up through this incision to the lower part of the cervical incision where the lower end of the esophagus projected. The esophagus was pulled down through the tunnel. At the point of the transverse incision it was attached to the skin edges of the incision using fine silk sutures. The approximation was rechecked to assure an airtight closure. The skin incision was closed and the patient repositioned on his right side. The temporary closure of the thoracic wound was reopened. The mediastinal pleura was closed. A catheter was introduced through the 9th intercostal space at the posterior axillary line. The chest was closed in anatomic layers. The intercostal tube was connected to a suction machine with underwater-seal drainage.

15 } *Urology*

Urology is a surgical specialty concerned with inflammatory and surgical lesions of the urinary tract in the male and female. It also extends to include diseases of the male genitalia. Diseases of the female genital system are managed by the gynecologist rather than the urologist. In both sexes the major anatomic structures of the urinary tract are comprised of the kidneys, renal pelves, ureters, urethra and urinary bladder.

The major male genital organs consist of the testes, epididymis, spermatic cord, vas deferens, seminal vesicles, prostate and the external genitalia consisting of the penis and scrotum.

In this chapter features of the urinary system and of the male genital system will be described, anatomic terms listed and representative operative reports presented to thoroughly familiarize the secretary with this phase of surgical terminology.

THE KIDNEYS AND URETERS

The kidneys are two in number, situated behind the peritoneum on either side of the spinal column, between the level of the third lumbar vertebra and the twelfth thoracic vertebra. The kidney and its vessels are situated in a fatty cushion referred to as the *adipose capsule* or *perirenal fat* which together with the kidney is enclosed in the *renal fascia*. The kidneys are not rigid structures but move freely with the diaphragm during respiration. They are maintained in their anatomic position by the renal fascia which attaches to the fascia of surrounding structures such as the diaphragm, Psoas major muscle and Quadratus lumborum muscle. The kidneys might be described as bean shaped with a cleft or depression in their mid-portion, facing the spinal column. This area is called the *hilum* (hilus) and serves as the point at which the ureter, blood vessels, nerves and lymphatic channels enter and leave the kidney. The hilus expands into a cavity called the *renal sinus* which contains the branched *calyces* and the upper part of the *renal pelvis*. The renal pelvis is a fanned out structure within the kidney which diminishes in caliber and continues as the ureter. The average length of the ureter, which extends from the kidney to the bladder, varies from 28 to 34 cm.

Diseases which cause irreversible major damage to the kidney resulting in a nonfunctioning, septic, toxic or malignant organ provide indications for its removal. Such an operation is termed a *nephrectomy*. Excision of the ureter is referred to as *ureterectomy*.

In dealing with terminology referable to the kidney, the secretary should keep in mind the Latin term for kidney (ren pl. renes). Structures pertaining to the kidney use the term ren-; e.g., renal pelvis, renal capsule, etc.

ANATOMIC STRUCTURES OF THE KIDNEYS, URETERS AND RELATED AREAS

Adipose capsule of the kidney
Arcuate arteries
Arcuate veins
Bowman's capsule
Bröedel's line
Calyx (pl. calyces)
Cortex of the kidney
Costovertebral angle
Diaphragm
Exsanguinated zone of Hyrtl
Fascia renalis
Genitocrural area
Genitofemoral area
Gerota's capsule
Glomeruli
Hilum
Hilus
Hypogastric artery
Iliocostal space
Iliohypogastric
Ilio-inguinal
Inferior vena cava
Inferior vesical artery
Infundibulum
Intercostal nerves
Interlobar arteries
Interlobar veins
Interlobular arteries
Internal spermatic vessels
Lamella
Medulla

Obturatorius internus muscle
Paranephric fat body
Pararenal fat
Parenchyma of the kidney
Pedicle
Pelvis
Perinephritic areolar tissue
Perirenal fat
Pole of the kidney
Psoas major muscle
Pyramids
Quadratus lumborum muscle
Renal artery
Renal fascia
Renal papillae
Renal pedicle
Renal pelvis (pl. pelves)
Renal plexus
Renal pouch
Renal sinus
Renal vein
Retroperitoneal space
Sacral plexus
Subserous fascia
Suprarenal area
Suprarenal glands
Transversus abdominis muscle
Ureter
Ureteropelvic junction
Vas deferens
Vesical artery

NEPHRECTOMY INSTRUMENTS

Also: See listings in Chapter 5

Blake stone forceps
Bozeman dressing forceps
Deaver retractor
Desjardin stone forceps
Guyon-Pean vessel clamp
Herrick pedicle clamp
Metzenbaum scissors

Moynihan probe
Moynihan scoop
Ochsner spiral probe
Ochsner trocar
Ockerblad kidney clamp
Randall stone grasping forceps
Rochester-Pean forceps
Walther kidney pedicle clamp
Young renal pedicle clamp

INCISIONS USED IN KIDNEY SURGERY

Bardenheuer (trap door)
Bergman-Israel (oblique)
Langenbeck
Lateral flank

Pararectus
Pean
Simon
Vertical

TECHNIQUES FOR NEPHRECTOMY

Abdominal
Israel's method
Lowsley ribbon gut method
Lumbar

Morcellement operation (piece-meal
  removal of the kidney)
Transperitoneal
Tuffier Morcellement

Nephrectomy

Under endotracheal general anesthesia, the patient was placed on the table in the decubitus position with the right flank elevated. The skin of the abdomen, flank and back was sterilely prepared and draped.

A right subcostal incision was made beginning at the costovertebral angle, extending downward onto the abdomen for a distance of approximately 12 cm. This incision was carried down through the subcutaneous tissue, extending through the external oblique, internal oblique and transversalis muscles. Gerota's fascia was identified and opened posteriorly.

Dissection revealed a markedly scarred, shriveled right kidney with the presence of pus within the upper collecting system. The upper ureter was obstructed by several calculi.

The kidney was freed with considerable difficulty owing to inflammatory adhesions. The vascular pedicle was freed, doubly clamped and divided. The stump of the pedicle was individually ligated with ties of No. 1 chromic catgut. The ureter was traced down with some difficulty for about half its length beyond which it became incased in impassable scar tissue. The ureter was exposed and freed to the extent possible. At the greatest possible depth of this dissection, it was doubly clamped, transected and its stump ligated with 0 chromic catgut. The wound was examined for hemostasis. This was satisfactory.

Two Penrose drains were placed into the wound, one in the renal fossa and the other in the ureteral area. These were brought out through the posterior angle of the wound.

The wound was closed in layers using interrupted 0 chromic catgut suture on individual layers. The subcutaneous tissues were closed with interrupted 00 plain catgut and the skin with interrupted 00 silk. A sterile dressing was applied.

TECHNIQUES FOR NEPHROPEXY (Suspension of the Kidney)

Deming's hammock method	Narath's method
Edebohl's	O'Conor operation
Hugh H. Young	Stanischeff operation
Kelly modification of Dodson	Vogel's method
Lowsley method with ribbon gut	Young technique

Nephropexy

After sterile preparation and draping, with the patient in the kidney position on his left side, a subcostal flank incision was made. The muscles were divided. The fatty capsule of the kidney was opened and retracted. An oblique incision, 1.5 cm. in length and parallel to the long axis of the kidney, was made on its posterior surface in the upper pole region. It penetrated the fibrous capsule to the parenchyma of the kidney. A similar incision was made through the fibrous capsule to the parenchyma, parallel to it, near the lateral border of the organ. Using a Kocher director, a connection was created between these two incisions. The 12th rib was insinuated through this tunnel. A few sutures were placed to attach the kidney to the periosteum of the rib. As a precaution against slipping, the 12th rib was fractured about 4 cm. from its end. After being reflected upward, it was attached to the periosteum of the contiguous rib with catgut sutures.

The fatty capsule was resutured over the kidney and the fractured rib. The adipose capsule was attached to the lumbar musculature with a few sutures.

The wound was closed in layers without drainage.

OTHER KIDNEY OPERATIONS

A variety of conditions may indicate the establishment of a temporary or permanent urinary opening from the kidney. Such a procedure is called a *nephrostomy*. It is a lifesaving procedure when the ureters are accidentally severed during surgery. It is a palliative procedure where malignancy or other disease process has obstructed the ureters. A temporary type nephrostomy is sometimes required preliminary to reconstructive surgery on the ureters.

This operation consists of the introduction of a nephrostomy tube into the kidney for purposes of drainage.

In order to familiarize the secretary with the terminology used in reporting this procedure, the following description of the operative proceedings is presented.

Nephrostomy

With the patient under general anesthesia, in the right decubitus position, and the kidney rest elevated, the operative field was prepared and draped.

A lateral flank incision was made just below the 12th rib. The muscles were divided. The transversalis fascia was divided. The kidney which had been palpated was freed of its perinephritic fat. It was brought into view. It measured approximately three times its normal size. Numerous adhesions binding it inferiorly, laterally and medially were lysed.

The first portion of the ureter was brought into view. It was freed by blunt dissection. Blunt dissection was carried upward until a small intrapelvic kidney pelvis was isolated. After the kidney was exposed, a pyelotomy incision was made between stay sutures of fine plain catgut. A curved clamp was then passed through this pyelotomy incision, into the lower calyx and through the parenchyma. The clamp was then used to grasp the end of the nephrostomy tube and bring it into the pelvis. Bleeding was controlled by placing a Halsted type of mattress suture of plain catgut through the renal parenchyma around the drain.

The pyelotomy wound was loosely approximated and the kidney replaced in the renal fossa. The nephrostomy tube was allowed to extend in a direct line from the wound. The lateral flank wound was closed in layers and a Penrose drain placed behind the kidney and brought out through a separate stab wound.

Nephrolithotomy and Pyelolithotomy (Removal of calculus from kidney and kidney pelvis)

After satisfactory general anesthesia, the patient was placed in the lateral decubitus position with the left side elevated by a kidney rest.

A 12 cm. curvilinear incision was made in the left subcostal area extending onto the anterior abdomen. The incision was deepened through the subcutaneous tissues and the Latissimus dorsi, external oblique, internal oblique and transversalis muscles. The lumbodorsal fascia was opened posteriorly and the retroperitoneal space entered. Gerota's capsule was identified and opened posteriorly. The left kidney was freed and exposed by blunt dissection.

Examination of the kidney revealed a healthy appearing organ except for a readily palpable stone in the lower pole and a suggestion of a second calculus in the infundibulum. A 2 cm. incision was made longitudinally over the left renal pelvis after appropriate freeing and exposure of this area. Using stone forceps, the infundibular calculus was grasped and removed. The calyceal stone could not be reached through the renal pelvis and therefore, a radial nephrotomy was performed over the palpable calyx. The stone was removed. Bleeding was controlled.

The incised renal parenchyma was closed with interrupted mattress sutures of 00 chromic catgut which controlled bleeding. The pyelotomy incision was loosely closed with interrupted 0000 chromic catgut.

One unit of blood was started during the procedure. A Penrose drain was placed into the perirenal space and the kidney was replaced in its usual anatomic position.

The wound was closed in layers using interrupted 0 chromic catgut sutures on the muscle layers, interrupted 00 plain on the subcutaneous tissues and interrupted 00 silk sutures for the skin. The drain was brought out posteriorly.

THE URINARY BLADDER

The urinary tract structures above the level of the urinary bladder are situated bilaterally in the body in a normal anatomic situation. Urine is secreted in the kidneys from whence it passes into the branched calyces, renal pelves and ureters into the urinary bladder. The bladder, a musculo-membranous sac, receives urine via both ureters and acts as a reservoir and medium by which the urine is eventually discharged from the body.

The urinary bladder is subject to many defects; congenital, developmental, and acquired. Fortunately, it is not an organ which is essential to life. Its removal in part or in toto is sometimes necessary. Such an operation is designated as a *cystectomy,* total or subtotal. In cases where complete cystectomy is indicated, urinary diversion by reimplantation of the ureters into the sigmoid (ureterosigmoidostomy), ileum (ure-teroileostomy) or skin (cutaneous ureterostomy) is performed prelimi-nary to the bladder excision.

Other operations on the bladder include incisions into the urinary bladder (cystotomy) for removal of lesions which cannot be successfully managed endoscopically; incision into the bladder for purposes of drain-age (cystotomy); and the frequently performed endoscopic examination, *cystoscopy,* which is used for bladder exploration, biopsy, fulguration and removal of calculi, foreign bodies and various lesions.

The Latin (B.N.A.) term for the bladder is vesica urinaria. It is from this designation that the use of "vesical" is derived in reference to bladder structures; e.g., vesical neck, perivesical fascia, etc. It should not be confused with the word "vesicle".

ANATOMIC FEATURES OF THE URINARY BLADDER AND URETHRA

Anterior abdominal wall
Bas-fond
Bladder reflection
Bladder wall
Bulbourethral
Cavernous portion of urethra
Cavum Retzii
Cellules
Detrusor urinae muscle
Dome of the bladder
Ductus deferens (deferentes)
External urethral orifice
False ligaments of bladder
Fossa navicularis urethrae
Fundus
Hypogastric arteries
Hypogastric plexus
Inferior fascia
Internal urethral orifice
Interureteric ridge
Intravesical space
Lacuna magna
Lacuna (pl. lacunae)
Lateral false ligaments
Lateral puboprostatic ligaments
Lateral umbilical folds
Medial puboprostatic ligaments
Membranous urethra

Middle umbilical fold
Middle umbilical ligament
Mucous membrane
Obliterated hypogastric arteries
Paraurethral glands
Paravesical fossa
Peritoneal reflection
Peritoneum (peritoneal)
Posterior false ligaments
Preperitoneal space
Prevesical space
Prostate
Prostatic area
Pubovesical ligaments
Pubovesicalis muscle
Rectovesical fascia
Rectovesical fold of peritoneum
Rectovesical pouch
Rectovesicalis muscle
Retzius space
Sacrogenital folds
Seminal vesicles
Skene glands
Space of Retzius
Sphincter vesicae
Summit
Torus uretericus
Trabeculations

ANATOMIC FEATURES OF THE URINARY BLADDER
AND URETRA (Continued)

Trigone
Trigonum vesicae
Urachus
Ureteral orifice(s)
Ureteric ridge
Urethra
Urethral crest
Urethral orifice(s)

Urogenital diaphragm
Uvula vesicae
Vas deferens
Vertex
Verumontanum
Vesical
Vesicouterine excavation
Viscus

BLADDER ARTERIES

Inferior gluteal
Inferior vesical
Internal iliac

Middle vesical
Obturator
Superior vesical

Operative reports, typical of those the surgeon's secretary will be required to transcribe, are presented here for the purpose of affording the secretary a reference of terms used in contextual form. This is intended to promote familiarity with the words and their usage.

CYSTOSCOPY

One of the most frequently performed urologic examinations is the cystoscopy. It consists of the examination of the urinary bladder by means of an instrument called a cystoscope or foroblique pan-endoscope, a type of cystoscope. By means of a lens system the interior of the urinary bladder can be examined. Attachments permit use of the cystoscope for: crushing and removal of bladder stones (litholapaxy); removal of new growths and biopsy specimens, evacuation of blood clots and debris; control of bleeding; irrigation of the bladder, renal pelves and ureters; instillation of diagnostic media; dilation of stenotic areas; collection of split urines and instillation of x-ray contrast media into the renal pelves by way of the ureters for retrograde pyelography studies. Very frequently the retrograde pyelogram is done with the cystoscopy. Pyelographic roentgen studies may also be done by injecting the contrast solution intravenously, through the arm, with study of the kidneys, ureters and renal pelves after these structures have been filled with the injected contrast material.

TYPES OF CYSTOSCOPES

Braasch direct catheterizing
Brown-Buerger
Butterfield
Kelly
Lowsley-Peterson
McCarthy-Peterson

McCarthy-Campbell miniature
McCarthy foroblique pan-endoscope
McCarthy miniature
National general purpose
Nesbit
Ravich convertible

Cystoscopy With Retrograde Pyelogram

After satisfactory general anesthesia with intravenous Surital, the patient was placed on the cystoscopy table in the lithotomy position. The skin of the perineum and genitalia was sterilely prepared and draped.

A #24 McCarthy Pan-Endoscope was introduced. Examination of the urethra revealed generalized chronic inflammatory change. No definite urethral polyps were noted. There was no evidence of vesical neck contracture.

The bladder was then surveyed with a #21 Brown-Buerger Cystoscope. A mild chronic inflammatory mucosal change was observed. No stones, foreign bodies or neoplastic growths were noted. The air bubble was in the midline situated at the dome of the bladder. There was a good bladder light reflex. No diverticulum of the bladder was seen. There were many large and small interlacing trabeculations with considerable cellule formation.

The ureteral orifices were well seen. There was a clear urinary spurt on the right. No definite urine reflux was seen on the left. No. 5 ureteral catheters were passed bilaterally with ease. There was no drainage from the left catheter.

Indigo carmine was given intravenously and excreted in $+++$ concentration in four minutes on the right. There was no demonstrable excretion on the left. Retrograde pyelography was done demonstrating a staghorn calculus on the left.

Endoscopic Bladder Litholapaxy (Crushing and Removal of Bladder Calculi)

The patient was prepared and draped in the dorsal decubitus position. Under local anesthesia of 5 cc. of 1:500 Nupercaine Solution with equal parts instilled into the posterior and anterior urethra, a lithotrite was introduced into the bladder. The instrument passed smoothly along the trigone to the base of the bladder. Following this, the instrument was unlocked and the male blades opened. The blades were closed over the stone which had been visualized through the lens at the beak of the instrument. The lithotrite was then locked and raised slightly off the base of the bladder. The male blade was screwed home thus crushing the stone. The lithotrite was unlocked and used again in a similar manner until all of the stones were crushed. The blades were then closed securely and the instrument withdrawn. The tiny fragments were evacuated from the bladder along with other debris by irrigation and an Ellik Evacuator.

Cystoscopy; Urethroscopy with Dilation and Transurethral Biopsy of Bladder and Urethra

After satisfactory spinal anesthesia was obtained, the patient was placed in the lithotomy position on the operating table. The skin of the perineum and genitalia was prepared and draped.

A #20 McCarthy Pan-Endoscope was passed but some obstruction was encountered in the bulbomembranous area of the urethra. Urethral dilation was carried out with metal sounds to 22 French caliber without difficulty. The pan-endoscope was reinserted without further obstruction.

The posterior urethra revealed evidence of mild urethral stricture in the obstructed area. The prostate was moderately enlarged and partially obstructing. There was a moderate bladder neck contracture. The remainder of the urethra was normal.

The urinary bladder was examined with a No. 21 Brown-Buerger Cystoscope. Examination disclosed a chronic inflammatory change throughout the vesical mucosa, most marked about the bladder floor. There were four or five slightly elevated lesions about the trigone and vesical neck. These raised areas were approximatly 1-1.5 cm. in their greatest diameter and were pale in appearance as contrasted with the surrounding mucosa. Using an Iglesias Resectoscope, biopsies were taken of the urethra and the bladder lesions.

#20 Foley catheter was left indwelling.

THE MALE GENITAL SYSTEM

Urology also encompasses the male genital system comprised of a pair of testes with paired seminal ducts, seminal vesicles, ejaculatory ducts and bulbourethral glands (Cowper's glands). The single structures in this system include the urethra, penis, scrotum and prostate gland.

In the fetus the two testes are contained in the abdominal cavity. Prior to birth they descend into the scrotum with a portion of their spermatic cord. Failure of this process to occur, either bilaterally or unilaterally, is known as *cryptorchism* (undescended testis). A corrective operation termed an *orchiopexy* (suspension of the testis) is performed in these cases. Spermatogenesis and testosterone production take place within the testes. In an undescended testis, body temperatures reduce and finally completely suppress spermatogenesis.

In a normal anatomic situation, the testes and a portion of their spermatic cords are suspended in a cutaneous pouch known as the *scrotum*. The testes consist internally of communicating chambers which contain the seminiferous tubules. These tubules unite and continue outside the testis as a tortuous tubule called the *epididymis*. This structure connects the testis with the *seminal duct* (ductus deferens; vas deferens) which is the excretory duct of the testis. The seminal duct follows a winding course to the base of the prostate where its caliber diminishes and it is joined by the duct of the seminal vesicle to form the *ejaculatory duct*. The ejaculatory duct opens into the prostatic area of the urethra near the orifice of the prostatic utricle. This is a bilateral process.

The seminal vesicles are two in number situated between the fundus of the bladder and the rectum. They secrete a fluid substance which is excreted into the seminal stream at the base of the prostate, where the two seminal vesicles converge, each uniting with its respective seminal duct to produce the ejaculatory duct. The ejaculatory ducts are two in number and extend to the urethra, into which they discharge their secretions.

The external male genitalia consist of the penis and scrotum. The penis serves as the copulatory organ of the male through which spermatozoa are injected into the vagina. The penis also contains the greatest portion of the urethra through which urine as well as semen are discharged to the outside of the body.

The penile shaft consists of three bundles of cavernous tissue. The lateral two masses are called the *corpora cavernosa penis* and the medial portion, containing the urethra, is known as the *corpus cavernosum urethrae*. The end of the corpus cavernosum consists of a cap-like structure which covers the tip of the penis. This is called the *glans penis*.

The penis is a flaccid organ attached at the front and sides of the pubic arch, just above the scrotum. In response to stimulation or sexual excitement, the venous spaces in the cavernous tissue become distended with blood causing the penis to become erect and rigid.

The prostate gland is surgically important because of its location. It is situated just below the internal urethral orifice and around the urethra in a doughnut shape. Since the urethra is surrounded by this gland, any enlargement of the prostate diminishes the urethral caliber. This often occurs in older men and ranges from narrowing of the urethra to complete obstruction with retention of urine. Enlargement of the prostate is termed *hypertrophy of the prostate* and although it is usually a benign process, malignancy must be ruled out because of the incidence of carcinoma in the prostate gland. Hypertrophy of the prostate is relieved by an operation known as a *prostatectomy* which can be performed from below as a transurethral resection of the prostate (TUR) with a resectoscope or through the abdominal route as a suprapubic prostatectomy.

The prostate secretes a fluid which further facilitates the flow of the spermatozoa.

Two additional glands of the male genital system consist of the *bulbourethral glands* (Cowper's). They are two pea-sized bodies located at either side of the membranous portion of the urethra, just below the prostate gland. Each of these glands secretes a fluid which is carried by an excretory duct emanating from each gland to the cavernous portion of the urethra, just before the urogenital diaphragm.

SURGERY OF THE PENIS

The circumcision (excision of redundant foreskin) is the most common surgical procedure performed on the penis and for this reason an operative report describing the operation is included here. Anatomic structures of the penis and related anatomy have been listed below in addition to those terms one might expect to use in a circumcision report.

ANATOMIC FEATURES OF THE PENIS AND RELATED STRUCTURES

Arcuate pubic ligament
Arteries:
  dorsal
  helicine
  internal pudendal
Buck's fascia
Bulb
Bulbus urethrae
Colle's fascia
Corona glandis
Corpora cavernosa penis
Corpus cavernosa urethrae
Corpus spongiosum
Crura
Crus penis
Dartos tunic
Deep dorsal vein
External perineal fascia
Foreskin
Frenulum
Glans penis
Ischiopubic rami
Lamina
Ligamentum fundiforme penis

Meatus
Median raphe
Muscles:
  Bulbocavernosus
  Ischiocavernosus
  Transversus perinei superficialis
Neck of penis
Prepuce
Preputial glands (Tyson)
Preputial space
Pubis (pl. pubes)
Pudendal nerve
Retroglandular sulcus
Scarpa's fascia
Scrotum
Septum of penis
Septum pectiniforme
Smegma (sebaceous material)
Superficial fascia
Suspensory ligament of penis
Urethra
Urethral mucous membrane
Urogenital diaphragm

Circumcision

Using an infiltration anesthetic of 2% Novocain and filling the preputial sac with a 4% solution of Novocain for five minutes, the area was prepared for surgery.

An artery forceps was used to engage the prepuce. A grooved director was passed beneath the prepuce over the head of the penis. A Gomco clamp was applied, the prepuce cut away and the clamp removed.

One blade of a scissors was passed between the glans penis and the inner layer of the mucous membrane which was divided back as far as the margin of the corona glandis. A cuff of mucous membrane was turned back. The mucosa was trimmed. The edges of the mucous membrane were united to the integumental border with interrupted catgut sutures. Coaptation was satisfactory.

SURGERY OF THE TESTES

Orchiopexy (suspension of an undescended testis) and orchiectomy (removal of the testis) are probably the most common operations performed on the testes.

Diseases and operations pertaining to the testes assume the prefix "orchi-" from the Greek term for the testes, "orchis." Inflammation of the testis is known as orchitis, pain in the testis is called orchialgia, etc.

Anatomic terms pertaining to the testes, their investing tissues and related structures have been listed below with several operative reports exemplifying procedures performed on these organs.

ANATOMIC FEATURES OF THE TESTES AND RELATED STRUCTURES

Ampulla
Appendix of epididymis
Areolar tissue
Arteries:
  cremasteric
  deep external pudendal
  int. & ext. spermatics
  superficial perineal
Cremasteric fascia
Cremasteric layer
Dartos tunic
Ductulus aberrans inferior
Ductulus aberrans superior
Ductus deferens
Ductus deferentes
Ejaculatory duct
Epididymis
  head (globus major)
  tail (globus minor)

External spermatic fascia
Fascia innominata of Gallaudet
Gubernaculum chorda
Infundibuloform fascia
Integument
Internal spermatic fascia
Mediastinum testis (corpus Highmori)
Paradidymis (organ of Giraldes)
Parietal lamina
Plexus pampiniformis
Prostate gland
Raphe
Rete testis
Rugae
Scrotum
Seminal duct
Seminal vesicles
Spermatic cord
Spermatic veins

ANATOMIC FEATURES OF THE TESTES AND
RELATED STRUCTURES (Continued)

Testicle

Testicular

Testis (pl. testes)

Trabeculae

Transversalis fascia

Tunica albuginea

Tunica Dartos

Tunica vaginalis

Tunica vasculosa

Vas aberrans of Haller

Vas deferens

Visceral lamina

Bilateral Orchiectomy (Removal of Testes)

The patient was prepared and draped in the supine position. A 6 cm. vertical midline scrotal incision was made. Dissection was then carried into the right scrotal compartment, through the various testicular tunics, to expose the testes and epididymis as well as the lower spermatic cord on the right. The lower cord was transected and its proximal stump doubly ligated with 00 chromic catgut. The testes, epididymis and lower cord were then removed. A similar procedure was carried out on the opposite side.

A Penrose drain was drawn through the wound and brought out through the lower corner. The incision was closed in two layers, using interrupted 00 chromic catgut. A sterile dressing was applied.

Orchiopexy (Torek Operation) First Stage

The patient was prepared and draped in the supine position. An incision was made in the inguinal canal providing good exposure. The testis was liberated from the cremaster muscle, gubernaculum and surrounding tissues. The spermatic cord was likewise stripped of its investments; however, the vas deferens and spermatic vessels were allowed to remain intact. Dissection of the vessels was carried out to the level of the transversalis fascia.

The liberated testis was laid on the thigh to the extent that it would reach. A point above this level was selected for the incision. A transverse incision was made, long enough to accommodate the length of the testis, and carried to the fascia of the thigh. Using two fingers, a pocket was created extending from the lower end of the inguinal incision to the bottom of the scrotum. An opening in the pocket was then made by an incision matching the incision in the thigh, in length as well as in direction. A strip of gauze was passed through the tunnel thus created.

The upper end of the wound of the thigh was approximated to the identical wound in the scrotum, passing the suture from surface to depth and from depth to surface. The knot was brought to lie on the skin surface. Interrupted sutures were used. The cut posterior lip of the scrotal wound was then approximated with the corresponding edge of the thigh wound using catgut sutures. The testis, which had been replaced in the inguinal wound, was delivered through the channel created. Two fine sutures of chromicized catgut were placed through the tunica albuginea and fascia of the thigh. Particular care was exercised to avoid the saphenous and femoral veins.

Fine silk was used to approximate the anterior lip of the scrotal wound to the lower lip of the wound in the thigh. Closure of the wound was carried out uniting the internal oblique and transversus muscle to Poupart's ligament. The aponeurosis of the external oblique was also approximated. Following this, the skin was closed and a strip of gauze drawn through the canal in the skin between the scrotum and thigh.

A second operation will be performed in three months to free the testis from the thigh and bury it in the scrotum.

Hydrocelectomy (Andrews Bottle Operation)

With the patient in the supine position on the operating table, the external genitalia were sterilely prepared and draped.

The tunica vaginalis was opened at its upper pole and its fluid contents expressed. The testicle was brought out of the scrotum, extruding it through the opening in the sac. The sac was everted without a suture. The blood supply to the testis was adequate. The testis and everted tunica vaginalis were reposited into the scrotum. The wound was closed without drainage.

SURGERY OF THE PROSTATE

One of the most frequently encountered surgical conditions of the prostate is benign prostatic hypertrophy. The prostate is also a common site of malignancy and when detected early enough can be eradicated by surgery.

Resection of the prostate is referred to as a *prostatectomy*. It may be perineal, radical, retropubic, suprapubic (transvesical) or transurethral in type. The transurethral method is referred to in the vernacular as a TUR and is performed with a resectoscope passed endoscopically through the urethra. The suprapubic and transurethral methods are employed more often than the other approaches mentioned.

ANATOMIC FEATURES OF THE PROSTATE AND ASSOCIATED STRUCTURES

Arteries:
  inferior vesical
  internal pudendal
  middle hemorrhoidal
Apex of prostate
Base of prostate
Bladder mucosa
Bladder neck
Capsule
Central tendon
Denonvillier's fascia
Ejaculatory ducts
External urethral sphincter
Internal urethral orifice
Isthmus
Lateral fossae
Lateral lobes of prostate
Levator ani muscles
Levatores prostatae

Median furrow
Membranous urethra
Middle lobe of prostate
Mucosal cuff
Paravesical spaces
Plexus of Santorini
Prostatic cavity
Prostatic fossa
Prostatovesicular junction
Puboprostatic ligaments
Rectourethralis muscle
Subtrigonal spheroids
Suprapubic sinus
Transverse perinei muscles
Trigone
Urethra
Urogenital diaphragm
Verumontanum
Vesical orifice

Suprapubic Prostatectomy

The patient was prepared and draped in a supine position. A transverse incision was made midway between the umbilicus and the symphysis pubis and carried through the subcutaneous tissues. A small Gelpi vaginal retractor was inserted. The anterior rectus sheath was incised transversely and the underlying rectus muscles separated in the midline and retracted laterally with a Farr retractor. Using moist gauze manipulation, the peritoneum was reflected upward from the dome of the bladder. The retropubic space was exposed.

The clamp on the urethral catheter was released by an assistant permitting the previously instilled sterile water to flow out of the urinary bladder. The catheter was removed from the bladder.

A transverse incision was made in the bladder wall 2 cm. above the prostatovesicular junction for approximately 4 cm. in length. A traction suture of 0 chromic was inserted through the bladder wall on both sides. A Judd retractor was then introduced into the bladder and inspection carried out under direct vision. No diverticuli, calculi or neoplastic growths were noted. Using a sharp scalpel, circumcision of the mucosa around the vesical neck was performed. The dissecting finger was steadied by two left fingers in the rectum which also pushed the prostate forward toward the suprapubic opening. The gland was shelled out en masse.

The prostatic cavity was tightly packed with three-inch gauze. Direct inspection was carried out of the bladder neck and floor. Bleeders were coagulated. Hemostasis was satisfactory. A No. 22 Foley bag was placed and inflated to 60 cc. at the vesical neck. A No. 32 right angle de Pezzer catheter was placed through a stab wound in the bladder and the bladder closed in two layers with 0 chromic catgut. Prior to closure of the muscle layers a split rubber drain was placed leading from the prevesical space.

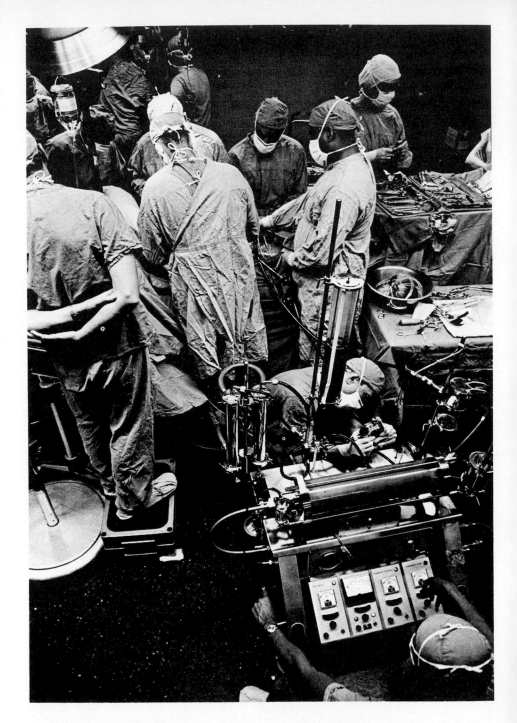

Heart and lungs machine shown in foreground in use during open heart surgery at the Montefiore Hospital and Medical Center, New York City, New York.

16 { *Vascular Surgery*

The specialty of vascular surgery concerns itself with the diagnosis, repair and reconstruction of the circulatory channels for the purpose of restoring normal circulation and blood supply to the tissues. Important diagnostic procedures performed in this specialty include aortography, angiography and arteriography for the study of circulation and vascular defects. Surgery performed in this specialty includes: repair of congenital, traumatic and developmental vascular defects; thromboendarterectomy for occlusive phenomena; the use of grafts to replace diseased arterial segments or to act as shunts for an occluded area, and other operations designed to restore circulation to the degree possible.

Vascular surgery is a highly specialized division of surgery which is usually confined to the larger teaching hospitals where necessary facilities and personnel trained to properly assist vascular operating teams are available. In the medium sized general hospital, surgery on the blood vessels is usually confined to saphenous ligations and stripping, intimectomy for removal of calcified plaques, arterial repairs following lacerations and work less highly specialized than that of vascular grafting, shunting, etc.

The secretary should be familiar with the terms peculiar to this specialty as well as the other phases of surgery if her background is to be comprehensive. Surgical reports which further illustrate the diagnostic and operative procedures performed in this branch of surgery are included here to assist her with this aspect of her training.

DIAGNOSTIC PROCEDURES

When one stops to consider the intricacy and margin for individual variation in the vascular network throughout the body, the importance of proper preliminary assessment and localization of vascular lesions becomes more apparent. X-ray evaluation of the vessels is of further value to the surgeon in determining the extent of the disease process and the possibility of coexisting pathology, such as arteriosclerosis, which might influence the course of treatment to be followed. These are but a few of the reasons for the preoperative x-ray work-up.

The format for recording these examinations should include the complete title of the procedure, the indication for it, a description of what was done, a report of any eventful occurrences during the examination and an immediate interpretation of the films, in addition to information completely identifying the patient by name, age, case number, room number and name of the attending physician.

The following examples demonstrate the format and context of typical reports exclusive of patient identification.

CONTRAST MATERIALS USED FOR VASCULAR X-RAY EXAMINATIONS

Angio-Conray	Hypaque 50%
Conray	Hypaque-M 75%
Conray-400	Hypaque-M 90%
Hypaque 20%	

Right Subclavian Arteriogram

Indications: Evaluation of arterial supply of the right arm in a patient with Buerger's Disease and gangrene.

Procedure:

The patient was placed on the x-ray table in the supine position. The skin over the right neck in the supraclavicular region was prepared and draped in the usual manner. The skin over the pulsating right subclavian artery was anesthetized with 1% Xylocaine.

A short 17 gauge needle was introduced into the right subclavian artery. Good backflow was obtained. A routine injection consisting of 20 cc. of 50% Hypaque was administered. The patient experienced minimal discomfort. These films were not satisfactory and it was felt to be partially due to insufficient contrast material. A second injection of 50% Hypaque was given with good film results. Pressure was maintained over the puncture site and hemostasis appeared to be satisfactory. This was followed by PA and lateral chest films.

Immediate Interpretation of Films:

1. Distal small artery disease with occlusion of the ulnar artery below the brachial artery bifurcation and the radial artery proximal to the level of the wrist.

Right Femoral Arteriogram

Indications: Right popliteal aneurysm

Procedure:

The patient was placed in the supine position. The right groin was prepared with Merthiolate and draped in the usual fashion. Using a special needle of the Rochester type, the femoral artery was entered. The metal stylet was withdrawn and a plastic catheter was then left in the right common femoral. One injection was made utilizing 20 cc. of Angio-Conray. Films were obtained in the AP position. A second run was then made with the leg in the lateral position using the same quantity of dye and again films were obtained at the usual rate.

Immediate Interpretation of Films:
1. Popliteal aneurysm with thrombosis of the wall; the aneurysm measuring approximately 1 inch in length.
2. Arteries normal with good outflow.

Aortogram

Indications: This 70 year old white male stepped on a nail 4 weeks ago, subsequent to which he developed an ulcer of the left foot followed by gangrene of the left first toe. Popliteal pulse on left diminished as compared with the right. Pedal pulses on the left very faint.

Procedure:

The patient was placed in the prone position and the lumbar area prepared and draped. 1% Xylocaine was infiltrated locally. A 17 gauge needle was introduced at a level below the renal arteries in the aorta with good backflow in all four quadrants. Two test films at two second intervals were obtained after injection of 10 cc. of Conray-400. The usual run of eight films at two second intervals after 25 cc. of Angio-Conray was obtained. The films were of good quality. The needle was withdrawn.

The distal arteries of the left extremity were not entirely visualized and a left femoral arteriogram was done.

Left Femoral Arteriogram:

With the patient in the supine position, the groin area was prepared with Merthiolate and 1% Xylocaine was infiltrated locally. A 17 gauge needle was introduced into the left common femoral artery with good backflow in all four quadrants. Eight films at two second intervals were taken after injection of 25 cc. of Angio-Conray. The films were of good quality. The needle was withdrawn.

Immediate Interpretation of Films:

1. Patent femoral system on left
2. High bifurcation of popliteal with takeoff of peroneal artery from left anterior tibial artery
3. Stenosis of the left posterior tibial and peroneal arteries
4. Low femoral (common) bifurcation on the left

Translumbar Aortogram

Indication: Postoperative aortic bilateral external iliac dacron bypass

Procedure:

With the patient in the prone position the back was prepared and draped in the usual manner. 1% Xylocaine was used to anesthetize the back area. A 17 gauge needle was then inserted into the aorta. A good backflow was demonstrated. A test dose of 8 cc. of Angio-Conray showed the needle to be in good position. A final run was then made using 20 cc. of Angio-Conray. A total of three runs were made, each using 20 cc. of Angio-Conray.

Immediate Interpretation of Films:
1. Patent aorto-iliac bypass

Right Open Transbrachial Arch Aortogram

Indications: Possible thoracic aneurysm on routine chest x-ray

Procedure:

The patient was placed on the aortogram table in the supine position. The skin of the right arm and shoulder was prepared and draped in the usual manner. The skin and subcutaneous tissues over the lower third of the right brachial artery were anesthetized with 1% Xylocaine.

A 4 cm. longitudinal incision was made and carried through the skin and subcutaneous tissues. The brachial artery was easily exposed. Bleeding points were clamped and ligated with 0000 Tevdek as encountered. The brachial artery was isolated for a distance of 2½ cm. and slung with cord tapes proximally and distally. It was necessary to clamp and ligate only a small arterial branch and this was done with 0000 Tevdek. The brachial artery was clamped proximally and 20 cc. of ½ mg. per cc. Heparin was injected into the distal arterial tree. The distal cord tape was tightened and an arteriotomy incision was made.

A No. 8 NIH catheter was passed into the ascending aorta under fluoroscopy using 50 cc. of 50% Hypaque. A test film was taken using 20 cc. of 50% Hypaque and this film was found to be of satisfactory quality. A routine injection with the patient in the oblique position was then made, the patient receiving 40 cc. of 90% Hypaque at a pressure of 600 lbs. per square inch. A second set of films was then taken with the patient in the straight PA position, using the same quantity of dye under the same injection technique. The catheter was withdrawn and the proximal and distal arterial tree flushed.

The arteriotomy incision was closed with a running suture of 000000 Mersilene with satisfactory hemostasis. The fascia and subcutaneous tissues were closed with interrupted 0000 Tevdek. The skin was closed with interrupted deep mattress sutures of the same material.

A dry sterile dressing was applied and the patient returned to his room in good condition with an easily palpable full right radial pulse.

Immediate Interpretation of Films:
1. Presence of thoracic aortic aneurysm noted

VASCULAR OPERATIONS

A considerable amount of investigation has been carried out on autogenous vein grafts particularly to bypass occluded portions of the peripheral arteries; however, because of the high incidence of postoperative aneurysm or thrombosis eventuating in failures, surgeons prefer synthetic vascular implants or arterial homografts. Because homologous arterial transplants (segments of artery taken from one individual and transplanted into another) do not act as true grafts, artificial prosthesis may be used just as well. Heterologous arterial transplants (vascular segments used from another species) were used successfully by Carrel in 1907; however, some authorities believe that they do not function as well as homologous transplants and are therefore unsatisfactory as vascular transplants. Experimental work is being done with bovine arterial segments in the hope that methods of preparation and preservation can be developed to permit successful use of this material.

The lack of readily available transplants for vascular grafts has long prompted investigators to seek suitable substitutes. Rigid materials were used initially but soon abandoned in favor of pliable tubes. The first successful use of such tubes for arterial replacement was introduced in 1952 by Voorhees, Jaretski, and Blakemore, using vinyon-N cloth. In the years which have followed, a variety of different materials have been tried experimentally. Dacron, Teflon and Terylene cloth are some of the more popular materials used today. The actual success of these vascular transplants can only be tested by time. The techniques for replacement and use of these fabrics will be better appreciated in a few years when studies can be based on significant survival rates.

Another factor being carefully observed by scientific investigators is the carcinogenic (cancer causing) potential of these foreign implants in the body. Experiments have demonstrated carcinomatous growths in mice at the site of implantation of some of these materials but it does not follow that an identical response will occur in man. Numerous substances exist which are carcinogenic in experimental animals and innocuous in man. Time holds the answer to this question also.

Some of the materials, types of prostheses and sutures used in vascular surgery have been listed here with typical operative dictations to acquaint the secretary with the terminology characteristic of this specialty.

VASCULAR PROSTHESES

Crimped dacron tube
No. 25 dacron bifurcation
DeBakey's
Edward's seamless bifurcated
Frozen arterial homograft
Helanca seamless tubes
Knitted

Nylon
Orlon
Starr-Edwards valve
Teflon
Terylene cloth
Woven tubes

SUTURES AND TECHNIQUES

Carrel method interrupted Lembert
Dacron
Deknatel silk
Halsted mattress
Mersilene

Metal bands
Silk
Tevdek
Transfixion silk

AORTIC VALVE PROSTHESES (total replacement)

Silastic bicuspid valve with compressed Ivalon rim
Silastic flap valve with compressed Ivalon base
Silastic impregnated Teflon felt three-cusp valve

VASCULAR OPERATIONS

For a complete listing of arteries and veins the secretary is referred to chapter 6.

Left Femoropopliteal Bypass and Autogenous Vein Graft

Indications: Patient is a 64 year old colored male with rest pain in his left foot secondary to superficial femoral artery (probably malignant) and small artery disease. Femoral arteriography revealed a patent popliteal stump of poor quality.

Technique:

With the patient on the operating table in the supine position, the entire left leg and groin were prepared and draped for surgery.

A groin incision was made over the fossa ovalis exposing the saphenous vein. Hemostasis was obtained throughout with fine Tevdek. The saphenous vein was isolated at one point, retained with a rubber band and by meticulous dissection, both distally and proximally, was freed from surrounding tissue. Its tributaries were ligated with 000 Tevdek and divided. The saphenous vein was of good quality although somewhat narrow. A satisfactory link was obtained from the fossa ovalis to below the knee. The skin did not need to be undermined to obtain the vein.

The popliteal artery was exposed in the customary fashion without cutting the pes anserinus. The popliteal artery was of poor quality and the bifurcation was therefore exposed revealing a discrete plaque at the branching of the anterior tibial and posterior tibial arteries. When a satisfactory link of artery had been obtained, a Pott's clamp was placed proximally and the artery was opened with a longitudinal incision. This incision was carried down to the bifurcation previously mentioned. Backflow was poor and therefore an endarterectomy was performed. The resulting backflow was improved to a sufficient degree to warrant grafting.

The lower portion of the incision was closed with a running 00000 Tevdek suture. A catheter was threaded down this artery and the distal limbs heparinized through this catheter. A Pott's clamp was placed across the artery where it had been sewn, isolating the area for anastomosis.

The vein was prepared, distended and irrigated. The proximal portion was prepared for anastomosis. This was performed in the usual manner with 000 Tevdek using an end-to-side anastomosis. The vein was passed up the thigh behind the Sartorius muscle, care being taken not to twist it. The distal part of the vein was prepared for proximal anastomosis. The common femoral artery was isolated including its bifurcation. Pott's clamps were placed across all of the major arteries. The distal limbs were heparinized. A longitudinal incision was made in the anterior portion of the common femoral artery. The artery was of excellent quality at this level. An anastomosis was carried out in an end-to-side manner. All clamps were removed. Flow was established and an excellent pulse was palpable in the distal popliteal artery, including its branches. One portion of the vein above the lower anastomosis ballooned out, weakened by removal of its adventitial layer. This was imbricated with a 0000 patching suture.

The anastomosis was checked and found to be leakproof. The wound was closed in layers with 000 and 0000 Tevdek on the deep fascia and 0000 Tevdek on the skin. A cotton dressing was applied.

Intimectomy of Right Common Femoral and Deep Femoral Arteries With Autogenous Vein Bypass From Right Common Femoral to Right Popliteal Artery

Indications:

Patient is a known diabetic with severe claudication and rest pain involving the right foot. Angiographic studies revealed complete occlusion of the superficial femoral and the deep femoral artery on the right side with a very narrow popliteal artery with no outflow noted. The operation was a desperate attempt to save the limb.

Technique:

The patient was placed in the supine position and the right leg was prepared and draped in the usual fashion using vi-drape and Tincture of Zephiran. An incision was made along the medial aspect of the lower leg posterior to the tibial ridge. The incision was extended downward until the saphenous vein was identified. It was in good condition. Dissection was carried down further through the crural fascia until the Gastrocnemius was identified and retracted posteriorly. Dissection was carried in the popliteal space where the popliteal vein and artery were identified. Dissection of the popliteal artery was carried out both upward and downward. The anterior tibial artery was noted to be occluded; however, the popliteal artery was thought to be in fairly good condition. The distal outflow tree was thought to be in rather poor condition. There was noted to be some slight amount of backflow through the popliteal artery after a clamp had been placed proximal to a needle injection in the distal popliteal. Attempts at irrigation and suctioning of the distal arterial tree were performed in an attempt to open up thrombosed channels.

The right groin was explored. The right common femoral was identified as well as the saphenous vein. The deep femoral artery and superficial arteries were isolated and slung individually. The incision was carried along the medial aspect of the leg in order to facilitate the dissection of the long saphenous vein. This was removed and its branches clamped and tied with a 0000 Tevdek suture. The vein was found to be in relatively good condition. It was removed and prepared in the usual fashion. Dissection of the groin was completed.

An incision was then made in the right common femoral which was found to be markedly involved with arteriosclerosis. The common femoral was endarterectomized and the deep femoral was identified. The wall of the deep femoral was incised and a large intimal plaque was removed from it. The deep femoral incision was then reconstructed. The saphenous vein was then approximated to the popliteal artery using 00000 Tevdek suture in an end-to-side fashion. After completion of the anastomosis, release of the clamps revealed a watertight anastomosis. The distal arterial tree had been previously heparinized.

A McDonald clamp was then applied to the saphenous vein after it had been flushed with Heparin. The vein was then passed beneath the crural fascia, beneath the tibial plateau, upward into the leg and into the right groin. The vein was then anastomosed to the right common femoral artery in an end-to-side fashion using 00000 Tevdek suture. The remaining incised portion of the common femoral was closed in a longitudinal manner. Distal and proximal clamps were all removed and hemostasis in the proximal anastomosis as well as the distal anastomosis was found to be hemostatic. The blood pulsation in the popliteal flow was quite evident.

The crural fascia was closed throughout its entirety using 000 Tevdek suture. The subcutaneous tissue was closed using interrupted 0000 Tevdek suture. The skin was then closed using an interrupted vertical mattress 00000 Tevdek suture. The groin was closed in a similar fashion.

A dry sterile dressing was applied. The leg was then wrapped in a bulky dressing and Ace bandage.

Crafoord Operation for Coarctation of the Aorta

The patient was placed on the operating table on his right side and sterilely prepared and draped. The left arm was used to raise the scapula anteriorly and upward. A blood transfusion was started.

An incision was made at the level of the 2nd rib and extended to the posterior axillary line, encircling the inferior scapular angle. The incision was deepened through the muscles. The scapula was transected and lifted. The 3rd rib was resected between the midaxillary line and the paravertebral portion. A small paravertebral bite was taken from the 2nd and 4th ribs. The intercostal nerves were resected and the intercostal vessels ligated.

A rib spreader was introduced to separate the ribs. The lung was collapsed and retracted downwards with wet pads.

The mediastinal pleura was incised over the aortic arch exposing the stenosed area. Further ligation of vessels leading to the esophagus and intercostal spaces was carried out. The aorta 4 cm. above and below the stenosis was then clamped with Kochers and the stenosed area resected. The stumps of the aorta were then aligned with the use of the clamps. The lumina of the stumps were washed out. Intima was approximated to intima. The anterior wall was sutured first. Two holding sutures were placed followed by interrupted mattress sutures. The Kochers were then rotated 180 degrees to bring the posterior wall into view. This was likewise sutured. A pressure packing was placed around the suture line and the Kochers released. After a few minutes the packing was removed and the anastomosis checked for leakage. None was found. The pleura was closed with a continuous suture and the wound closed in anatomic layers. A catheter was inserted at the 9th intercostal space just prior to closure of the chest.

Arteriotomy with Removal of Emboli

The operation was begun under 1% Xylocaine. The femoral vessels were exposed through a longitudinal incision. The profunda femoris at the junction with the common femoral artery was identified. There was no pulsation at this point of the artery. The artery did not appear to be in spasm. Its wall was soft and pliable. It was therefore decided that the embolus was higher in the common femoral area, possibly at the bifurcation of the aorta.

The patient was repositioned and spinal anesthesia administered. After redraping the operative field, the incision was carried superiorly, coursing through the inguinal area with division of the fascia and muscles until the retroperitoneal space was reached. The iliac artery was then identified and noted to be pulsating to the point of junction with the hypogastric artery on the right side. At this site, a small induration, thought to represent an embolus, was found. After isolating the artery and freeing it with tape, the artery was clamped with bulldogs. An arteriotomy was done immediately above the bulge at the junction. A 1 X 2 cm. clot was extruded. The inferior clamp was then removed but reconstitution was unobtainable. There was good reconstitution from the hypogastric artery. By gently milking the femoral artery, two small clots were evacuated through the arteriotomy wound. The reconstitution of blood was brisk. The clamps were reapplied and the artery was irrigated with Heparin solution.

The arteriotomy was closed longitudinally with a continuous running 00000 silk suture. There were no leaks through this closure after the clamps were removed. The femoral pulses became readily palpable at the termination of the procedure. The wound was closed in layers with interrupted chromic. The skin was reapproximated with interrupted cotton.

Intimectomy for Leriche's Syndrome

Under spinal anesthesia the patient was prepared and draped in the supine position.

A right pararectus incision was made. The skin was incised from the xiphoid to the pubis. The anterior rectus sheath was incised and the rectus muscle was retracted. The posterior sheath was opened. The aorta was exposed.

Upon palpation of the aorta there was an impulse present approximately 3 inches below the renal artery and distal to that point. The colon and small bowel were grasped and herniated out of the abdomen and retracted superiorly.

An incision along the peritoneum of the aorta and the iliac arteries bilaterally was made with the reflection of the peritoneum away from the vessels. An incision through the anterior portion of the external and internal iliacs was then made in three places bilaterally. One was just proximal to the femoral canal; the other was in the mid-portion of the external iliac; and the other was just proximal to the bifurcation of the iliacs. Following the incisions, the intimectomy knife was used to remove the large calcified plaques present in the center of these vessels. It was noted that pulsations were present in both of the iliacs to the level of the femoral canal after removal of the intima and plaques.

The small and large bowels were packed back into the abdomen. The posterior sheath and peritoneum were closed with 00 continuous lock stitch anteriorly, No. 30 wire double loop suture for the anterior rectus sheath, and 00 chromic interrupted for the subcutaneous tissues. The skin was closed with 000 cotton mattress suture.

Saphenous Vein Ligation and Stripping

Under spinal anesthesia with the patient in a supine position, the lower extremities were prepared and sterilely draped.

A subinguinal incision was made over the fossa ovalis. By blunt and sharp dissection the greater saphenous vein was isolated and its tributaries transected and ligated with 000 silk to the edge of the foramen ovale. The saphenous vein was transected and tied with one 000 cotton. A stick tie of 000 cotton was placed over its base. Beginning at the medial aspect of the ankle, the saphenous vein was unroofed and stripped in a retrograde fashion.

In the area of the knee of the left leg two incisional areas were used to tie off the perforating branches. On the right leg one incision on the medial aspect was made to tie off the perforating branch. Minimal bleeding was encountered.

The fossa ovalis was closed with a purse-string of 000 silk. The subcutaneous tissues were closed with 000 intestinal chromic and the skin was closed with a mattress 000 chromic suture.

Ligation of the External Carotid Artery

The area of the neck was prepared and draped in a sterile manner. It was decided to ligate the external carotid artery between the lingual and the superficial temporal branches of the artery, just below the digastric muscle.

A three inch incision parallel to the course of the artery along the anterior border of the sternocleidomastoid muscle was made. The center of the incision was at the level of the hyoid bone.

Identification was carried out of the hypoglossal nerve and the posterior belly of the digastric muscle. The apex of the great cornu of the hyoid bone was exposed under which the sheath of the artery was incised. The superior laryngeal nerve was identified and avoided immediately below the artery. The external jugular vein and its anastomosis with the facial was likewise identified and avoided. The sternocleidomastoid muscle was identified as was the stylomandibular ligament. After all structures were identified with certainty, a ligature was placed around the external carotid artery and tied.

The wound was closed in layers.

17 ⟩ *The Language of Medicine*

Fluency with a language requires lifelong study and dedicated effort. Thousands of words are being added to the dictionary annually. Advances in the sciences have contributed significantly to this growth with medicine figuring prominently in the development.

Medicine has a language of its own. It is a highly technical and extremely specialized mode of communication. Knowledge of one phase of this language does not assure comprehension of its other subdivisions. How many M.D.'s or D.O.'s would have any suspicion of what a doctor of veterinary medicine might be referring to when he declared that an animal was "fardel-bound with a distended omasum and inflamed abomasum."?

There is a fundamental division of terminology which constitutes the foundation basic to all divisions of medicine. This level of the language includes terms relative to anatomic position, direction and location in addition to commonly used combining forms, prefixes and suffixes. From this beginning it is possible to build a vocabulary of more particularized terms.

Initial exposure to medical terminology might prove discouraging to the student until an orderly system is introduced into the plan of study. The degree of application necessary to develop any proficiency with the language requires the same interest and determination necessary for the study of a foreign language. The element of "want to" must prevail over the element of "have to" in the student's approach to the subject. With continued study, an intelligent curiosity about unfamiliar words and liberal use of the dictionary, the language of medicine eventually becomes comprehensible.

After the student has mastered the rudiments of terminology presented in the following pages, the next step consists of learning human anatomy and physiology. The application of anatomic terms has been demonstrated in the preceding pages. Several excellent textbooks on the subject of anatomy and physiology are available. One of the most popular of such references is ANATOMY AND PHYSIOLOGY by Kimber, Gray, Stackpole and Leavell. Following a study of anatomy, the student will have sufficient background and orientation to develop her vocabulary further in terms of the technical information presented in this book.

364

In the space allotted here, it is impossible to do more than introduce the student to terminology and recommend steps toward further development of this knowledge. The extent to which her vocabulary will grow depends largely upon the effort and energy expended to this end.

Anatomic Position

The anatomic position consists of the body erect, facing us, with the arms at the sides and palms turned toward us. The soles of the feet are comparable anatomically to the palms of the hand and we must therefore imagine the soles of the feet turned upward facing us as are the palms. The aspect of the foot we look down on from above is actually the back of the foot although it is continuous with the front of the body. The front view of the body is regarded as the anterior or ventral aspect and yet the view of the foot continuous with it is the dorsum of the foot rather than the ventral aspect. A stationary uniform position is necessary for the development of references indicating position, direction and aspect.

The suffix -ad is used to indicate direction toward; e.g., caudad, cephalad, anteriad, posteriad, etc.

Basic to the knowledge of medical terminology is proper orientation relative to position and direction. Some of the more frequently used references are listed here with their antitheses.

POSITION REFERENCES

Anterior .... Front view of the body; same as ventral view or face surface.
Posterior .... Back view of the body; same as hind or dorsal aspect.

Inferior .... Located or directed below a point of reference.
Superior .... Located or directed above a point of reference.

Medial (mesial) .. Middle or toward the middle.
Lateral .... Away from the middle, toward the outside aspect.

Distal .... Furthest point from a point of reference.
Proximal .... Nearest point to a point of reference.

Caudal .... Direction away from the head; caudad.
Cranial .... Toward the head or in the region of the head; craniad.

Dorsal .... Back or hind aspect.
Ventral .... Front or face aspect.

Internal .... Inside   Supine .... Lying face up
External .... Outside   Prone .... Lying face down

In addition to the terms listed above, various compounded combinations of these words may be used by dropping the ending of the first word, adding the combining -i or -o and attaching the second word; e.g., mediolateral (median lateral), anterolateral (anterior lateral), posteromedial (posterior medial), dorsoposterior (dorsal posterior), etc.

Elements of Terminology

Medical terms may be analyzed into their component parts consisting of roots, stems, prefixes, infixes, suffixes, combining forms and inflectional endings. In order to build a medical vocabulary the student need not make a study of philology or even etymology, but recognition of the divisions in word structure can do much to promote facility with usage of the language.

Roots constitute the basic word element from which words are derived by one or more extensions comprised of prefixes, suffixes or inflectional changes. The stem is that portion of the word which remains unchanged throughout a given inflection. The root and stem are sometimes identical, although the stem is more often derived from the root with some formative suffix. With the aid of such suffixes, word endings are changed to indicate distinctions of case, gender, mood, person, tense, etc. These changes are called inflectional endings.

Combining forms are used so extensively throughout medical terminology that familiarity with them can assist the student immeasurably in understanding new terms. They consist of a word or word element combined with another word or word element to form a compound. These compounds may assume the form of a simple union between two words; e.g., eyebrow, workman, earache, etc. Compound words may also consist of word unions where o or i have been added to Greek or Latin stems; e.g., abdomino-anterior, abdominohysterectomy, uterosacral, etc.

Prefixes consist of one or more letters placed at the beginning of a word to modify its meaning. Infixes are inserted within the word and suffixes are placed at the end of the word to provide an inflectional, derivative or formative function.

A knowledge of commonly used prefixes and suffixes is basic to the understanding of medical terminology. Those which should prove most helpful have been listed below with some of the more important combining forms.

PREFIXES AND COMBINING FORMS	MEANING	EXAMPLE
a-, an-	negative	avascular (without vessels)
a-, ab-, abs-	away from	abstain
ad-	toward	adduct (bring toward)
aer-	air	aeremia
alb-	white	albino (without pigment)
alge-	pain	algesia (pain sensitivity)
all-	other	allaxis (exchange)
amb-	both	ambidextrous
amph-	all around	amphibious
an-, ana-	up; increase	anabolism (build up)
angio-	blood vessels	angiospasm (vessel spasm)
ante-	before	antepartum (before birth)
anti-	against	antibiotic
apo-	from	aponeurosis (expansion from tendon)
auto-	self	automatic
bi-, bis-	two; double	bistratal (in two layers)
brachy-	short	brachybasia (short steps)
brady-	slow	bradycardia (slow heartbeat)
cardi-	heart	cardiogram (heart test)
cat-, cata-	down	catabolism (breakdown)
cephal-	pert. to head	cephalalgia (headache)
chole-	gallbladder	cholecystitis (inflamed gallbladder)
chrom-	color	chromogenic (producing color)
circum-	around	circumcision
co-, com-, con-	together	combine
contra-	against	contraindicate (warn against)
cyst-	bladder	cystocele
dacry-	tears	dacryocystitis (inflamed tear sac)
dactyl-	fingers	dactyledema (edema of fingers or toes)
de-	from	deduce
demi-	half	demigauntlet (half bandage)
dent-	pert. to teeth	dentist
derma-	skin	dermatology
di-	double; in two forms	dimorphous (two forms)
dia-	between	diaphragm
diplo-	double	diplopia (seeing double)
dis-	negative; double	disjoint
dys-	difficult	dystocia (difficult childbirth)

PREFIXES AND COMBINING FORMS	MEANING	EXAMPLE
en-	in	encapsulated (in a capsule)
endo-	within	endoceliac (within the abdomen)
entero-	intestine	enterocolitis (inflamed intestine)
epi-	upon	epineural (upon neural arch)
eu-	well	euphoria (well-being)
ex-	out	exophthalmos (bulging eyes)
extra-	beyond; outside	extraocular (outside the eye)
fore-	in front of	foreskin
galact-	milk	galactocele (cyst of milk gland)
gastro-	stomach	gastrotomy (stomach incision)
glosso-	tongue	glossoplegia (tongue paralysis)
hemato-	pert. to blood	hematology (study of blood)
hemi-	half	hemiplegia (paralysis on one side)
hepa-	liver	hepatitis (liver infection)
hetero-	dissimilar	heterogenous
holo-	all; entire	holocephalic (entire head)
homo-	same	homogenous
hydro-	water	hydrocephalus (fluid in head)
hyper-	over; above	hypertension (elevated blood pressure)
hypo-	under; below	hypothyroidism (decreased thyroid)
idio-	peculiar to one	idiosyncrasy
ileo-	pert. to ileum	ileocecal
in-	in; into	internal
infra-	beneath	infraorbital (below orbit)
inter-	between	intermittent
intra-	within	intra-abdominal
iso-	equal	isotonic
juxta-	close by	juxtaposition
kera-	hard	keratosis (horny growth)
laryng-	larynx	laryngoscope
latero-	side	laterodeviation
leuko-	white	leukorrhea (white discharge)
lith-	stone	lithiasis
macro-	large; long	macrostomia (large mouth)
mal-	poor; inadequate	malabsorption

PREFIXES AND COMBINING FORMS	MEANING	EXAMPLE
medi-	middle	medicommissure
mega-	large	megacolon (enlarged colon)
melan-	black	melanoma (black neoplasm)
meso-	middle	mesocardia (heart in midline)
meta-	beyond	metaphysics
micro-	small	microscope
mono-	single	monograph
multi-	many	multilobular (many lobed)
myo-	muscle	myositis (inflamed muscle)
myelo-	marrow	myelocystocele
neo-	new	neonate (newly born)
nephro-	kidney	nephrolithiasis (kidney stone)
neuro-	nerve	neurosurgery
non-	not	nonunion
ob-	closing	obstruction
oculo-	eye	oculopathy (eye disease)
odont-	teeth	odontology
omo-	shoulder	omodynia (shoulder pain)
oophoro-	ovary	oophorocystectomy (excision of ovarian cyst)
orchi-	testicle	orchitis (inflamed testis)
ortho-	straight	orthopedics
os-	mouth	ostium (a mouth)
oss-	bone	osseous (bony)
osteo-	bone	osteomyelitis (bone infection)
pan-	all; entire	panhysterectomy (total removal of uterus)
para-	beyond; beside	parahepatic (beside the liver)
path-	disease	pathology
pend-	hang down	pendulous
per-	through	percussion (through tapping)
peri-	around	periosteum (bone covering)
phleb-	vein	phlebothrombosis (vein clot)
pneu-	air	pneumothorax (air in chest)
poly-	many	polychromatic (multicolored)
post-	after	postpartum (after childbirth)
pre-	before	prenatal (before delivery)
pro-	before	prophylactic (preventive)
proct-	anus	proctoscope
pseudo-	false	pseudocyesis (false pregnancy)

PREFIXES AND COMBINING FORMS	MEANING	EXAMPLE
psych-	mind	psychiatry
pyo-	pus	pyosalpinx (pus tubes)
re-	again; back	regain
ren-	kidneys	renal
retro-	backward	retrograde
rhino-	nose	rhinoplasty (nose repair)
sacro-	sacrum	sacrolumbar
salpingo-	tube	salpingitis (inflamed tubes)
sclero-	hard	sclerosis
semi-	half	semilunar (half moon)
sub-	under	subcutaneous (under skin)
super-; supra-	above	superficial
tact-	touch	tactile
thyro-	thyroid	thyrocele (thyroid cyst)
tox-	poison	toxicology
trans-	across	transverse
tri-	three	trilobar (three lobed)
trich-	hair	trichopathic (hair disease)
uni-	one	unilateral (one side)
uro-	urine	urogenital
vaso-	vessel	vasoconstrictor
vesic-	bladder	vesicotomy (bladder incision)
xanth-	yellow	xanthochromic (yellow colored)

SUFFIXES

The prefixes frequently indicate the site of the disease process, operation or point of reference. The suffixes more often indicate the pathology, type of operation or phenomena occurring at the site.

-algesia	pain	analgesia (loss of pain)
-cele	cyst; hernia	cystocele (hernia of bladder wall)
-cide	to kill	germicide
-cyte	cell	lymphocyte
-dynia	pain	coccygodynia (pain in coccyx)
-ectomy	cutting out	splenectomy (cutting out spleen)

-emesis	vomiting	hyperemesis (excessive vomiting)
-emia	blood	uremia (urinary elements in blood)
-esthesia	feeling	anesthesia (without feeling)
-flect	divert	reflect
-form	form	malformed
-fuge	flee; repel	centrifuge
-genetic	form; originate	cytogenic (producing cells)
-gogue	to flow	hemagogue (favoring discharge of blood)
-gram	tracing; graph	electrocardiogram
-iasis	pathologic	amebiasis (amebic infection)
-ism	condition	alcoholism
-itis	inflammation	glossitis (inflamed tongue)
-ize	to treat	adrenalectomize (to remove adrenals)
-kinesis	motion	hyperkinesia (increased mobility)
-lith	stone	cholelith
-logy	study of	hematology (study of blood)
-lysis	separation	enterolysis (separating intestines)
-megaly	very large	acromegaly (enlarged bones)
-meter	measure	centimeter (unit of measure)
-oid	shape	scaphoid (boat-shaped)
-oma	tumor; neoplasm	hepatoma (liver tumor)
-osis	disease	sclerosis
-ostomy	incision into	gastrostomy (stomach incision) with drainage
-otomy	cutting into	ileotomy (incision into ileum)
-pellent	drive	repellent
-penia	deficiency	pancytopenia (deficiency of cell components of the blood)
-phobia	fear	agoraphobia (fear of wide open areas)
-phylaxis	protection	prophylaxis
-plasty	restoration	cineplasty (muscle restoration)
-plegia	stroke; paralysis	hemiplegia (paralysis on one side)
-rhagia	flow	hemorrhage; menorrhagia
-rhaphy	repair	herniorrhaphy
-rhea	discharge	rhinorrhea (nasal discharge)
-sclerosis	hardness	arteriosclerosis
-scopy	to view	cystoscopy (viewing of bladder)
-stomosis	form a mouth	anastomosis
-tomy	cutting	vagotomy (cutting vagus nerves)
-uria	urine	hematuria (blood in urine)

COMMONLY USED MEDICAL ABBREVIATIONS AND SYMBOLS

A_2 .... aortic second sound
abort. .... abortion
a.c. .... before meals
AJ .... ankle jerk
A-P .... anteroposterior
A-P & Lat .... anteroposterior and lateral
A-V .... arteriovenous
abd .... abdomen
accom. .... accommodation
acid p'tase .... acid phosphatase
ad. lib .... at pleasure
alk. p'tase .... alkaline phosphatase
adm. .... admission
alb .... albumin
amp .... ampule
ant. ax line .... anterior axillary line
aort. regurg .... aortic regurgitation
aort. sten .... aortic stenosis
aur. fib. .... auricular fibrillation

b.i.d. .... twice a day
bis .... twice
BM .... bowel movement
BMR .... basal metabolic rate
BP .... blood pressure
BRP .... bathroom privileges
BSP .... bromsulphalein
BUN .... blood urea nitrogen
baso .... basophile
bili .... bilirubin
bl. cult. .... blood culture
br. sounds .... breath sounds

c .... with
CC. .... chief complaint
cc. .... cubic centimeter
cap. .... capsule
CA .... carcinoma
ca .... calcium
cath. .... catheter
CHO .... carbohydrate
chol. .... cholesterol
chol. est. .... cholesterol esters
Cl .... chloride
cldy .... cloudy
cm. .... centimeter (2.5 cm = 1 inch)

COMMONLY USED MEDICAL ABBREVIATIONS AND SYMBOLS

cmpd .... compound
cont .... continued
cta .... catamenia
D & C .... dilation & curettage
DL .... danger list
DIE .... died in Emergency Rm.
DOA .... dead on arrival
decr .... decreased
DERM .... dermatology
diag .... diagnosis
dil .... dilute
dim .... one half (ss)
disch .... discharge
div .... divide
dr. .... dram
EKG .... electrocardiogram
EDC .... estimated date of confinement
EEG .... electroencephalogram
ENT .... ears, nose and throat or **Ear, Nose & Throat** specialty
EOM .... extraocular movement
emul .... emulsion
epith .... epithelium
expir. .... expiration; expiratory
F .... Fahrenheit temperature
FH .... family history
FB .... foreign body
fract. .... fracture
F.U.O. .... fever of undetermined origin

Fetal Position & Presentation:

LOA	left occiput anterior
LOT	left occiput transverse
LOP	left occiput posterior
ROA	right occiput anterior
ROT	right occiput transverse
ROP	right occiput posterior
LSA(RSA)	left sacrum anterior (rt.)
LST(RST)	left sacrum transverse (rt.)
LSP(RSP)	left sacrum posterior (rt.)
LFA(RFA)	left fronto-anterior (right)
LFT(RFT)	left frontotransverse (rt.)
LFP(RFP)	left frontoposterior (rt.)
LMA(RMA)	left mento-anterior (right)
LMT(RMT)	left mentotransverse (right)
LMP(RMP)	left mentoposterior (right)

COMMONLY USED MEDICAL ABBREVIATIONS AND SYMBOLS

GBS .... gallbladder series
G.I. .... gastrointestinal
G.U. .... genito-urinary
Gm. .... gram
gr .... grain
Grav. I .... pregnancy one
gtt. .... drops
Gyn. .... Gynecology

(H) .... per hypo
Hct .... hematocrit
Hgb .... hemoglobin
hpf .... per high powered field
h.s. .... at bedtime

I^{131} .... radioactive iodine
I & D .... incision and drainage
IM .... intramuscular
IQ .... intelligence quotient
IV .... intravenously
IVP .... intravenous pyelogram
incr. .... increase
inspir .... inspiration

K .... potassium
KJ .... knee jerk
KUB .... kidney, ureter & bladder (X-ray =plain film of the
                        abdomen)
Kg. .... kilogram

L .... left
LLL .... left lower lobe (lung)
LUL .... left upper lobe (lung)
LLQ .... left lower quadrant of the abdomen
LUQ .... left upper quadrant of the abdomen
LMP .... last menstrual period
LNMP .... last normal menstrual period
lot .... lotion
LP .... lumbar puncture
l & w .... living and well
lab .... laboratory
lat .... lateral
lb .... pound
lymphs .... lymphocytes

M_1 .... mitral first
mEq .... milliequivalents
mg .... milligram

COMMONLY USED MEDICAL ABBREVIATIONS AND SYMBOLS

med ....medicine
Mg ....magnesium
mg% ....milligrams per 100 milliliters
mitt ....send
ml ....milliliter
mm. ....millimeter
Mn ....manganese
mono ....monocyte

Na ....sodium
NB ....newborn
NB: ....note well
NPN ....nonprotein nitrogen
NPO ....nothing by mouth
NS ....Neurosurgery
noct ....nocturnal

OB ....Obstetrics
O_2 ....oxygen
O_2 cap. ....oxygen capacity
O_2 sat. ....oxygen saturation
O.D. ....right eye
OR ....operating room
O.S. ....left eye
OT ....old tuberculin
O.U. ....both eyes
Ortho. ....Orthopedics

P ....phosphorus
P_2 ....pulmonic second
heart sound
P-A ....postero-anterior
PBI ....protein bound iodine
pc ....after meals
PE ....physical examination
PH ....past history
pH ....hydrogen ion concentration—pH 7.00 = neutral;
pH below 7.00 is acid and above is alkaline
PI ....present illness
p.o. ....by mouth
p.r. ....per rectum
prn ....as often as necessary
Para I ....woman with one child
Ped ....Pediatrics
P & A ....percussion & auscultation
P.T. ....Physical Therapy

COMMONLY USED MEDICAL ABBREVIATIONS AND SYMBOLS

polys .... polymorphonuclear
                  leucocytes
prep. .... preparation
prot .... protein
pro. time .... prothrombin time
pt. .... patient
Pelvic Measurements

(pelvimetry)

    DC .... diagonal conjugate
    OC .... obstetrical conjugate
    bisp .... bispinous diameter (interspinous diameter)
    IT .... intertuberous
    Ant. Sag .... anterior sagittal diameter
    Post. Sag .... posterior sagittal diameter
    A-P D .... anteroposterior diameter
    Trans D .... transverse diameter

PSP .... phenolsulfonphthalein

q .... every
q AM .... every morning
q d .... every day
q.i.d. .... four times daily
q.n. .... every night
q.s. .... as much as suffices
q.n.s. .... quantity not sufficient
q 2 h .... every two hours
q 3 h .... every three hours
quant. .... quantity

rbc .... red blood cell
RBC .... red blood count
Rh .... Rhesus blood factor
RRE .... round, regular and equal
Rx .... therapy
R/O .... rule out

s .... without
SB .... stillborn
SC .... subcutaneous
SH .... social history
sol .... solution
s.o.s. .... repeat once if urgent need exists
SR .... review of systems
ss enema .... soap suds enema
sed. rate .... erythrocyte sedimentation rate

COMMONLY USED MEDICAL ABBREVIATIONS AND SYMBOLS

sp. gr .... specific gravity
spec .... specimen
Staph .... Staphylococcus
stat .... immediately
Strep .... Streptococcus
subling .... under the tongue
SURG .... Surgery; surgical
sympt .... symptoms

tab .... tablet
T & A .... tonsillectomy and adenoidectomy
t.i.d. .... three times per day
TPR .... temp, pulse & resp.
TBC .... tuberculosis

URI .... upper respiratory infection
Urol. .... Urology

vag .... vaginal
VD .... venereal disease

WD, WN .... well developed and well nourished
wbc .... white blood cell
WBC .... white blood count
wt .... weight

MEDICAL SYMBOLS

℥ .... dram
℥ .... ounce
> .... greater than
< .... less than
♀ .... female
♂ .... male

18 } *Style Guide*

Some of the most perplexing problems which beset the secretary have to do with three items classified in the category of style. These include punctuation, capitalization and hyphenization. Many rules have been set down by many authorities with listings of exceptions which always outnumber the rules. There is no universal concurrence on the subject of style. Seldom do two authorities agree completely in all respects. Usage has a great nullifying effect on rules. The degree to which usage is recognized as an important enough factor to warrant exception to a rule likewise varies with authorities.

Those rules which most readily apply to common transcription problems have been listed here.

Formation of Plurals

Numerous situations exist in medical terminology where irregular plural endings are used. The singular and plural endings are given here with medical terms which illustrate these endings.

SINGULAR ENDING	PLURAL ENDING	EXAMPLES (SINGULAR AND PLURAL FORMS)
a	ae	aorta-aortae; verruca-verrucae ampulla-ampullae; pleura-pleurae vertebra-vertebrae; intima-intimae
ax	aces	thorax-thoraces
en	ina	foramen-foramina; lumen-lumina tegmen-tegmina; flumen-flumina
ex	ices	cortex-cortices; vertex-vertices
is	es	anastomosis-anastomoses; testis-testes pubis-pubes; unguis-ungues

SINGULAR ENDING	PLURAL ENDING	EXAMPLES (SINGULAR AND PLURAL FORMS)
is	ides	iris-irides; epulis-epulides
ix	ices	appendix-appendices; varix-varices
on	a	phenomenon-phenomena
u	ua	cornu-cornua; genu-genua
um	a	dorsum-dorsa; curriculum-curricula frenulum-frenula; medium-media infundibulum-infundibula
ur	ora	femur-femora
us	i	annulus-annuli; meniscus-menisci; embolus-emboli; fundus-fundi; alveus-alvei; fungus-fungi; (but: crus-crura)
x	ces	calyx-calyces; falx-falces
y	ies	anomaly-anomalies; biopsy-biopsies; deformity-deformities

Capitalization

We cannot attempt to list rules to cover every conceivable situation where a question regarding the use of a capital letter might arise; however, a list has been prepared to cover the usual instances where problems develop.

Capitalize the First Letter of:

1. Proper nouns (name of a particular person, place or thing) and proper adjectives in English and Latin.
2. Trade-mark names; e.g., Pyrex tube, Ethicon sutures, Teflon, and trade names of drugs.
3. Scientific Latin names but not their English derivatives; e.g., Obliquus abdominis internus (but: internal oblique muscle).
4. Names of genera but not of species; e.g., Escherichia coli, Aerobacter aerogenes, Staphylococcus pyogenes.
5. Derivatives of proper names; e.g., Foley catheter; Jurasz laryngeal forceps; Cantor tube.
6. Abbreviated forms of proper names and titles of tests; e.g., NPN, PBI, IVP, VDRL.

Do Not Capitalize:

1. A common noun or adjective standing in the place of a proper noun; e.g., acid-fast bacilli
2. Words derived from proper nouns which have developed specialized meanings; e.g., platonic, cesarean section, pasteurize, bunsen burner, fallopian tube
3. Usage sanctions the lowercasing of some proper names. When in doubt, consult the dictionary.
4. Units of measurement; e.g., centimeter (cc); ounce (oz.)

Hyphenation

Use of the hyphen is another phase of style which often proves perplexing to the secretary. In recent years the tendency has been away from hyphenation, to the extent possible, but there remain instances when it must be used to prevent misunderstanding or difficulties with pronunciation.

Rules designed to guide the secretary with the use of hyphens in medical and scientific terminology follow.

The Hyphen Is Used:

1. When the first part of the word is a capital letter.

X-ray	Y-incision	Z-plasty
T-tube	U-shaped	S-flap

2. Between three word segments.

cul-de-sac	end-to-end	back-to-back
felo-de-sac	side-to-side	Roux-en-Y

3. To avoid tripling a consonant or doubling a vowel.

grill-like	anti-insulin	intra-abdominal
shell-less	supra-axillary	infra-auricular

4. Between word elements in which the first ends in a vowel and the second begins with a vowel, except the combination of *iu.*

   intero-inferiorly
   para-umbilical   (but: periumbilical)

5. In compound numerals *under 100* when written out.

   forty-five
   six-and-thirty   (but: one hundred and five)

6. Between words expressing fractions when used as adjective modifiers.

    one-half size   one-quarter section

7. With two or more compounds having a common base and used in sequence. The hyphen may be used and the base omitted except for the last word.

    pre- and postoperative   in- and outpatients

The Hyphen Is Not Used:

1. After some prefixes unless followed by a proper noun or proper adjective.

bi-	non-	re-
co-	over-	sub-
ex-	post-	super-
in-	pre-	un-
inter-	pro-	under-

    EXAMPLE: international   BUT: inter-American

2. In chemical terms used as adjectives.

    sodium chloride solution
    hydrochloric acid test

3. In diagnoses or operative titles except as indicated under rules governing use of hyphens.

    gastroenterostomy   NOT: gastro-enterostomy
    panhysterectomy   NOT: pan-hysterectomy

    BUT: salpingo-oophorectomy
             Roux-en-Y anastomosis
             Z-plasty

Problems which cannot be solved with the use of these rules may be resolved with the aid of a dictionary. There are a number of sanctioned uses of hyphenation which are not covered by any of the rules. The occurrence of unwieldy word combinations should alert the secretary to the possibility of hyphenation.

GLOSSARY OF OPERATIVE TITLES

ABBE FLAP—Technique for repair of the lip.

ABDOMINAL PARACENTESIS—Direct drainage of the abdominal cavity with the aid of a trocar and cannula. Technique used to withdraw ascitic fluid accumulating in the abdomen as a result of diseases such as cirrhosis of the liver and carcinoma of the ovary.

ADENOIDECTOMY—Excision of adenoidal tissue from the nasopharynx.

ADRENALECTOMY—Removal of the adrenal gland(s).

ALBEE—Technique for spinal fusion.

ALVEOLECTOMY—Removal of the dental alveolus (tooth socket).

AMPUTATION—Removal of a projecting part of the body such as a limb, penis, breast, fingers or toes.

ANASTOMOSIS—Restoration of continuity to a passage or tube by suturing it in an end-to-side, end-to-end, or side-to-side manner.

ANEURYSMECTOMY—Surgical removal of a sac-like defect from the wall of a blood vessel.

ANEURYSMORRHAPHY—Surgical closure of the sac of an aneurysm.

ANGIECTOMY—Excision of a portion of a blood vessel.

ANGIOPLASTY—Repair and reconstruction of a blood vessel.

ANGIORRHAPHY—Suture of a blood vessel.

ANGIOTOMY—Incision into a blood vessel.

ANOPLASTY—A plastic repair of the anus.

ANOSCOPY—Examination of the anus with a proctoscopic speculum (anoscope).

ANTROTOMY—Incision through the wall of a cavity (antrum)

AORTOTOMY—Incision into the aorta.

APICECTOMY—Excision of the apex of a tooth root.

APICOLYSIS—Artificial collapse of the upper portion of the lung by divesting it of its parietal pleura.

APPENDECTOMY—Removal of the vermiform appendix situated at the distal tip of the cecum.

APPENDICOSTOMY—Incision into the intestine via the vermiform appendix for the purpose of emptying the cecum.

ARGYLL ROBERTSON—Strap operation for ectropion of the eyelid.

GLOSSARY OF OPERATIVE TITLES (Continued)

ARLT—Operation on the eyelid for symblepharon and internal tarsorrhaphy.

ARTERIECTOMY—Excision of segment of an artery.

ARTERIOPLASTY—Repair of an artery.

ARTERIOTOMY—Incision into an artery.

ARTHRECTOMY—Excision of a joint.

ARTHROCENTESIS—Incision into a joint and insertion of a needle for withdrawal of fluid.

ARTHRODESIS—Surgical immobilization of a joint.

ARTHROPLASTY—Repair and reconstruction of a joint.

ARTHROSTOMY—Temporary opening made in a joint.

ARTHROTOMY—Incision into a joint.

ARYTENOIDECTOMY—Excision of arytenoid cartilage of the larynx.

ARYTENOIDOPEXY—Surgical fixation of arytenoid cartilage.

ASPIRATION—Withdrawal of fluid, purulent matter, etc.

ASTRAGALECTOMY—Removal of astragalus (bone of ankle joint).

BAFFES—Inferior vena cava and right pulmonary vein transplant.

BALANOPLASTY—Plastic operation on the glans penis.

BANCROFT-PLENK—Operation for peptic ulcer.

BANKART—Corrective procedure for chronic shoulder dislocation.

BASIOTRIPSY—Crushing operation on the skull of a fetus for delivery when a live infant is impossible.

BASSINI—Technique for inguinal herniorrhaphy.

BAUDELOCQUE—Cutting into posterior cul-de-sac of the vagina for the purpose of removing an ovum in ectopic pregnancy.

BECK—Cardiopericardiopexy.

BECK-JIANU—Gastrostomy for stomach carcinoma.

BEER—Cataract flap operation.

BELFIELD—Cutting into deferent duct.

BERGENHEM—Implantation of ureter into rectum.

BERKE—Ptosis operation on the eyelid.

BILLROTH I—Resection of the pylorus with end-to-end anastomosis of the duodenum and stomach.

BILLROTH II—Resection of the pylorus and most of the lesser curvature of the stomach; closure of open ends of stomach and duodenum with a posterior gastrojejunostomy.

BIOPSY—Removal of a sample of tissue for pathologic examination.

BISCHOFF'S—Abdominal removal of a pregnant uterus.

BLAIR-BROWN—Intermediate skin graft.

BLALOCK (Blalock-Taussig)—Anastomosis of carotid artery, right or left subclavian or innominate artery to the pulmonary artery to increase pulmonary circulation in certain congenital cardiovascular conditions.

BLEPHARECTOMY—Resection of the eyelid.

BLEPHAROPLASTY—Plastic repair or reconstruction of the eyelid.

BLEPHARORRHAPHY—Repair or suturing of an eyelid; (tarsorrhaphy).

BLEPHAROTOMY—Incision into an eyelid.

BLOODGOOD—Technique for inguinal herniorrhaphy.

BONNET—Enucleation of the eyeball.

BORTHEN—Stretching operation of the iris.

BOUILLY—Partial excision of the mucous membrane of the cervix uteri.

BOWMAN—Double needle operation on a cataract, making an opening through the lens at its center and separating the membrane into two halves. Also: slitting of canaliculus of the eye.

BOZEMAN—Operation for uterovaginal fistula.

BRAILEY—Stretching of supratrochlear nerve.

BRAUN—Pinch graft technique.

BRAUER—Breaking up adhesions of the pericardium around the heart.

BRENNER—Inguinal herniorrhaphy technique utilizing the cremaster muscle for support.

BRETT—Osteoperiosteal iliac bone graft.

BROCK—Transventricular valvotomy.

BRONCHOPLASTY—Plastic repair of the bronchus.

BRONCHORRHAPHY—Repair of the bronchus.

BRONCHOSCOPY—Endoscopic examination of the bronchus utilizing a bronchoscope (viewing instrument).

GLOSSARY OF OPERATIVE TITLES (Continued)

BRONCHOSTOMY—Incision into the bronchus with aspiration or removal of contents.

BRONCHOTOMY—Incision into the bronchus.

BROWN-BLAIR—Intermediate split skin graft.

BRUNSCHWIG—Pancreatoduodenectomy; excision of pancreas and a portion of the duodenum adjacent to it.

BUROW—Flap operation used to cover a lip defect.

BURSECTOMY—Excision of a bursa.

CALDWELL-LUC—Window operation; opening made in the canine fossa for removal of contents from maxillary antrum.

CANTHOPLASTY—Plastic repair of the canthus which is the angle where the lids meet on either side of the eye.

CANTHORRHAPHY—Repair of the canthus.

CANTHOTOMY—Splitting operation of the canthus used for lengthening the palpebral fissure (opening between the upper and lower eyelids).

CAPSULECTOMY—Excision of a capsule such as that found on the lens or around the kidney. This also applies to the joint capsule.

CAPSULORRHAPHY—Repair of a capsule, especially a joint capsule.

CAPSULOTOMY—Incision into a capsule.

CARDIOCENTESIS—Surgical puncture of the heart.

CARDIOPLASTY—Repair or plastic reconstruction of the cardiac portion of the stomach; esophagogastroplasty.

CARDIORRHAPHY—Suture repair of the heart muscle.

CARDIOTOMY—Incision into the heart. Incision into the cardia of the stomach.

CARPECTOMY—Excision of carpal bones of the wrist.

CASTRATION—Removal of the testicles in the male or ovaries in the female resulting in sterility.

CATHETERIZATION—Insertion of a narrow tube into a cavity for drainage.

CATTELL—Method of reconstruction in pancreaticoduodenectomy.

CAVERNOSTOMY—Opening made in a cavity to promote drainage. (speleostomy)

CECECTOMY—Resection of the cecum; typhlectomy.

GLOSSARY OF OPERATIVE TITLES (Continued)

CECOCOLOSTOMY—Creation of a communication between the cecum and colon.

CECO-ILEOSTOMY—Creation of a communication between the cecum and ileum.

CECOPEXY—Fixation or securing operation of the cecum.

CECOSIGMOIDOSTOMY—Creation of a connection between the cecum and sigmoid.

CECOSTOMY—Creation of a fistula in the cecum.

CECOTOMY—Incision into the cecum.

CELIOTOMY—Exploratory laparotomy.

CELSUS—Lithotomy operation by cutting of the stone; amputation operation performed with a single circular maneuver of the knife.

CERVICECTOMY—Amputation of the cervix; also called a trachelectomy.

CESAREAN SECTION—Removal of fetus through an abdominal incision and direct incision into the uterus.

CHEILOPLASTY—Plastic repair of the lip.

CHOLECYSTECTOMY—Excision of the gallbladder.

CHOLECYSTODUODENOSTOMY—Creation of a direct connection between the gallbladder and duodenum.

CHOLECYSTOGASTROSTOMY—Creation of a connection between the gallbladder and stomach.

CHOLECYSTORRHAPHY—Repair or suture of the gallbladder.

CHOLECYSTOSTOMY—Incision and drainage of the gallbladder.

CHOLECYSTOTOMY—Incision into the gallbladder, usually for removal of a calculus.

CHOLEDOCHECTOMY—Surgical excision of a portion of the common bile duct.

CHOLEDOCHODUODENOSTOMY—Creation of a communication between the duodenum and common bile duct.

CHOLEDOCHOENTEROSTOMY—Creation of a communication between the common bile duct and a part of the intestine.

CHOLEDOCHOLITHOTOMY—Cutting into the common bile duct for removal of a calculus.

GLOSSARY OF OPERATIVE TITLES (Continued)

CHOLEDOCHOPLASTY—Plastic repair on the common bile duct.

CHOLEDOCHORRHAPHY—Repair of the common bile duct.

CHOLEDOCHOSTOMY—Incision into the common bile duct, usually for drainage.

CHOLEDOCHOTOMY—Incision into the common bile duct for exploration and/or removal of calculus.

CHONDRECTOMY—Excision of a cartilage.

CHOPART—Amputation of the foot through the midtarsal bones.

CHORDOTOMY—Transection of a cord nerve tract for relief of pain.

CIRCUMCISION—Male: Excision of foreskin or prepuce of glans penis. Female: Clitoridotomy.

CLARK—Technique used with subscleral implant for scleral buckling in cases of retinal detachment.

CLAVICOTOMY—Surgical division of the clavicle (collar bone).

CLEIDOTOMY—Separation of the collar bones of the fetus to facilitate delivery.

CLITORIDECTOMY—Excision of the clitoris in the female.

CLITORIDOTOMY—Female circumcision.

CLOSED REDUCTION—Reduction of a fracture or dislocation without incision.

COAKLEY—Frontal sinus operation with scraping of the mucous membrane.

COCCYGECTOMY—Excision of the coccyx (tail bone).

CODIVILLA—Use of tibial osteoperiosteal grafts for insertion around a pseudarthrosis.

COLECTOMY—Resection of the large bowel.

COLOCOLOSTOMY—Surgical formation of a continuity between two anatomically noncontinuous portions of the colon.

COLOPROCTOSTOMY—Creation of a continuity between the rectum and a section of colon not continuous with the rectum anatomically; colorectostomy.

COLOSIGMOIDOSTOMY—Formation of a connection between a portion of the colon and sigmoid.

COLOSTOMY—Formation of an artificial anus by making an opening in the colon and bringing it up through the abdominal wall.

GLOSSARY OF OPERATIVE TITLES (Continued)

COLOTOMY—Incision into the colon.

COLPECTOMY—Excision of the vagina; vaginectomy.

COLPOCLEISIS—Obliteration of the vaginal canal.
COLPOPERINEOPLASTY—Repair of the perineum and vaginal wall.

COLPOPERINEORRHAPHY—Reconstruction of the perineum and vaginal wall.

COLPOPEXY—Suspension of a prolapsed vagina by attachment to the abdominal wall.

COLPOPLASTY—Plastic repair of the vagina; elytroplasty.

COLPORRHAPHY—Tightening of a relaxed vaginal wall and excision of redundant tissue performed as an anterior repair for a cystocele and a posterior repair for a rectocele.

COLPOTOMY—Incision into the vagina; elytotomy.

COMMISSUROTOMY—Surgical division of a fibrous band.
Mitral—Division of scar tissue around the mitral orifice by insertion of a finger with an attached scalpel blade into the mitral orifice.

CONDYLECTOMY—Excision of a condyle (rounded prominence at the articular surface of the bone).

CONJUNCTIVOPLASTY—Plastic repair of the mucous membrane which covers the anterior surface of the eyeball.

CORDOPEXY—Fixation to a side of one or both vocal cords for the relief of laryngeal stenosis.

COREOPLASTY—Plastic repair of a deformed pupil.

COTTING—Excision of tissue on either side of a persistent ingrowing toenail.

COSTECTOMY—Excision of a rib.

COSTOTRANSVERSECTOMY—Excision of the transverse process of a vertebra with its adjacent rib.

CRANIECTOMY—Excision of a section of the skull (cranium).

CRANIOCLASIS—Crushing of the fetal skull to facilitate removal of the dead fetus from the uterus.

CRANIOPLASTY—Plastic repair of a defect of the cranium (skull).

CRANIOTOMY—(Trephination). Boring of a hole in the skull for purposes of decompression, biopsy, aspiration of the brain, etc.

GLOSSARY OF OPERATIVE TITLES (Continued)

CRICOTRACHEOTOMY—Incision separating the cricoid cartilage and the upper rings of the trachea for emergency respiratory relief because of occlusion of the glottis.

CRITCHETT—Resection of anterior eyeball.

CROSBY-COONEY—Drainage of ascites (fluid accumulation) in the abdomen by means of a glass tube.

CURETTAGE—A scraping operation performed within a cavity for purposes of cleaning, debriding or biopsy.

CYCLODIALYSIS—Formation of a connection between the anterior chamber of the eye and the suprachoroidal space to relieve pressure within the eye.

CYCLODIATHERMY—Electrocoagulation of the ciliary body of the eye by use of heat produced by a high frequency current.

CYSTECTOMY—Resection of the bladder, usually the urinary bladder; (gallbladder removal—cholecystectomy); removal of a cyst.

CYSTOLITHOTOMY—Endoscopic removal of a calculus with a cystoscope.

CYSTOPLASTY—Surgical repair of a bladder defect.

CYSTORRHAPHY—Bladder repair.

CYSTOSCOPY—Endoscopic (viewing instrument with lighted tip) examination of the urinary bladder. With various attachments the cystoscope may be used for biopsy, crushing of calculi, fulguration of tumor, etc.

CYSTOSTOMY—Surgical opening made into a bladder for purposes of drainage through an abdominal incision.

CYSTOTOMY—Incision into the bladder, usually suprapubic, through the abdominal wall.

CZERNY—Radical herniorrhaphy.

DACRYOADENECTOMY—Excision of the lacrimal gland.

DACRYOCYSTECTOMY—Excision of the lacrimal sac.

DACRYOCYSTORHINOSTOMY—Formation of a communication between the lacrimal sac and nasal cavity to facilitate drainage.

DACRYOCYSTOSTOMY—Drainage of the lacrimal sac.

DACRYOCYSTOTOMY—Incision into the lacrimal sac.

DANA—Resection of the posterior spinal nerve roots for alleviation of pain.

DAVIEL—Incision into the capsule of the lens for removal of a cataract.

GLOSSARY OF OPERATIVE TITLES (Continued)

DAVIS GRAFT—Thick pinch graft of skin.

DEBRIDEMENT—Freshening and cleansing of a wound by removal of all friable, necrotic and nonviable tissue.

DECOMPRESSION—Relief of pressure.

DECORTICATION—Removal of the outer layer of an organ, usually the lung.

DEPAGE-JANEWAY—Gastrostomy for carcinoma of the stomach.

DESMOTOMY—Incisional division of a ligament.

DIAPHYSECTOMY—Partial removal of a bone, particularly the shaft of a long bone.

DICKEY—Operation for ptosis of the eyelid.

DIEFFENBACH-WARREN—Technique for palatoplasty.

DILATION—Enlargement of a canal by stretching with the aid of a dilator. Also: dilatation.

DISARTICULATION—Removal of a limb through a joint without incision through a bone.

DISCISSION—Needling as a destructive procedure, usually used in soft cataract over the lens.

DIVERTICULECTOMY—Excision of a diverticulum (abnormal pouch) in the contour of an organ such as the intestine or bladder.

DOUGLAS GRAFT—Full thickness sieve skin graft.

DRAGSTEDT—Accordion skin graft.

DRUMMOND-MORISON—Operation for the formation of anastomosis between portal venous and systemic circulation to relieve ascites.

DUDLEY—A splitting operation on the cervix uteri; suspension operation on the uterus with shortening of the round ligaments.

DÜHRSSEN INCISION—Three surgical incisions into the cervix at 2, 6 and 10 o'clock for purposes of rapid dilation to facilitate delivery of the infant.

DÜHRSSEN'S OPERATION—Fixation of the uterus to the vagina.

DUODENECTOMY—Resection of the duodenum (first portion of small intestine).

DUODENOCHOLEDOCHOTOMY—Cutting into the common bile duct and proximal duodenum.

GLOSSARY OF OPERATIVE TITLES (Continued)

DUODENOCHOLEDOCHOSTOMY—Formation of a communication between the common bile duct and the duodenum.

DUODENODUODENOSTOMY—Formation of a communication between two noncontinuous portions of the duodenum.

DUODENOENTEROSTOMY—Formation of a communication between the duodenum and another portion of the intestine such as the jejunum, ileum, duodenum, etc.

DUODENORRHAPHY—Repair of the duodenum following perforation or tear.

DUODENOSTOMY—Incision into the duodenum, usually for drainage.

DUODENOTOMY—Cutting into the duodenum, usually for exploration.

DUPUY-DUTEMPS—Technique of dacryocystorhinostomy.

DURAPLASTY—Plastic repair of the outer layer (dura mater) enveloping the brain.

ECK'S—End-to-end anastomosis between portal vein and inferior vena cava.

EDEBOHLS—Stripping of kidney capsule to promote better vascular supply.

ELECTROCOAGULATION—Passage of high frequency current through tissue producing coagulation of tissue cells and also destruction of tissue.

ELLIOT—Trephination of the eyeball for relief of tension as associated with glaucoma.

ELLIS—Bilateral vagotomy plus procedure for excision of esophageal stricture and esophagogastric junction with resection of distal end of stomach with antrum and reconstruction of continuity by esophagogastrostomy and gastroduodenostomy of Schoemaker, Billroth I type.

EMBOLECTOMY—Incision into a blood vessel for removal of an embolus (plug usually made up of portion of a blood clot which has broken off a thrombus).

EMMETT—Operation for suture of the cervix.

ENDOSCOPY—Examination of a body cavity by introduction of a scope with a lighted tip; includes specific examinations such as bronchoscopy, laryngoscopy, cystoscopy, proctoscopy, etc.

ENTERECTOMY—General term for resection of a portion of the intestine (enteron); specifically it may be a duodenectomy, jejunectomy, ileectomy, etc.

ENTEROENTEROSTOMY—General term for an anastomosis formed surgically between two noncontinuous sections of the intestine; more specifically, it may be a duodenoduodenostomy, jejunojejunostomy, etc.

GLOSSARY OF OPERATIVE TITLES (Continued)

ENTEROLYSIS—Division of adhesions between intestines.

ENTEROPEXY—Suspension or attachment, for purposes of fixation, of a portion of intestine to the abdominal wall.

ENTERORRHAPHY—Suturing of an intestine for closure purposes.

ENTEROSTOMY—Formation of an orifice for excretion of feces through the abdominal wall by bringing the intestine up through the wall and making an opening; specifically, called a colostomy, ileostomy, etc.

ENTEROTOMY—Incision into an intestine.

ENUCLEATION—Shelling out of an organ, cyst or tumor in toto.

EPIDIDYMECTOMY—Removal of the epididymis (portion of the excretory duct of the testes).

EPIDIDYMOTOMY—Incision into the epididymis.

EPIDIDYMOVASOSTOMY—Formation of a communication between the epididymis and vas deferens when obstruction occurs in the ductus deferens leading from the epididymis to the prostatic urethra.

EPIGASTRIC HERNIORRHAPHY—Repair of a defect in the wall of the middle upper region of the abdomen.

EPIGLOTTIDECTOMY—Excision of the epiglottis (cartilaginous plate which closes over the windpipe opening in the process of swallowing).

EPILATION—Extraction of hair from the eyelid, face etc. (depilation)

EPIPLOECTOMY—Excision of omentum (epiploon).

EPIPLOPEXY—Suturing of the omentum to the abdominal wall.

EPIPLORRHAPHY—Suturing of the omentum.

EPISIOTOMY—Incision of the vulva prior to delivery to facilitate delivery and prevent laceration.

ESOPHAGECTOMY—Resection of the esophagus.

ESOPHAGODUODENOSTOMY—Surgical formation of a continuity between the esophagus and the duodenum.

ESOPHAGOGASTROSTOMY—Surgical formation of a communication between the stomach and esophagus.

ESOPHAGOPLASTY—Plastic repair of the esophagus.

ESOPHAGOSCOPY—Endoscopic (use of scope) examination of the esophagus.

ESOPHAGOTOMY—An incision into the esophagus.

GLOSSARY OF OPERATIVE TITLES (Continued)

ESSER—Operation for epithelial inlay.

ESTES—Therapeutic operation for sterility consisting of implantation of an ovary into a uterine cornu.

ESTLANDERS—Operation performed for empyema (accumulation of pus in pleural cavity) in which ribs and involved pleura are excised to permit collapse of the abnormal cavity.

ETHMOIDECTOMY—Resection operation of the ethmoid sinuses.

EVERBUSCH—Procedure for correcting ptosis of the eyelid.

EXCISION—Cutting out; surgical incisional removal.

EXENTERATION—Surgical removal of the contents (anatomic) of an organ or cavity; procedure for bringing the bowel up through the abdominal wall.

EXPLORATORY—Procedure performed in search for pathology; exploratory laparotomy of the abdomen.

EXTERIORIZATION—Temporary exposure of a viable organ by bringing it outside the body cavity, e.g., exteriorization of bowel.

EXTIRPATION—Removal of a structure or mass in toto.

EXTRACTION—Process of removal by drawing or pulling out.

FALK-SHUKURIS—Hysterectomy with cornual excision by means of a transverse fundal incision.

FARABEUF—Surgical division of the ischiopubic ramus and ascending ramus of the pubes.

FASCIECTOMY—Excision of fascia.

FASCIODESIS—Suturing of fascia to a skeletal attachment.

FEHLING—Operation on the anterior vaginal wall for prolapse of the uterus.

FEMORAL HERNIORRHAPHY—Repair of a femorocele or bulging defect in the crural or upper thigh region.

FENESTRATION—Formation of a window or opening; operation to improve hearing in cases of otosclerosis by making an opening into the labyrinth.

FERGUSON REPAIR—Technique for repair of an inguinal hernia.

FERGUSSON—Excision of the upper jaw bone (maxilla).

FINNEY—Formation of an enlarged opening between the stomach and duodenum. Finney modification of von Haberer-Billroth I.

GLOSSARY OF OPERATIVE TITLES (Continued)

FINOCHIETTO—Method of Billroth I.

FINSTERER—Modification of Billroth II.

FINSTERER-HOFMEISTER—Gastric resection in gastric carcinoma or duodenal ulcer.

FISTULECTOMY—Excision of a fistula (abnormal communication between two cavities or a hollow organ and the abdominal wall).

FISTULOTOMY—Incision into a fistula.

FOERSTER—Operation performed in locomotor ataxia which involves transsection intradurally of the 7th, 8th and 9th dorsal nerve roots.

FOERSTER-PENFIELD—Removal of scar tissue from the brain in an attempt to treat traumatic epilepsy.

FOLEY—Procedure for relief of ureteropelvic junction stricture consisting of a Y-plasty operation.

FOTHERGILL—Suspension of the cardinal ligaments for relief of uterine prolapse. Manchester operation.

FOWLER—Decortication of the lung in pulmonary empyema.

FOX—Operation for senile entropion.

FRANCO—Incision into the urinary bladder via an abdominal route.

FRANK—Gastrostomy with formation of a communication of the stomach and chest wall through which a tube is inserted.

FRANKE'S—Removal of intercostal nerves in cases of tabes.

FREDET-RAMSTEDT—Pyloroplasty consisting of a longitudinal incision of the thickened serosa and muscularis in cases of pyloric stenosis.

FREUND'S—Total removal of the uterus for cancer; surgical division of cartilage in funnel chest deformity.

FREYER'S—Suprapubic enucleation of prostate.

FRIEDRICH'S—In cases of unilateral tuberculosis, removal of ribs on one side of chest to cause collapse of the lung. Pleuropneumonolysis.

FROMMEL'S—Operation for correcting the retrodisplacement of the uterus by shortening the uterosacral ligaments.

FROST-LANG—Insertion of a gold ball prosthesis for cosmetic purposes following enucleation of the eyeball.

FUCH'S—Technique for tarsorrhaphy.

FUKALA—Lens removal in severe nearsightedness.

GLOSSARY OF OPERATIVE TITLES (Continued)

FULGURATION—Utilization of sparks from a d'Arsonval current for destruction of tissue.

FUSION—Operation for uniting two structures as in spinal fusion where an immobilization of two segments of the bony spine is formed.

GALBIATI'S—Bilateral ischiopubiotomy performed on a fetus to facilitate delivery in contracted pelvis.

GANGLIONECTOMY—Excision of a ganglion which may be a collection of nerve cells or may manifest the form of a cystic tumor of a tendon sheath.

GANT'S—Division of the shaft of the long thigh bone below the lesser trochanter to cause ankylosis of the hip joint.

GASTRECTOMY—Resection of the stomach.

GASTRODUODENOSTOMY—Surgical formation of a communication between the stomach and the duodenum.

GASTROGASTROSTOMY—Communication formed surgically between the pylorus and cardiac portion of the stomach.

GASTROJEJUNOSTOMY—Formation of a communication between the stomach and the jejunum.

GASTROMYOTOMY—Incision through the muscular wall of the stomach (pylorus).
GASTRORRHAPHY—Repair of a stomach wound.

GASTROSCOPY—Examination of the interior stomach by means of a scope inserted via the mouth and esophagus.

GAUNTLET FLAP—A plastic procedure using a piece of tissue connected at one end to its original site. Used to cover a defect of the hand and fingers.

GENYPLASTY—Plastic operation on the cheek (of the face).

GERSUNY—Operation performed on the rectum for incontinence of feces; performed also on female urethra for urinary incontinence.

GIFFORD—Incision into the cornea.

GIFFORD-PUNTENNY—Procedure for correcting ptosis of the eyelid.

GIGLI—Sectioning of the os pubis with a Gigli chain saw to facilitate delivery of the fetus.

GILL—Insertion of a wedge of bone to limit plantar flexion in cases of foot drop (paralysis of dorsiflexor muscles of foot causing toes to drag in walking).

GILLIES GRAFT—A tube graft.

GLOSSARY OF OPERATIVE TITLES (Continued)

GILLIAM—Operation on the round ligaments for suspension of the uterus in cases of uterine retroversion.

GILLIES OPERATION—Use of an epithelial flap to form skin of the eyelid in ectropion of the eyelid.

GINGIVECTOMY—Excision of a section of the gums of the mouth.

GOEBEL-STOECKEL—Suspension of the uterus.

GLOSSECTOMY—Resection of the tongue.

GOFFE—Operation for correction of cystocele (defect in anterior vaginal wall).

GONIN—In cases of retinal detachment, closure of the laceration by electrocautery.

GONIOTOMY—Operation performed in certain cases of glaucoma consisting of the opening of Schlemm's canal under direct vision.

GOTTSCHALK—Shortening of uterosacral ligaments suspending uterus via the vaginal route.

GRABER-DUVERNAY—Boring holes leading to the center of the femoral head for the purpose of promoting circulation.

GRAFT—Implantation of skin, bone, tissue, etc. for the purpose of correcting a defect.

GRANT'S—Operation for excision of tumor of the lip and reapproximating the lip edges cosmetically.

GRATTAGE—Removal of diseased tissue by scraping or abrasion.

GRITTI-STOKES—Supracondylar amputation of the femur with preservation of the patella.

GROSSMAN—Operation for treatment of retinal detachment by withdrawal of subretinal fluid and injection of warm salt solution into the vitreous.

GUSSENBAUER—Cutting through an esophageal stricture from an esophagotomy made above the obstruction.

GUYON—Amputation of the foot.

HAGNER—Epididymotomy for purposes of drainage.

HAHN—Gastrotomy with correction of gastric stenosis.

HALPIN—Operation for removal of lacrimal gland in toto.

HALSTED—Technique for inguinal herniorrhaphy.

HANCOCK—Amputation of the foot at the ankle joint.

GLOSSARY OF OPERATIVE TITLES (Continued)

HANDYSIDE—Ovariotomy.

HARTLEY-KRAUSE—Removal of gasserian ganglion and its roots.

HAYNES—Drainage of cisterna magna in meningitis.

HEATH—An operation performed in the mouth with division of the ascending rami of the lower jaw for ankylosis.

HEATON—Technique for inguinal herniorrhaphy.

HEGAR—Technique for perineorrhaphy.

HEINE—Operation for relieving pressure in glaucoma. (cyclodialysis)

HEINEKE—Operation for cancer of the rectum.

HEINEKE-MIKULICZ—Technique for pyloroplasty.

HEISRATH—Operation for trachoma of conjunctiva and cornea by excision of the tarsal folds.

HELLER—Esophagocardiomyotomy.

HEMIGLOSSECTOMY—Resection of half of the tongue.

HEMILAMINECTOMY—Resection of laminae of the vertebra of one side only.

HEMILARYNGECTOMY—Resection of a half of the larynx.

HEMINEPHRECTOMY—Resection of a part of the kidney.

HEMITHYROIDECTOMY—Subtotal resection of the thyroid.

HEMORRHOIDECTOMY—Excision of infected rectal varices.

HEPATECTOMY—Resection of a portion of the liver.

HEPATICODUODENOSTOMY—Formation of a communication between the hepatic duct and the duodenum.

HEPATICOGASTROSTOMY—Formation of a communication between the hepatic duct and the stomach.

HEPATICOLITHOTOMY—Cutting into the hepatic duct for the purpose of removing calculi.

HEPATICOSTOMY—Opening made into the hepatic duct.

HEPATORRHAPHY—Repair of the liver.

HERBERT—Formation of a filtering cicatrix in glaucoma using a displaced wedge-shaped portion of sclera.

GLOSSARY OF OPERATIVE TITLES (Continued)

HERNIORRHAPHY—Repair of a weakened body wall which has permitted bulging of cavity contents.

HERNIOTOMY—Operation for repair of hernia; kelotomy, celotomy.

HEWETT—Ligation of the oviduct in three sections for the purpose of producing sterility.

HEY—Foot amputation with the incision made just before the tarsometatarsal joint.

HIBBS—Operation performed for stabilizing the spine or hip. Hibbs spinal fusion; Hibbs arthrodesis of the hip.

HOCHENEGGE—Rectal operation for carcinoma.

HOFFA (Hoffa-Lorenz)—Operation for congenital dislocation of the hip.

HOFMEISTER-FINSTERER—Gastric resection with gastrojejunostomy.

HOFMEISTER-POLYA—Antecolic gastrojejunostomy.

HOLMES—Operation for excision of the os calcis.

HOLTH—Punch operation for removal of sclera of the eye.

HORSLEY—Method of Billroth I and pyloroplasty.

HOTCHKISS—Plastic repair of facial defect in the cheek region.

HOTZ-ANAGNOSTAKIS—Procedure for correcting entropion of the eyelid.

HUGGINS—Castration operation performed for carcinoma of the prostate.

HUGHES—Operation for lower lid repair.

HUGIER—Right lateral incision into the colon.

HUNT—Technique of inguinal herniorrhaphy.

HUNTER—Operation for relief of aneurysm with ligation of the vessel proximal to the defect.

HUNT-TONSLEY—Repair of ptosis of the eyelid.

HYMENOTOMY—Incision with enlargement of the hymenal ring in an imperforate hymen (membranous tissue covering the external vaginal orifice).

HYPOPHYSECTOMY—Excision of the pituitary body.

HYSTERECTOMY—Removal of the uterus, totally or partially, either through an abdominal or vaginal route.

HYSTEROTOMY—Incision into the uterus.

GLOSSARY OF OPERATIVE TITLES (Continued)

ILEECTOMY—Surgical resection of the distal portion of the small intestine (ileum). DO NOT CONFUSE WITH ILIUM (hip bone).

ILEOCECOSTOMY—Formation of a surgical communication between the ileum and cecum.

ILEOCOLOSTOMY—Formation of a surgical communication between the ileum and colon.

ILEOILEOSTOMY—Formation of a communication between two parts of the ileum.

ILEOSIGMOIDOSTOMY—Formation of the communication between the ileum and sigmoid flexure.

ILEOSTOMY—A surgical opening made into the ileum.

IMPLANT OPERATION—Insertion of a prosthesis to simulate a normal anatomic structure or contour.

IMRE—Procedure for correcting ectropion and repair of lid notch.

INCUDECTOMY—Surgical removal of the incus (one of the three ossicles of the middle ear, often referred to as the "anvil").

INDIAN OPERATION—Plastic operation for covering a nasal defect with a flap taken from the forehead.

INGUINAL HERNIORRHAPHY—Repair of a hernia in the groin.

ITALIAN OPERATION—Plastic operation for repair of a nasal defect with a flap taken from the arm.

INTERCRICOTHYROTOMY—Inferior laryngotomy; incision into the larynx through the cricothyroid membrane.

INTERPOSITION—Suspension operation on the uterus for correction of a positional defect; hysteropexy.

IRIDECTOMY—Excision of a portion of the iris (pigmented circular band around the pupil).

IRIDENCLEISIS—Displacement of the pupil by constriction of a portion of the iris in an incision of the cornea.

IRIDODIALYSIS—Detachment of the outer edge of the iris from its ciliary attachment.

IRIDOTASIS (Borthen Operation)—Stretching operation of the iris performed in glaucoma.

IRIDOTOMY—Incision into the iris.

GLOSSARY OF OPERATIVE TITLES (Continued)

ISCHIATIC HERNIOPLASTY—Repair of a hernia in the hip region.

ISTHMECTOMY—Excision of the isthmus of the thyroid gland; median strumectomy.

JABOULAY—Interpelvi-abdominal amputation.

JACOBAEUS—Endoscopic examination for pleural adhesions followed by lysis of adhesions with electrocautery.

JANSEN—Operation on the frontal sinus with scraping of the mucous membrane.

JARVIS—Snare removal of hypertrophic area on the lower turbinate.

JASCHE-ARLT—Procedure for entropion repair.

JAYAPATHY—Repair of tympanic membrane perforation.

JEJUNECTOMY—Resection of all or a portion of the small intestine known as the jejunum.

JEJUNOCECOSTOMY—Formation of a communication between the jejunum and the cecum.

JEJUNOCOLOSTOMY—Formation of a communication between the jejunum and the colon.

JEJUNOILEOSTOMY—Formation of a surgical communication between continuous portions of the jejunum.

JEJUNOJEJUNOSTOMY—Formation of a communication between two non-continuous portions of the jejunum.

JEJUNORRHAPHY—Repair of a wound or perforation of the jejunum.

JEJUNOSTOMY—Formation of a surgical opening into the jejunum through the abdominal wall.

JEJUNOTOMY—Incision into the jejunum.

JELK—Incisions made on both sides of the anus with incision of the rectum for relieving rectal stricture.

JIANU-BECK—Gastrostomy for carcinoma of the stomach.

JOBERT de LAMBELLE—Closure of vesicovaginal fistula.

JOLY—Total hysterectomy (panhysterectomy) for uterine prolapse.

JONNESCO—Excision of sympathetic ganglion on both sides of the neck for exophthalmic goiter.

JUDD—Pyloroplasty.

GLOSSARY OF OPERATIVE TITLES (Continued)

JUMP GRAFT—Transferring a pedicle graft from one location to another in stages.

JUDIN—Closure of duodenal stump.

KADER—Gastrostomy for carcinoma of the stomach.

KADER-SENN—Surgical formation of a gastric fistula.

KEEGAN—Plastic operation for reconstruction of the nose utilizing tissue from one side of the forehead for the flap.

KEEN—Excision of the umbilicus (navel).

KEHR—Resection of the gallbladder and cystic duct followed by drainage of the hepatic duct.

KEHRER—Correction of an inverted nipple.

KELLY—Fixation of the uterus to the anterior abdominal wall for correction of retroversion.

KERATECTOMY—Excision of a portion of the cornea of the eye.

KERATOCENTESIS—Puncture of the cornea.

KERATOPLASTY—Plastic operation on the cornea; e.g., corneal grafting, trephination, tissue replacement, etc.

KERATOTOMY—Surgical incision into the cornea.

KILLIAN—Operation on the frontal sinus with removal of the anterior wall, mucous membranes and ethmoid cells. The upper wall of the orbit is also removed with formation of a communication to the nose.

KING—Fixation of the arytenoid cartilage or muscle.

KIRMISSON—Operation for clubfoot with transplantation of the Achille's tendon to the Peroneus longus muscle.

KIRSCHNER—Operation for ruptured spleen.

KJELLAND—Cystocele repair.

KNAPP—Cataract removal without iridectomy.

KOCHER—Excision of ankle joint with suturing of the peroneal tendons.

    Resection of pylorus.
    Thyroidectomy technique.
    Reduction of dislocated humerus.
    Resection of the tongue.
    Resection of the wrist.

GLOSSARY OF OPERATIVE TITLES (Continued)

KOCK—Corrective operation for uterine prolapse or retroversion with shortening of the base of the broad ligament via a vaginal approach.

KOEBERLE—Fixation of the uterus to the anterior abdominal wall for the correction of retroversion.

KONDOLEON—Therapeutic operation in elephantiasis consisting of removal of strips of subcutaneous connective tissue.

KÖNIG—Operation for correction of congenital dislocation of the hip with reduction of the dislocation and formation of a ring-like projection on the upper border of the acetabulum, fashioned from osteoperiosteal flap taken from the ilium.

KÖRTE-BALLANCE—Operation for relief of facial paralysis consisting of anastomosis of the hypoglossal and facial nerves.

KORTZEBORN—Lengthening of extensor tendons of thumb and formation of a fascial attachment of the thumb to the ulnar side of the hand to relieve "ape hand" deformity.

KRASKE—Surgical approach to the rectum by resection of the coccyx and portion of the sacrum.

KRAUSE—Gasserian ganglionectomy in trigeminal neuralgia.

KRAUSE-WOLFE GRAFT—Full-thickness skin graft.

KRIMER—Palatoplasty; uranoplasty.

KRÖNLEIN—Removal of a portion of the lateral wall of the orbit for removal of tumor without sacrificing the eye.

KUHNT—Frontal sinus operation with resection of the anterior wall and scraping of the mucous membrane.

KUHNT-HELMHOLD—Repair of atonic ectropion of the eyelid.

KUHNT-SZYMANOWSKI—Operation for repair of atonic ectropion of eyelid.

KUSTER—Drainage procedure in mastoiditis with exposure of the antrum, attic and tympanum.

LABBE—Incision into the stomach utilizing a parietal incision along the border of the lowest left rib.

LABYRINTHECTOMY—Excision of the internal ear (labyrinth).

LAGLEYZE—Eyelid repair.

LAGRANGE—Establishment of a filtering scar in glaucoma through a combination sclerectomy and iridectomy.

GLOSSARY OF OPERATIVE TITLES (Continued)

LAHEY—Anterior gastrojejunostomy.

LAMINECTOMY—Excision of the flattened posterior aspect of the vertebral arch from which the spinous processes project.

LANDOLT—Plastic construction of the lower eyelid, the upper eyelid acting as the donor site for the skin graft.

LANE—A short-circuit type operation in which the ileum is attached to the lower portion of the sigmoid, circumventing the colon.

LANE-LANNELONGUE—Decompression of the brain with removal of sections of the bone from the roof of the skull.

LANGE—Implantation of silk strands to simulate tendon transplantation.

LANNELONGUE—Method of craniotomy employed where the head is abnormally small.

LANZ—Insertion of strips of fascia lata into the femur for relief of elephantiasis of the leg.

LAPAROTOMY—Incision through the abdominal wall usually performed for exploration of the abdominal contents.

LAROYENNE—Incision into the uterosacral excavation (pouch of Douglas) for the purpose of permitting drainage of purulent matter.

LARRY—Operation for amputation of the arm by disarticulation of the humerus at the shoulder joint.

LARYNGECTOMY—Removal of the larynx (voice organ).

LARYNGOCENTESIS—Incision into the larynx.

LARYNGOPHARYNGECTOMY—Excision of the larynx and pharynx.

LARYNGOPLASTY—Plastic repair of the larynx.

LARYNGOSCOPY—Endoscopic examination of the inner larynx by means of a laryngoscope.

LARYNGOTRACHEOTOMY—Surgical incision of the larynx and the respiratory tube (trachea) situated just below it.

LATZKO—Extraperitoneal cesarean section.

LAUREN—Plastic closure of defect remaining following mastoidectomy.

LEFEVRE—Method of esophagojejunostomy.

LEFORT—Operation for correction of prolapse of the uterus.

GLOSSARY OF OPERATIVE TITLES (Continued)

LEGG—Tensor fascia transplantation into the femur.

LENNANDER—Operation for dissecting out the inguinal glands.

LERICHE—Periarterial sympathectomy.

LEUCOTOMY—Prefrontal lobotomy of the brain.

LEXER—Resection of gasserian ganglion of the trigeminal nerve.

LIGATION—Operation for tying off a segment of a vascular channel or tubular structure.

LIPECTOMY—Excision of adipose tissue.

LISFRANC—Amputation of the foot with incision between the tarsus and the metatarsus.

LISTON—Method of resection of the upper jaw.

LITHOLAPAXY—Crushing of a calculus within the bladder with a cystoscopic approach followed by irrigation and flushing out of the fragments.

LITHOTOMY—Incision into an organ for removal of a calculus.

LITHOTRIPSY—Procedure for crushing a calculus in the bladder or urethra.

LITHOTRITY—Procedure for crushing a stone situated in the urinary bladder or urethra.

LITTRE—Method of incision into the colon through an inguinal incision.

LIZAR—Operation for resection of the upper jaw.

LOBECTOMY—Excision of a projecting part of an organ or gland such as a lobe of the lung or lobe of the thyroid gland.

LOBOTOMY—Cutting into a nerve tract in the cerebrum of the brain. An incision into a lobe.

LONGMIRE—Surgical connection of an intrahepatic biliary duct to the jejunum after partial removal of the left lobe of the liver to relieve obstruction of the hepatic duct or common bile duct.

LONGUET—Transplantation operation of testicle in the presence of varicocele and hydrocele.

LORENZ—Operation for congenital dislocation of the hip consisting of reduction of dislocation and fixing femur in position until a proper socket can be formed in the acetabulum.

LORETA—Gastrotomy with dilation of stenotic stomach opening. Also: Treatment of aneurysm by insertion of wire and electrolysis.

GLOSSARY OF OPERATIVE TITLES (Continued)

LOSSEN—Resection of the second division of the fifth nerve.

LUC (Caldwell-Luc Operation)—Incision into the maxillary sinus antrum (antrum of Highmore) for the purpose of drainage.

LUND—An operation for correcting a clubfoot (talipes) deformity by removal of the talus bone (astragalus or ankle bone).

LUDLOFF—An operation for correcting a hallux valgus deformity by an oblique incision into the first metatarsal bone.

LYMPHATICOSTOMY—Surgical opening made into a lymphatic duct.

LYON-HORGAN—An operation performed for the relief of angina pectoris consisting of severance and ligation of the superior and inferior thyroid arteries, bilaterally.

MACDOWELL—Resection of an ovary by abdominal section.

MACEWEN—An operation for knock-knee consisting of supracondyloid incision into the femur.

MACHEK-BLASKOVICS—Procedure for correcting entropion.

MACHEK-GIFFORD—Procedure for correction of ptosis of the eyelid.

MACKENRODT—Corrective operation for retrodisplacement of the uterus involving vaginal fixation of round ligaments.

MADELUNG—Incision into the colon through a lumbar incision with detachment and invagination of the distal colon.

MADLENER—Ligation of the oviducts and removal of the fimbriated ends in the female for the purpose of sterilization.

MAKKA—Utilization of the cecum as a bladder and the appendix as the ureter in cases of ectopia of the urinary bladder.

MAMMECTOMY—Excision of the breast.

MAMMILLIPLASTY—Plastic operation of the breast nipple; thelyplasty.

MAMMOTOMY—Incision into the breast.

MANCHESTER—Operation for correcting a prolapsed uterus by amputation of the cervix and fixation of the cardinal ligaments (Fothergill operation).

MARCKWALD—Operation to relieve stenosis of the external os of the uterus by excision of wedge-shaped pieces of tissue from opposite sides of the vaginal section of the cervix.

MARIAN—An operation through a median perineal route for urinary bladder calculus removal.

GLOSSARY OF OPERATIVE TITLES (Continued)

MARSHALL-MARCHETTI—Plication of the urethra for correction of urinary stress incontinence.

MARSUPIALIZATION—Incision into a cystic lesion with evacuation of its contents and approximation of the walls of the cyst to those of the external incision to permit drainage and closure by granulation of the wound.

MARWEDEL—Gastrotomy.

MASTECTOMY—Amputation of the breast.

MASTOIDECTOMY—Scraping of the mastoid area of the temporal bone and curetting out the osseous partitions which form the mastoid cells.

MASTOPEXY—Plastic corrective operation for sagging breasts; mazopexy.

MASTOPLASTY—Plastic operation of the breast; mammoplasty.

MATAS—Corrective operation for aneurysm consisting of opening the defect and resuturing the walls in such a manner as to restore a normal cylindrical lumen.

MAXILLARY ANTROTOMY—Incision into the maxillary antrum (antrum of Highmore).

MAYDL—Colostomy operation in which an open wound is maintained until adhesions are formed. A glass rod is placed beneath the exteriorized colon while it remains out of the abdominal cavity.

MAYO—Technique for posterior gastrojejunostomy involving excision of the pylorus and closure of the proximal end of the duodenum.
Also: Bunionectomy with arthroplasty of 1st metatarsophalangeal joint.

MCARTHUR—Catheterization of the common bile duct.

MCBURNEY—Technique for radical cure of inguinal hernia.

MCGILL—Suprapubic prostatectomy technique.

MCKEEVER—Arthrodesis for correction of hallux rigidus or hallux valgus of the metatarsophalangeal joint of the great toe.

MCREYNOLD—Procedure for correction of strabismus.

MEATOTOMY—Incision to enlarge the external opening of the urethra or meatus; porotomy.

MELLER—Operative technique for excision of the tear sac.

MENGE'S—Resection of the fallopian tube brought out through an inguinal incision and eventuating in sterilization of the female.

MENISCECTOMY—Excision of the fibrocartilage of the knee joint.

GLOSSARY OF OPERATIVE TITLES (Continued)

MERCIER'S—Prostatectomy technique.

MESOPEXY—Attachment or fixation of an incised or torn mesentery (mesenteriopexy).

METATARSECTOMY—Excision of the metatarsus, that portion of the foot skeleton situated between the toes and instep, consisting of five long bones.

MIKULICZ—An operation performed for wry neck (torticollis) involving excision of the sternocleidomastoid muscle.

MIKULICZ-VLADIMIROFF—Resection of the ankle which includes excision of the talus and calcaneus plus removal of the articulating surfaces of the tibia, fibula, cuboid and scaphoid. The patient thereafter has to walk on tiptoe.

MILES'—Proctosigmoidectomy; abdominoperineal resection of the rectum for carcinoma.

MINGAZZINI-FOERSTER—Cutting the 7, 8 and 9th dorsal nerve roots intradurally for locomotor ataxia.

MIRAULT—Cleft lip repair.

MOORE'S—Operation for producing coagulation in an aortic aneurysm by means of a small wire coil inserted into the aneurysmal sac.

MORESTIN'S—Intracondyloid division of the femur with disarticulation of the knee.

MOSCHCOWITZ'S—Femoral herniorrhaphy via an inguinal incision.

MOTAIS'S—An operation performed for ptosis of the eyelid in which the middle third of the tendon of the superior rectus muscle of the eyeball is transplanted into the upper lid, for the purpose of augmenting the action of the levator muscle.

MOYNIHAN—Anterior gastrojejunostomy.

MULE'S—Enucleation of the eyeball followed by insertion of a prosthesis.

MULLER'S—Technique for vaginal hysterectomy.
Sclerectomy performed for detachment of the retina.

Technique for cesarean section-involving an incision into the uterus after it is brought up out of the pelvis.

MUSTARD'S—Transfer of the Iliopsoas muscle.
MYECTOMY—Resection of a muscle.

MYOMECTOMY—Excision of tumors with muscular tissue components, most commonly used to refer to excision of myomas of the uterus.

GLOSSARY OF OPERATIVE TITLES (Continued)

MYOPLASTY—Plastic operation on a muscle.

MYORRHAPHY—Repair of a muscle.

MYOTENOTOMY—Division of the tendon of a muscle.

MYOTOMY—Incision into a muscle.

MYRINGOTOMY—Surgical incision of the tympanic membrane.

NAFFZIGER'S—Operation for exophthalmos (protrusion of eyeballs) which includes resection of the super and lateral orbital walls for decompression.

NARATH'S—Operation performed in portal obstruction for the purpose of creating a collateral circulation. This is accomplished by means of fixation of the omentum to the subcutaneous tissue of the abdominal wall.

NEBINGER-PRAUN'S—Operation on the frontal sinus with removal of the anterior bony wall.

NEEDLING OF LENS—An operation for opening the capsule and breaking up the soft or secondary cataract; discission of lens.

NELATON'S—Utilization of a transverse incision to remove the shoulder joint.

NEPHRECTOMY—Excision of the kidney.

NEPHROLITHOTOMY—Removal of a kidney calculus.

NEPHROLYSIS—Lysis or breaking up of the adhesions formed about the kidney.

NEPHROPEXY—Fixation or suspension of a mobile kidney.

NEPHRORRHAPHY—Suture of the kidney.

NEPHROSTOMY—Creation of an opening from the kidney pelvis to the outside of the body.

NEPHROTOMY—Incision into the kidney.

NEUBER—Operation for obliterating a bone cavity with skin flaps developed from the sides of the wound.

NEURECTOMY—Resection of a segment of nerve.

NEUROLYSIS—Lysis or destruction of perineural adhesions.

NEUROPLASTY—Plastic repair of a nerve.

NEURORRHAPHY—Suture of a nerve.

NEUROTOMY—Surgical division of a nerve.

GLOSSARY OF OPERATIVE TITLES (Continued)

NEUROTRIPSY—Operation for crushing of a nerve.

NICOLA—Operation for dislocated shoulder.

OBER'S—Cutting of a joint capsule; capsulotomy.

OBERST'S—An operation for providing drainage of abdominal ascites by burying an abdominal wall skin flap in the abdomen.

OGSTON'S—An operation for the development of an arch in flatfootedness by removing a wedge of the tarsus bone.
An operation for relieving knock-knee by excision of the inner condyle of the femur.

OGSTON-LUC—Frontal sinusotomy.

OLLIER-THIERSCH—A very thin skin graft including the epidermis and some of the dermis.

OLSHAUSEN'S—A corrective operation for retroversion of the uterus consisting of fixation of the uterus to the abdominal wall.

OMBREDDANE—Transscrotal suspension of the testes.
A corrective operation for hypospadius (defect where urethra opens on the undersurface of the penis).
An operative procedure wherein the structures operated upon are exposed to the air.

OMENTECTOMY—Resection of the omentum (membrane enclosing the bowels).

OMPHALECTOMY—Excision of the umbilicus.

ONYCHECTOMY—Removal of a toenail or fingernail.

ONYCHOTOMY—Cutting into a fingernail or toenail.

OOPHORECTOMY—Excision of one or both ovaries.

OOPHOROPEXY—Fixation of a wandering ovary; oothecopexy.

OOPHOROPLASTY—Plastic repair of an ovary.

OOTHECECTOMY—Removal of an ovary.

OPEN REDUCTION—Reduction of a fracture by manipulation performed after incision of the tissues overlying the fracture.

ORBITOTOMY—Surgical entry into the orbit.

ORCHIDECTOMY—Removal of one or both testes.

ORCHIDORRHAPHY—Suspension of the testes in the scrotum by suturing; orchiopexy.

GLOSSARY OF OPERATIVE TITLES (Continued)

ORCHIDOTOMY—Incision into the testis.

ORCHIECTOMY—Same as orchidectomy.

ORCHIOPEXY—Suspension of undescended testis or testes.

ORCHIOPLASTY—Plastic surgery on the testes; orcheoplasty.

ORD'S—An operation for division of fresh adhesions in a joint.

OSSICULECTOMY—Removal of the small bones of the middle ear (incus, malleus or stapes); otectomy.

OSTECTOMY—Removal of a portion of a bone.

OSTEOPERIOSTEAL GRAFT—Graft involving bone and the underlying periosteal membrane.

OSTEOPLASTY—Plastic operation on a bone.

OSTEORRHAPHY—Repair of a bone by wiring the fragments.

OSTEOSYNTHESIS—Bringing pieces of a fractured bone into apposition.

OSTEOTOMY—Cutting into a bone.

OTOPLASTY—Plastic surgery of the auricle (external projection of the ear on each side of the head).

OTOSCOPY—Examination of the ear by means of an instrument (scope).

OVERHOLT'S—Thoracoplasty with replacement of inverted ribs.

PACI'S—Modified Lorenz operation for reduction of congenital dislocation of the hip.

PALATOPLASTY—Plastic repair of the palate (uraniscus) which is the roof of the mouth. Uranoplasty; uraniscoplasty.

PALLIATIVE—A noncurative operation designed for relieving the severity of symptoms.

PANAS'—An operation for ptosis (drooping) of the upper eyelid wherein the upper eyelid is attached to the Occipitofrontalis muscle.
An operation for incision into the rectum.

PANCOAST'S—Transection of the 5th cranial nerve (trigeminal) at the level of the foramen ovale.

PANCREATECTOMY—Resection of the pancreas, a gland which secretes pancreatic juices containing enzymes discharged into the digestive tract and also secretes insulin.

GLOSSARY OF OPERATIVE TITLES (Continued)

PANCREATICODUODENOSTOMY—Creation of a surgical continuity between the pancreas and the duodenum.

PANCREATICOGASTROSTOMY—Continuity established between the stomach and a fistula of the pancreas.

PANCREOLITHOTOMY—Removal of a calculus of the pancreas; pancreatolithotomy.

PANHYSTERECTOMY—Removal of the uterus with the cervix. If salpingo-oophorectomy was also performed, this should be specified since the term panhysterectomy does not include removal of the tubes and ovaries.

PARATHYROIDECTOMY—Resection of the parathyroid glands situated adjacent to the thyroid gland.

PAROTIDECTOMY—Resection of the parotid or salivary gland situated in the upper neck, behind the lower ear.

PEAN'S—Vaginal hysterectomy performed in a piecemeal fashion.
Operation for amputation of the lower extremity at the hip joint.

PEDICLE GRAFT—Preparation of skin for grafting by forming a tubular structure which may be moved to another site on the body which requires the graft.

PERICARDIECTOMY—Resection of a portion of the membrane enveloping the heart particularly in cases where the membrane is constricting the heart as following pericarditis. Pericardectomy.

PERICARDIOCENTESIS—Incision into the pericardium (membrane enveloping the heart) for the purpose of removing purulent secretions. Pericardiostomy.

PERIER'S—Removal of an everted uterus utilizing an elastic ligature.

PERINEOPLASTY—Plastic repair of the perineum. Perineorrhaphy.

PERIOSTEAL GRAFT—Graft consisting of the fibrous membrane which covers the bone.

PERIOSTEOTOMY—Incision through the membranous covering of the bone.

PERITECTOMY—Excision of the pannus (ring of conjunctiva) surrounding the cornea. Peritomy.

PERITONEOCENTESIS—Aspiration of ascitic fluid from the abdomen. Paracentesis; abdominoparacentesis.

PHARYNGECTOMY—Resection of the pharynx (portion of digestive canal situated above the esophagus).

GLOSSARY OF OPERATIVE TITLES (Continued)

PHELP'S—An operation for correcting clubfoot.

PHLEBECTOMY—Resection of a segment of vein.

PHLEBORRHAPHY—Repair of a vein.

PHLEBOTOMY—Incision into a vein usually for the purpose of withdrawing blood.

PHRENICECTOMY—Resection of a portion of phrenic nerve for permanent interruption.

PHRENICO-EXERESIS—Excision of phrenic nerve.

PHRENICOTRIPSY—Crushing operation on the phrenic nerve. Phrenemphraxis.

PHYSICK'S—Iridectomy with removal of a circular section of iris.

PINCH GRAFT—Insertion of small bits of skin into a denuded area.

PINEALECTOMY—Excision of the pineal body.

PIROGOFF AMPUTATION—Technique for amputation of the foot.

PLEURACOTOMY—Incision into the pleural cavity for drainage purposes.

PLEURECTOMY—Resection of the serous membrane covering the lungs.

PLEUROCENTESIS—Puncture of the pleura.

PLEUROLYSIS—Separating the pleura from the fascia of the thoracic wall to permit collapse of lung.

PLICOTOMY—Incision into the plica membranae tympani (posterior tympanic membrane).

PNEUMONECTOMY—Total or partial resection of a lung.

PNEUMONOLYSIS—Same as pleurolysis.

PNEUMONOTOMY—Incision into the lung.

POLLOCK—Amputation at the level of the knee leaving the patella.

POMEROY—Sterilization operation on the female with ligation and resection of the fallopian tubes.

PONCET—Operation for relief of talipes equinus (walking on the toes) by lengthening of the Achilles tendon.

PORRO—Technique for cesarean section with hysterectomy. Celiohysterectomy.

GLOSSARY OF OPERATIVE TITLES (Continued)

PORTACAVAL ANASTOMOSIS—Formation of a communication between the portal and caval veins surgically.

POTTS—Aorticopulmonary shunt (diverting operation).

POTTS-SMITH-GIBSON—Operation performed in pulmonary stenosis consisting of an anastomosis between the pulmonary artery and aorta.

PRESACRAL NEURECTOMY—Resection of a nerve plexus (hypogastric) located before the sacral promontory.

PROCTECTOMY—Resection of the rectum.

PROCTOPEXY—Fixation operation designed to correct prolapse of the rectum.

PROCTOPLASTY—Plastic repair of the rectum and/or anus.

PROCTORRHAPHY—Suture repair of the rectum.

PROCTOSCOPY—Endoscopic examination of the rectum with the aid of a scope.

PROCTOSIGMOIDECTOMY—Resection of the sigmoid colon and rectum.

PROCTOSTOMY—Establishment of an opening into the rectum.

PROCTOTOMY—Incision into the rectum or anus.

PROSTATECTOMY—Resection of the prostate gland.

PROSTATOLITHOTOMY—Incision into the prostate for removal of a calculus.

PROSTATOTOMY—Incision into the prostate gland.

PTYALECTASIS—Dilation of a salivary duct.

PUBIOTOMY—Surgical division of the pubic bone.

PUUSSEPP—Surgical treatment of syringomyelia by division of the central canal of the spinal cord.

PUTTI-PLATT—Capsulorrhaphy of the shoulder.

PYELOLITHOTOMY—Removal of calculus from the renal pelvis.

PYELOPLASTY—Plastic operation of the kidney pelvis.

PYELOSTOMY—Incision into the renal pelvis and drainage of urine by a route other than the ureter.

PYELOTOMY—Incision into the kidney pelvis.

GLOSSARY OF OPERATIVE TITLES (Continued)

PYLOROMYOTOMY—Incision of the muscles of the pylorus; Ramstedt operation.

PYLOROPLASTY—Plastic revision of the pylorus, particularly enlarging a stenotic opening.

PYLOROSTOMY—Surgical opening created through the abdominal wall and pyloric portion of the stomach for feeding purposes.

QUAGLINO—Sclerotomy.

QUENU-MAYO—Resection of the rectum and local lymph glands in cases of malignancy.

RACHIOCENTESIS—Spinal tap.

RADICOTOMY—Surgical division of nerve roots; rhizotomy.

RAMSTEDT—Incision of the muscles of the pylorus performed for congenital pyloric stenosis. Same as Fredet-Ramstedt.

REGNOLI—Excision of the tongue.

REVERDIN GRAFT—Graft utilizing epidermis.

RHINOPLASTY—Plastic repair or reconstruction of the nose.

RHINOSCOPY—Examination of the nose with a speculum.

RHIZOTOMY—Division of the roots of the spinal nerves.

RIDELL—Resection of the walls (anterior and inferior) of the frontal sinus for chronic sinusitis.

RIGAUD—Repair of urethral fistula.

ROBERTS—Pinning operation for correction of a deviated nasal septum.

ROSE—Gasserian ganglionectomy.

ROUGE—Operation for entering the nasal cavities (sinuses).

ROUX-en-Y—Anastomosis between the stomach and distal end of the severed jejunum. The proximal end of the jejunum is anastomosed to jejunum below the first anastomosis.

SAENGER—Technique for cesarean section.

SALPINGECTOMY—Resection of the fallopian tube(s).

SALPINGO-OOPHORECTOMY—Resection of the tube and ovary unilaterally or bilaterally.

SALPINGOPLASTY—Plastic repair of the fallopian tube (oviduct).

GLOSSARY OF OPERATIVE TITLES (Continued)

SALPINGOSTOMY—Incision and drainage of the fallopian tube.

SAUCERIZATION—Formation of a saucer-like depression in a bone.

SCALENECTOMY—Excision of the scalenus muscle.

SCANZONI—Obstetrical forceps delivery of an infant from an occiput posterior position.

SCAPULOPEXY—Fixation of the scapula to the ribs.

SCHAUTA—Vaginal hysterectomy for carcinoma of the cervix uteri.

SCHAUTA-WERTHEIM—Cystocele repair.

SCHUCHARDT—Hysterectomy (removal of uterus) using a paravaginal incision.

SCHWARTZE—Operation performed for drainage of matter in cases of mastoiditis.

SCHWARTZE-STACKE—Operation for mastoiditis.

SCLERECTOMY—Excision of the sclera of the eye.

SCLEROPLASTY—Plastic repair of the sclera covering the eye.

SCLEROSTOMY—Surgical opening through the sclera in glaucoma.

SCROTECTOMY—Resection of a portion of the scrotum.

SEPTECTOMY—Removal of a portion of the nasal septum.

SEQUESTRECTOMY—Removal of a fragment of dead bone which has broken off the normal bone.

SHUNT OPERATION—An operation performed for the purpose of diverting the flow of blood, urine or other body fluid through a route other than the normal anatomic one.

SIALOADENECTOMY—Excision of a salivary gland.

SIALODOCHOPLASTY—Plastic repair of the salivary ducts.

SIALOLITHOTOMY—Removal of calculus from the salivary gland.

SIGMOIDECTOMY—Resection of the sigmoid colon.

SIGMOIDOPEXY—Fixation of the sigmoid to the abdominal wound for repair of rectal prolapse.

SIGMOIDOPROCTOSTOMY—A surgical opening made at the junction of the sigmoid colon and rectum.

SIGMOIDORECTOSTOMY—Same as sigmoidoproctostomy.

GLOSSARY OF OPERATIVE TITLES (Continued)

SIGMOIDOSCOPY—Endoscopic examination of the sigmoid colon.

SIGMOIDOSIGMOIDOSTOMY—Formation of a connection between two parts of the sigmoid colon.

SIGMOIDOSTOMY—Formation of an opening into the sigmoid colon.

SPENCER-WATSON—Operation to relieve ingrowing eyelashes.

SPHENOID SINUSOTOMY—Incision into the sphenoid sinus, one of the accessory sinuses communicating with the nasal cavity.

SPHINCTEROPLASTY—Surgical repair of a circular constricting muscle situated at the mouth of natural orifices such as the bladder, anus, pylorus, ampulla of Vater, etc.

SPHINCTEROTOMY—Incision or division of a sphincter.

SPINAL FUSION—Surgical immobilization of the spine through formation of a bony union; spondylosyndesis.

SPINELLI—Restoration of a prolapsed uterus.

SPLANCHNICECTOMY—Resection of the greater splanchic nerve; splanchnic neurectomy.

SPLENECTOMY—Removal of the spleen.

SPLENOPEXY—Attachment of a mobile spleen to the abdominal wall for purposes of immobilization.

SPLENORENAL ANASTOMOSIS—Surgical connection of the renal vein and splenic vein.

SPLENORRHAPHY—Repair of injury to the spleen.

SPLENOTOMY—Incision into the spleen.

STACKE—Removal of the contents of the middle ear and the mastoid.

STAPEDECTOMY—Removal of the stapes, one of the three tiny bones of the middle ear.

STERNOTOMY—Incision into or through the sternum (breast bone).

STOMATOPLASTY—Plastic operation of the mouth (stoma).

STREATFIELD-SNELLEN—Operation for repair of cicatricial entropion of the eyelid.

STURMDORF—Technique for amputation of the cervix.

SUBMUCOUS RESECTION—Resection of the nasal septum; septectomy.

GLOSSARY OF OPERATIVE TITLES (Continued)

SUSPENSION—Suturing or fixation of a structure to an anatomic site such as the abdominal wall for the purpose of restoring normal anatomic position and relieving malposition or ptosis.

SYMPATHECTOMY—Division of sympathetic nervous pathway.

SYMPATHICOTRIPSY—Crushing operation performed on a ganglion, nerve or plexus of the (involuntary) sympathetic nervous system.

SYNCHONDROTOMY—Incision or division of an articulation which has no appreciable motility and in which cartilage is the intervening connective tissue.

SYNOVECTOMY—Excision of the membrane lining the joint capsule (synovial membrane).

TAIT—Utilization of flaps for closure of a perineal laceration.

TARSECTOMY—Excision of the tarsal bones located in the heel area of the foot.
Excision of the tarsal cartilage of the eyelid.

TARSOPLASTY—Plastic repair of the tarsus (firm outline of the eyelid which gives it shape) of the eyelid.

TARSORRHAPHY—Suturing together, partially or totally, the upper and lower eyelid margins.

TENODESIS—Suturing of the proximal portion of a tendon to the bone or reattachment of it at another site.

TENOPLASTY—Plastic operation of the tendons.

TENORRHAPHY—Restoration of continuity to a severed tendon.

TENOSYNOVECTOMY—Resection of a tendon sheath.

TENOTOMY—Incomplete or complete division of a tendon.

THELEPLASTY—Plastic revision or reconstruction of the nipple of the breast.

Also: thelyplasty or mammilliplasty.

THIERSCH-OLLIER GRAFT—Thin split skin graft.

THORACOPLASTY—Plastic surgery of the chest (thorax).

THORACOTOMY—Surgical incision of the chest wall.

THROMBECTOMY—Excision of a blood clot from a vein.

THYMECTOMY—Resection of the thymus gland situated in the anterior mediastinal cavity.

GLOSSARY OF OPERATIVE TITLES (Continued)

THYROCHONDROTOMY—Incision into the thyroid cartilage.

THYROCRICOTOMY—Surgical opening into the trachea made through the cricothyroid membrane.

THYROIDECTOMY—Resection of the thyroid gland.

THYROIDOTOMY—Surgical incision into the thyroid.

TONSILLECTOMY—Removal of the tonsils.

TOPECTOMY—Removal of a small area of the frontal cortex in the therapy of mental disease.

TOREK—Suspension of an undescended testicle.

TORKILDSEN—Ventriculocisternostomy utilizing plastic tubing.

TOTI—Dacryocystorhinostomy; passage of a probe through the lacrimal sac and into the nasal cavity for purposes of drainage.

TRACHELECTOMY—Excision of the cervix uteri.

TRACHELOPLASTY—Plastic repair of the cervix uteri.

TRACHELORRHAPHY—Suturing operation of the cervix uteri.

TRACHEOPLASTY—Plastic operation on the trachea.

TRACHEORRHAPHY—Suturing operation of the trachea.

TRACHEOSTOMY—Surgical opening into the trachea made through the neck for relief of severe respiratory distress.

TRACHEOTOMY—Surgical opening made in the trachea.

TRACTOTOMY—Division of a nerve tract.

TRANSDUODENAL CHOLEDOCHOLITHOTOMY—Removal of a common duct stone through a duodenal incision.

TRANSURETHRAL RESECTION OF PROSTATE—Resection of the prostate gland from below with a resectoscope. Also: TUR.

TRENDELENBURG—Excision of varicose veins.

TREPHINATION—Opening made in the skull with an instrument called a trephine. Also: craniotomy.

TURBINECTOMY—Excision of turbinated bone.

TYMPANOPLASTY—Plastic repair of the tympanic membrane and structures of the middle ear. Classified as Type I, II, III, IV and V.

TYMPANOTOMY—Surgical rupture of the tympanic membrane.

418

GLOSSARY OF OPERATIVE TITLES (Continued)

UMBILECTOMY—Excision of the navel (umbilicus).

UMBILICAL HERNIORRHAPHY—Repair of hernia in the umbilical region.

URACHUS LIGATION—Closure of a passage through the umbilicus, from the urinary bladder to the outside. This passage is present in the fetus and closes off after birth. Sometimes its lumen remains patent requiring surgical closure.

URANOPLASTY—Plastic repair of the palate (roof of the mouth). Also: palatoplasty.

URETERECTOMY—Resection of the ureter, a tube-like structure extending from the kidney to the urinary bladder for the passage of urine.

URETEROCENTESIS—Aspiration or drainage of a ureter.

URETEROCOLOSTOMY—Interruption of the normal course of the ureter to the urinary bladder and implantation of the ureter into the colon.

URETEROCYSTOSTOMY—Reimplantation of the ureter from its normal site to another site in the bladder. Also: ureteroneocystostomy.

URETEROLITHOTOMY—Removal of a calculus from the ureter.

URETEROLYSIS—Freeing (lysis) of adhesions of the ureter.

URETEROPLASTY—Plastic operation on the ureter.

URETEROPYELOSTOMY—Creation of a surgical passage from the renal pelvis to the ureter. Also: ureteroneopyelostomy.

URETERORRHAPHY—Suturing of the ureter for closure of a defect in its wall.

URETEROSIGMOIDOSTOMY—Implantation of the ureter into the sigmoid colon.

URETEROSTOMY—Surgical opening made in the ureter for drainage of urine.

URETEROTOMY—Incision into the ureter.

URETEROURETEROSTOMY—Connection of interrupted segments of the same ureter or one ureter to another.

URETHROPLASTY—Plastic operation on the urethra.

URETHRORRHAPHY—Surgical repair of the urethra.

URETHROSCOPY—Examination of the inside of the urethra with the aid of a scope.

GLOSSARY OF OPERATIVE TITLES (Continued)

URETHROSTOMY—Surgical opening made in the urethra for passage of urine in cases of persistent stricture.

URETHROTOMY—Incision into the urethra for surgical treatment of urethral stricture.

VAGINOTOMY—Incision of the vaginal wall.

VAGOTOMY—Division or partial transection of the vagus nerves. This operation is used in the treatment of duodenal ulcer.

VALVOTOMY—Incision of a valve.

VALVULOTOMY—Same as valvotomy.

VAN MILLINGEN—Entropion operation of the eyelid.

VARICOCELECTOMY—Resection of a portion of the scrotum and enlarged veins for relief of varicocele (varicose veins of the spermatic cord).

VASECTOMY—Resection of the vas deferens (excretory duct of the testicle).

VASOLIGATION—Ligation of the vas deferens. Sterilization operation on the male.

VASOTOMY—Incision of the vas deferens.

VENECTOMY—Resection of a vein. Also: phlebectomy.

VENOTOMY—Puncture or incision into a vein.

VENOVENOSTOMY—Connection of one segment of a vein with another.

VENTRAL HERNIORRHAPHY—Repair of a hernia of the belly wall.

VENTRICULOCISTERNOSTOMY—Surgical connection of the third ventricle of the cerebrum and the cisterna.

VENTRICULOSTOMY—Operation used in the treatment of hydrocephalus in which an opening is formed between the third ventricle floor and the cisterna situated just below it.

VENTROFIXATION—Fixation of the displaced uterus to the abdominal wall.

VERSION—Change in direction of the fetus within the uterus from an abnormal plane to a normal one for purposes of delivery.

VESICULECTOMY—Resection of the seminal vesicle. Sterilization operation on the male.

VESICULOTOMY—Incision into the seminal vesicles.

VESTIBULOTOMY—Opening made in the vestibule of the inner ear.

GLOSSARY OF OPERATIVE TITLES (Continued)

VON HABERER—Method of Billroth I gastrectomy.

VON HABERER-AGUIRRE—Method of Billroth I gastrectomy.

VON HABERER-FINNEY—Method of Billroth I.

VON HACKER—Posterior gastrojejunostomy.

VON EISELBERG—Modification of Billroth II gastrectomy.

VULVECTOMY—Resection of the vulva (external female genitalia).

WARDILL—Technique for palatoplasty.

WATKINS—Interposition operation for correction of uterine prolapse and procidentia uteri.

WATKINS-WERTHEIM—Suspension of the uterus.

WEIR—Operation on the nose performed with a rhinoplasty.

WEIS—Lid fracturing operation.

WERTHEIM—Radical hysterectomy (removal of the uterus, adjacent tissues and wide portion of the vagina) performed for uterine malignancy.

WHARTON-JONES—V-Y procedure for cicatricial ectropion.

WHIPPLE—One stage pancreaticoduodenectomy.

WICHERKIEWICZ—Upper eyelid reconstruction.

WITZEL—Gastrostomy for carcinoma of the stomach.

WÖLFLER—Anterior gastrojejunostomy.

Z-PLASTY—Relaxing incision used for correcting contractures; made in the shape of a Z.

INDEX

A

Abbreviations, medical, 371-376
Abdominal perineal resection, 187-188
Abell-Gilliam suspension, 261
Abraders, 47
Acetone, urinary, 26
Addis count, 26
Adenotomes, 47
Albumin
    blood, 21
    urinary, 26
Amniotomes, 47
Amputations, 272-274
    A-K, 273
    humerus, 273
    partial finger, 274
    revision, finger, 274
    techniques, 272
Amylase, serum, 21
Anal sphincterotomy, 187
Anastomoses
    bowel types, 177-178
    closed methods, 178
    open methods, 178
    types listed, 177-178
Anatomic position, 364
Anchors, 47
Andrews bottle operation, 347
Anesthetic agents, 35-36
  eyelid surgery, 311
    modes of induction, 37
    ophthalmic, 36
    preparations used with, 36
Angiotribes, 47
Anorectal anatomy, 185
Anoscopes, 47
Anus
    anatomic features, 185
    circulation, 185
Aortic valve prostheses, 356
Aortogram, 353
    transbrachial, 354-355
    translumbar, 354
Aortography, 31
A & P colporrhaphy, 264-265
Appendectomy, 183
    incisions, 184
    operative report, 184

terms used in, 184
Applicators, 48
Arteries, listing, 118-121
Arterial grafts, 355-356
Arteriogram
    femoral, 32, 353
    subclavian, 352
Arteriotomy, 360-361
Arthrodesis, 274
    Brittain technique, 276
    Charnley, 275
    Harrington spinal, 278-280
    Hibbs modified, 277-278
    hip, 276
    ischiofemoral, 276
    sacrum to L-4, 277
    shoulder, 276-277
Arthroplasty, 280
    Austin-Moore, 281-282
    knee, 280-281
    Magnuson, knee, 282-283
Arytenoidectomy, 216-217
Aschheim-Zondek test, 26
Ascorbic acid
    blood, 21
    urinary, 26
Aspirators, 48
Austin-Moore hip prosthesis, 281-282
Autografts, skin, 301
Awls, 48

B

Band neutrophiles, 20
Bandages, 45-46
Bands, 48
Bankart shoulder operation, 287
Barium enema, 31
Bars, 48
Basiotribes, 48
Basophiles, 20
Bassini inguinal repair, 152
Bence-Jones protein, 26
Bilirubin, 22
Billroth I, 167, 169
Billroth II, 167, 170-172
Blepharoplasty, 309, 311-312
Blood
    components, 19-21
    examinations, 19-25

formation, 19
hematocrit, 20
hemoglobin, 19-20
platelets, 21
pressure, 118
red blood count, 19
volume, 19, 118
white cell differential, 20
BMR, 29
Bolts, 48
Bone grafts, 283, 304
  femoral, 284
  removal, tibial, 285
  techniques, 284
  tibial, 285
  types, 284
Bones, 123-125
  illustrated, 126-127
Bougies, 48-49
Braces, 49
Brain
  anatomic features, 242-243
  arteries of, 243
Breasts, 159-160
  anatomic features, 159
  arterial supply, 159
  incisions, 160
  operative reports, 160
  biopsy, 160
  radical mastectomy, 160
  silastic implants, 320-321
Brittain hip arthrodesis, 276
Bronchial tree, 326
Bronchogram, 31
Bronchoscopes, 49, 327
Bronchoscopy, 326-327
BSP, 22
BUN, 22
Bunionectomy, 291
Burs, 49
Business letters
  alignment, 9
  carbon copies, 9
  complimentary close, 9
  corporation name, 9
  enclosures, 9
  form types, 5-8
  punctuation, 5, 13-17
  second page, 10

spacing, 9
typist's initials, 9

C

Calcium
  blood, 22
  urinary, 26
Caldwell-Luc, 221, 222
Calipers, 50
Cannulas, 50
Canthoplasty, 233
Capitals, use of, 17, 378-379
Carbon dioxide
  combining power, 22
Cardiac massage, 331
Cardioangiogram, 31
Carotid angiography, 31
Carotid ligation, 362
Cartilage grafts, 304
Cataract extraction
  extracapsular, 228-229
  with iridectomy, 229
Catheters, 50-51
Cautery units, 51-52
Cephalin flocculation, 22
Cerebral artery clipping, 249
Cerebrospinal fluid
  pressure readings, 28
  tests on, 29
  volume, 28
Cervical hemilaminectomy, 240
Cervical sympathectomy, 250
Cervix
  electrocoagulation, 262
  incompetent, 261-262
  Lash operation, 262
  radium insertion, 262-263
  Shirodkar operation, 261-262
  Sturmdorf amputation, 263
Cesarean section, 266-267
Chalazion excision, 231
Charnley arthrodesis, 275
Cheiloplasty
  anatomy in, 313
  techniques, 313
Chisels, 52
Chlorides
  blood, 22
  spinal fluid, 29

INDEX (Continued)

urinary, 27
Cholangiogram, 31-32
Cholecystectomy, 190
Cholecystogram, 32
Cholesterol
  blood, 22
  esters, 22
Chordotomy, 248
Circulation
  anatomy of, 117-118
  circuit, 117-118
  pressure, 118
  time, 118
Circumcision, 344-345
Cistern puncture, 253
Clamps, 52-55
Cleft palate, 317
  operations, 318-320
Clips, 55
Coagulation time, 22
Colectomy, segmental, 183
Colloidal gold, 29
Colocolostomy, 178
Colon, 181-189
  anatomic features, 182
  arterial supply, 182
Colporrhaphy, 264-265
Common duct stone removal, 190
Conjunctival flap, 230
Contractors, 55
Coombs
  direct, 22
  indirect, 22
Corneal grafts, 304
Costotomes, 55
Counterbores, 55
Crafoord operation, 359-360
Cranial nerves, 143
Craniectomy, 247-248
Cranioclasts, 56
Craniotomes, 56
Craniotomy, 244
  exploratory, 247
  instruments, 244-245
  temporal, 246
C-reactive protein, 23
Creatine
  blood, 23
  urinary, 27

Creatinine
  blood, 23
  urinary, 27
Curettes, 56-57
Cutters, 57
Cystoscopes, 57, 340
Cystoscopy, 340, 341-342
Cystotomes, 57

D

Dacryocystorhinostomy, 233
D & C, 258-259
  instruments, 259
Decompression, subtemporal, 249
Decortication, lung, 330-331
Dermabraders, 57
Dermabrasion, 321
Dermatomes, 57
Diacetic acid, 27
Diaphragmatic herniorrhaphy, 154
Dilators, 58
Directors, 58
Discission of lens, 232
Dislocations, 286
  ankle, 287
  operations for, 286
  shoulder, 287
Dissectors, 59
Drains, 59
Dressings, 45-46
Drills, 59-60
Drivers, 60
Dyspareunia
  Hirst operation, 266

E

Ear
  external, 308-309
    anatomic features, 308
    operations, 308-309
  middle, 199
    anatomic features, 199-200
    operations, 199-212
Electrocoagulation, cervix, 262
Electrodes, 60
Electrodiaphakes, 61
Electrotomes, 61
Elevators, 61-62

Endolymphatic-subarachnoid shunt, 201
ENT surgery, 197-222
Enteroenterostomy, 177-181
Enucleator, 62
Eosinophiles, 21, 25
Erisophakes, 62
Esophagectomy, 331-332
Esophagogastroscopy, 173
Esophagoscopes, 62, 172-173
Esophagoscopy, 174
Ethmoidectomy, 222
Evacuators, 62
Excavator, 62
Exploration, extracerebral, 247
Expressors, 62
Extractors, 62-63
Eye
    abbreviations, 227
    accessory structures, 224
    anatomic features, 223-227
    bank, 305
    evisceration, 232
    illustration, 225
    implants, 63
    medications, 227
    operations, 234-236
    prostheses, 63
        insertion, 232
        removal of, 232
Eyelids, 224-227, 309
    anatomic features, 310
    anesthetics, 311
    dressings, 311
    ptosis operations, 311
    repairs, 310

F

Face
    dermabrasion of, 321
    lift, 322
Facial fracture appliance, 63
Fallopian tube excision, 265
Fascia grafts, 305
Fascia lata graft, 307
Fascia stripper, 107
Female genitalia, 255-256
Femoral arteriography, 32, 353
Femoral herniorrhaphy, 153-154

    anatomy of, 153
    technique, 153-154
    types of repair, 153
Femoral intimectomy, 358-359
Femoropopliteal by-pass, 357
Fenestration
    semicircular canal, 211-212
Fibrinogen, 23
Flanges, 63
Forceps, 63-71
Formats
    business letters, 8-10
    operative report, 3-4
    release form, 10-11
Fractures, 288-291
    defined, 288
    reduction, 289
Frames, 72
Friedman test, 27
Frog test, 27

G

Gags (SEE: mouth gags), 80
Gallbladder, 189
    anatomic features, 190
    operations, 190-191
Gastrectomy, 167-172
    anatomic features, 169
    instruments, 168-169
    operative reports
        Billroth I, 169-170
        Billroth II, 170-172
    techniques defined
        anterior Polya, 168
        Billroth I, 167
        Billroth II, 167
        Hofmeister, 168
        posterior Polya, 168
        Schoemaker, 167
Gastroduodenostomy, 169, 175
Gastrojejunostomy, 170-172
    178-180
    anatomic features, 179
    anterior, report, 179-180
Gastroscopes, 72, 172
Gastroscopy, 172
    description, 172
    operative report, 173
Gastrostomy, 174

INDEX (Continued)

operative report, 175
  techniques, 174
Gauze packers, 72
General surgery, 149
Genitalia
  female, 255-256
  male, 342-344
Gilliam hysteropexy, 260-261
Globulin, 23
Glucose
  blood, 23
  spinal fluid, 29
Glucose tolerance, 23
Goniometers, 72
Gouges, 72
Grafts
  arterial, 355-356
  bone, 304
  cartilage, 304
  cornea, 304-305
  fascia, 305
  hair bearing, 305
  mucous membrane, 305
  nerve, 305
  tendon, 305
Groin dissection, 155-156
Guides, 73
Guillotines, 73
Gynecology, 255-269
  operations listed, 267-269

H

Hair grafts, 305
Halters, 73
Hammer toe correction, 291, 292
Harelip repair, 314
Harrington spinal fusion, 278
Hauser operation, 293
Hematocrit, 20
Hemilaminectomy
  cervical, 240
  lumbar, 239
Hemoglobin, 19, 20
Hemorrhoidectomy, 186
Hemostatic agents
  in neurosurgery, 245
Hemostatic bags, 73
Hemostats, 73
Hernia, 149-155

diaphragmatic, 154
femoral, 153
  anatomy of, 153
  operative report, 153
  repairs, 153
inguinal, 150
  anatomy of, 150-151
  Bassini repair, 152
  McVay repair, 151
  techniques, 150
transthoracic, 154
types, 149
umbilical, 155
Heterophile antibody, 23
Hippuric acid, 27
Hirst operation, 266
Homografts, 301
Hooks, 74-75
Hydrocelectomy, 347
Hyphens, use of, 379-380
Hypospadias, 323
  Cecil procedure, 323
  repair techniques, 323
Hysterectomy, 256
  abdominal, 257-258
  types, 256
  vaginal, 257
Hysteropexy
  Abell-Gilliam, 261
  techniques, 260
Hysterosalpingogram, 32

I

Icterus index, 23
Implant materials, 75
Incision and drainage
  buttocks, 158
  hand, 158
Incisions, 39-41
Inguinal herniorrhaphy, 150-153
  anatomy in, 150-151
  Bassini, 152-153
  McVay, 151-152
Intimectomy, femoral, 358
Inverters, 75
Iridectomy, 227-228
Iridencleisis, 228
Ischiorectal abscess, 185-186
Isografts, 301

INDEX (Continued)

J

Jejunostomy, 180
  description, 180
  Marwedel, 180-181
  purpose of, 180
  techniques, 180
Joints, bony, 125-128

K

Keratomes, 75
Keratoplasty, 231
17-ketosteroids, 27
Kidneys, 333-338
  anatomic features, 334
  incisions, 335
Knives, 76-78
Kuhnt-Szymanowski operation, 230

L

Lab exams, 19-29
  blood, 19-25
  spinal fluid, 28-29
  urine, 26-28
Labyrinthotomy, transmeatal, 201-202
Lactic acid, 23
Langenbeck, von, palatoplasty,
    318-319
Laryngectomy, 215
Laryngoplasty, 216-217
Laryngoscopes, 78, 214
Laryngoscopy, 215
Larynx, 213
  anatomic features, 213
  instruments, 214
  muscles, 213
  tubes, 214
Lash operation, 262
Latex slide agglutination, 23
Lens expressors, 78
Lens loupes, 78-79
L.E. test, 24
Lead, urinary, 27
Lens discission, 232
Letter writing, 5-9
  forms, 5-8
  punctuation in, 5, 13-17
  spacing, 9
Leukotomes, 79
Lid everters, 79

Ligaments, 129-132
Lights, 79
Lipase, serum, 23
Lipids, serum, 24
Lips, 312-314
  anatomic structures, 313
  arteries, 313
  deformities, 313
  operations on, 313
Litholapaxy, 341
Lithotriptoscopes, 79
Lithotrites, 79
Lobectomy of lung, 328
Loops, 79
Lottes nailing, 289
Lumbar sympathectomy, 250-251
Lymphocytes, 21

M

Magnet, 79
Magnuson arthroplasty, 282-283
Malar silastic implant, 320
Malaria slide, 24
Mallets, 79-80
Mammoplasty, augmentation, 320-321
Marwedel jejunostomy, 180-181
Mastectomy, 160
Mastoidectomy, 209
Mastoid searcher, 80
McLaughlin, canthoplasty, 233
McVay repair, 151
Meatoscope, 80
Meatotomes, 80
Mechanical finger, 80
Medical terminology, 363-376
Meniscectomy, medial, 294
Meniscotome, 80
Microscope, operating, 80
Miles operation, 187-188
Monocytes, 21
Mouth gags, 80
Mucotome, 81
Mucous membrane graft, 305
Muscles, 132-142
  illustrated, 138-139
  list by name, 133-137
  list by region, 137-142
Musculoplasty, 208-209
Myelocytes, 21

Myelogram, 32
Myringotomy, 208

N

Nails, 81
Nails, fingers and toes, 157
  anatomic features, 157
  diseases of, 157
  operative report, 157
Nasal polypectomy, 221
Nasolabial full flap, 306
Nasopharyngoscopes, 81
Neck dissection, 215
Needles, 81-82
Nephrectomy, 334-336
  instruments, 335
  operative report, 335-336
  techniques, 335
Nephrolithotomy, 337-338
Nephropexy, 336
  operative report, 336
  techniques for, 336
Nephrostomy, 337
Nerve graft, 305
Nerves, listed, 143-145
  cranial, 143
Nervous system, 142-145
Neurosurgery, 237-253
Neurotome, 83
Neutrophiles, 20, 21
Nose
  anatomic structures, 220, 314-315
  arteries of, 220, 315
  nerves of, 221, 315
  sinuses of, 220, 315
NPN, 24

O

Ocular muscle recession, 229-230
Open reduction
  hip, 290-291
  humerus, 290
  tibia, 289
Operative report, 4
  format for, 3-4
Ophthalmology, 223-236
Ophthalmodynamometer, 83
Orchiectomy, 346
Orchiopexy, 346-347

Orthopedic operations, 296-299
Orthopedic surgery, 271-299
  approaches, 271
Osteoclast, 83
Osteotomes, 83
Otolaryngology, 197-222
Otoplasty, 309
  techniques, 308
Otoscopes, 83

P

Palate
  anatomic features in, 317-318
  instruments, 318
  repair techniques, 318-320
Palatoplasty
  von Langenbeck, 318-319
  Wardill, 319
Pancreatoduodenectomy, 191
  techniques, 192
  Whipple technique, 192-193
Pan endoscope, 83
Paranasal sinuses, 220, 314-315
Parotid gland, 162-163
  anatomic features, 163
  circulation, 164
Parotidectomy, 164-165
PBI, 24, 29
Pedicle skin graft, 302
Pelvimeters, 83
Penis, 344-345
  anatomic features, 344
Perforators, 84
Periosteal elevators, 84
Periosteotomes, 84
Pessaries, 85
Pharynx, 317
  anatomic features, 317-318
Phenylketonuria, 27
Phosphatase
  acid, 24
  alkaline, 24
Phosphorus, 24
Physicians' Desk Reference, 1
Picks, 85
Pilonidal cyst excision, 158
Pins, 85
Plastic surgery, 301
Platelets, 21

Plates, 85-86
Pliers, 85
Plurals, formation of, 377-378
Pneumoencephalogram, 32
Pneumonectomy, 329-330
Pneumothorax apparatus, 86
Polya gastrectomy, 168
Polya-Hofmeister gastrectomy, 168
Polys, 21
Porphyrins, 27
Positions
    anatomic, 364
    references to, 364
    surgical, 37-39
        illustrated, 38
Potassium
    blood, 24
    urinary, 27
Prefixes, 366-369
Probes, 86-87
Proctoscopes, 87
Proctosigmoidectomy, 187-188
Profilometers, 87
Prostate
    anatomic features, 348
Prostatectomy, 348-349
Prostheses
    aortic valves, 356
    eye, 63
    materials, 75
    orthopedic, 87
    vascular, 356
Protein bound iodine, 24, 29
Proteins
    blood, 24
    spinal fluid, 29
Prothrombin time, 24
PSP test, 27
Pterygium transplant, 231
Punches, 87-88
Punctuation, 13-17
    apostrophe, 13
    brackets, 16, 17
    capitals, 17, 378-379
    colon, 15
    comma, 14
    exclamation point, 17
    interrogation, 17

marks defined, 13
    parentheses, 16
        with brackets, 16
    quotation marks, 16
        single, 16
        with other punctuation, 16
    semicolon, 15
Purines, 28
Pyelogram
    intravenous, 32
    retrograde, 33
Pyelolithotomy, 337-338
Pylorus
    anatomic features, 175
Pyloromyotomy, Ramstedt, 176
Pyloroplasty techniques, 175

R

Radioiodine uptake, 29, 194
Radioisotopes, 194
Radium to cervix, 262-263
Ramstedt pyloromyotomy, 176
Raspatory, 89
Rasps, 88-89
Reamers, 90
Rectal polypectomy, 186
Rectum, 185-189
    anorectal anatomy, 185
    circulation, 185
Red blood count, 19
Red cell fragility, 24-25
References, essential, 1
Request form letter, 10-11
Resectoscopes, 90
Retinoscopes, 90
Retinal reattachment, 231
Retractors, 90-94
Rhinoplasty, 315-316
Rhizotomy, trigeminal, 245
Rib contractors, 95
Rib cutters, 95
Rib shears, 95
Rib spreaders, 95
Rods, 95
Rongeurs, 95-97
Rulers, 97
Rush rod to humerus, 290

INDEX (Continued)

S

Salivary glands, 162-167
 parotid, 162-165
 sublingual, 166-167
 submaxillary, 166
Saphenous ligation, 361-362
Saws, 97
Scar excision, 306
Schoemaker modification
 of Billroth I, 167-168
Scissors, 97-99
Sclerotomes, 99
Scoops, 99-100
Screw drivers, 100
Screws, 100
Sedimentation rate, 25
Segs, 21
Separators, 100
Semicircular canal
 fenestration, 211-212
Serology tests
 blood, 25
 spinal fluid, 29
Serum transaminase, 25
SGOT, 25
Shears, 101
Shirodkar operation, 261
Shunt, endolymphatic subarachnoid,
 201
Sickle cell anemia, 25
 in Negroes, 25
Sickle cell test, 25
Sigmoidoscopes, 101
Sigmoidoscopy, 186
Sinuses, paranasal, 219-220
Skeletal anatomy, 123-125
 illustrated, 126-127
Skids, 101
Skin graft
 chessboard, 302
 free graft, 302
 full thickness, 302
 pedicle, 302
 pinch, 302
 split thickness, 295, 302, 306
 techniques, 303
 types, 302-304

Skin flaps, 303-304
Skull fracture elevation, 248
Slings, 46
Small bowel, 177-181
Smith-Petersen hip nailing, 290
Smithwick's technique
 thoracolumbar sympathectomy, 251
SMR, 221
Snares, 101
Sodium
 blood, 25
 urinary, 28
Sounds, 102
Spatulas, 102
Specula, 102-104
Sphenoidotomy, 222
Sphincterotomes, 104
Sphincterotomy
 anal, 187
 of Oddi, 190-191
 of pylorus, 176
Spinal cord, 238
 anatomic features, 238-239
Spinal fluid, 28-29
 tests, 29
Spinal fusion
 Harrington, 278-280
 Hibbs modified, 277
 multilevel, 278-280
Spleen, 161-162
 anatomic features, 161
Splenectomy
 operative report, 161-162
 techniques, 161
Splints, 104-105
Spoons, 105-106
Spreaders, 106
Spuds, 106
Spur crushers, 106
Stabs, 20
Stapedectomy techniques, 210
 operative report, 210-211
Stapes, 210
Staples, 106
Stomach surgery, 167-172
Stone dislodgers, 106
Strabismus correction, 229-230
Strippers, 107

INDEX (Continued)

Stripping vocal cords, 215
Sturmdorf amputation, cervix, 263
Style guide, 377-380
Subclavian arteriogram, 352
Sublingual gland, 166-167
    anatomic features, 167
    circulation, 167
Submaxillary gland
    anatomic features, 166
    circulation, 166
Submucous resection, 221, 315-316
Subtemporal decompression, 249
Suction tubes, 107
Suffixes, 369-370
Sulkowitch test, 26
Surgical reports, 3-4
    context of, 3
    format, 3-4
    illustrated, 4
    requirements, 3
Suture materials, 41-42, 356
Suture techniques, 42-45
Symbols, medical, 376
Sympathectomy
    cervical, 250
    lumbar, 250
    Smithwick's, 251-252
    thoracolumbar, 251-252

T

T & A, 218-219
Takata-Ara test, 25
Tamps, 107
TBI index, 29
Telescopes, 107
Tenaculums, 107-108
Tendon graft, 294-295, 305
Tendon passers, 108
Tendon strippers, 108
Tendon tuckers, 112
Tennison harelip repair, 314
Tenorrhaphy, 294
Tenotomes, 108
Testes, 345-347
    anatomic features, 345-346
Thermopores, 108
Thoracic surgery, 325-332
Thoracolumbar sympathectomy, 251
Thoracoscopes, 108

Thoracotome, 108
Thoracotomy, 328, 331
Thorn test, 25
Thrombocytes, 21
Thymol turbidity, 25
Thyrobinding index, 29
Thyroid gland, 193-195
    anatomic features, 193-195
    circulation, 194
    radioactive uptake, 194
Thyroidectomy, subtotal, 194
Tissue banks, 305-306
    eye bank, 305
Tissue transplants, 301-305, 351
Toenail excision, 157
Tong, traction, 108
Tongue depressors, 109
Tonometers, 109
Tonsillectomes, 109
Tonsillectomy, 219
T & A, 218
Torek operation, 346-347
Toti operation, 233
Tourniquets, 109
TPI test, 25
Trachea, 217
    instruments, 218
    tubes, 218
Tracheotomy, 218
Traction bows, 109
Tractors, 110
Transilluminators, 110
Transplant of pterygium, 231
Transverse carpal ligament
    section, 295
Trephination, 246
Trephines, 110
Trocars, 110-111
Tube pedicle graft, 302
Tubes, 111-112
Tuckers, 112
Turnbuckle, 112
Tympanoplasty, 202-208
    operative reports
        type I, 203
        type II, 204
        type III, 204
        type IV, 207
        type V, 207

INDEX (Continued)

types defined, 202-203
Typing speed, 2

U

Umbilical herniorrhaphy, 155
Urea, 28
Ureters, 333-334
Urethroscopy, 341-342
Uric acid
  blood, 25
  urinary, 28
Urinary bladder, 338-342
  anatomic features, 339-340
  arteries, 340
Urine
  rate of excretion, 26
  tests on, 26-28
Urobilinogen, 28
Urology, 333-349
Uterine prolapse, 259
  Gilliam suspension, 260-261
  operations for, 260
Uterus
  prolapse operations, 259-260
  suspension of, 260-261

V

Vagotomy, abdominal, 176-177
Valvulotomes, 112
Van den Bergh, 22
Vascular surgery, 351-362
  prostheses in, 356

sutures, 356
VDRL, 25
Vein grafts, 357
Vein ligation, saphenous, 361
Veins listed, 121-123
Ventriculogram, 33
  posterior, 252
von Langenbeck palatoplasty, 318
Vulsellum, 112

W

Wardill palatoplasty, 319-320
Watson-Jones operation, 287
Weir nose operation, 316
Wharton's duct, 166
Whipple operation, 192-193
Whistle, 112
White blood count, 20
White cell differential, 20
Work volume measurement, 2
Wrenches, 112

X

X-ray
  examinations, 30-33
    vascular, 352-355
  media, 30
    vascular, 352

Z

Zinc flocculation, 25
Zoografts, 302